W9-AWJ-887

VETERINARY DENTAL TECHNIQUES

FOR THE SMALL ANIMAL PRACTITIONER

VETERINARY DENTAL TECHNIQUES

FOR THE SMALL ANIMAL PRACTITIONER

STEVEN E. HOLMSTROM, DVM
Diplomate, American Veterinary Dental College
Belmont, California

PATRICIA FROST, DVM
Diplomate, American Veterinary Dental College
North Highlands, California

RONALD L. GAMMON, DVM, MS
Diplomate, American Veterinary Dental College
Martinez, California

Illustrations by Leo Hagstrom

W. B. SAUNDERS COMPANY
Harcourt Brace Jovanovich, Inc.
Philadelphia □ London □ Toronto
Montreal □ Sydney □ Tokyo

W. B. SAUNDERS COMPANY
Harcourt Brace Jovanovich, Inc.

The Curtis Center
Independence Square West
Philadelphia, Pennsylvania 19106

Library of Congress Cataloging-in-Publication Data

Holmstrom, Steven E.

Veterinary dental techniques for the small animal practitioner /
Steven E. Holmstrom, Patricia Frost, Ronald L. Gammon.

p.   cm.

Includes index.

ISBN 0–7216–3234–3

1. Veterinary dentistry.   2. Dogs—Diseases—Treatment.
3. Cats—Diseases—Treatment.   I. Frost, Patricia.
II. Gammon, Ronald.   III. Title.

QL992.M68H65   1992

636.7'08976—dc20   91–15457

Editor: Linda Mills
Designer: Maureen Sweeney
Production Manager: Ken Neimeister
Manuscript Editor: Holly Lukens
Illustration Coordinator: Cecilia Roberts
Indexer: Roger Wall
Cover Designer: Michelle Malone

Veterinary Dental Techniques
for the Small Animal Practitioner   ISBN 0–7216–3234–3

Copyright © 1992 by W. B. Saunders Company.

All rights reserved.   No part of this publication may be reproduced or transmitted in any form or
by any means, electronic or mechanical, including photocopy, recording, or any information storage
and retrieval system, without permission in writing from the publisher.

Printed in Mexico.

Last digit is the print number: 9   8   7   6   5   4   3   2   1

PREFACE

Our hope in writing this text is to give veterinarians, animal health technicians, and students an understanding of dental equipment, instruments, materials, and techniques. Our goal and that of individuals practicing veterinary dentistry should be to obtain predictable results by following established protocol. This text is intended to supplement other texts, both veterinary and human dental, that discuss such topics as anatomy, pathogenesis, and theory.

The personal economic benefits that may be derived from adding dentistry to the veterinary practice must be countered with the realization that our obligation to our clients and patients goes far beyond simple disease prevention, relief of pain, treatment of disease, and performing tasks. Our duty is to perform a service that will respect the patient's need. Treatment plans also must be presented to the client with suitable alternative treatments, depending on the patient's needs and the client's desires and (unfortunately) ability to pay for these services. Our commitment is based on trust, and this trust must be upheld when we are performing all phases of our veterinary practice, including dentistry.

We hope that through the use of this text, all components of the veterinary triangle of patient, client, and veterinarian will benefit.

STEVEN E. HOLMSTROM, DVM, Dipl AVDC
PATRICIA FROST, DVM, Dipl AVDC
RONALD L. GAMMON, DVM, MS, Dipl AVDC

ACKNOWLEDGMENTS

We would like to thank Stephen John, DDS, and Carol Weldin, RDH, for their review of the periodontic chapters; James Guttman, DDS, and the Brasseler Company for coordinating the review of the endodontic chapter; and Kay Gammon and Laurie Holmstrom, RDH, for review of the manuscript. Special thanks to our illustrator, Leo Hagstrom, for his talent and for his patience during our revisions.

We are grateful to the following dentists who have contributed to our dental knowledge: Toby A. Burgess, DDS; Stephen John, DDS; Ronald Osiek, DDS; Morgan Powell, DDS; Charles L. Neubauer, DDS; Lynn Oakleaf, DDS; Nick Sabbia, DDS; Ronald Tosch, DDS; and Walter E. Tweedie, DDS.

We would like to thank our colleagues in the Academy of Veterinary Dentistry and the American Veterinary Dental College for their contributions to veterinary dentistry. Many of their techniques have become part of the "public domain" knowledge from which this text has been drawn.

We would also like to thank the American Dental Association and the California Dental Association for their generosity in admitting interested veterinarians to their annual meetings and symposia. Without the sharing of knowledge, veterinary dentistry would not have progressed so rapidly.

CONTENTS

chapter 1
DENTAL RECORDS 1

chapter 2
DENTAL EQUIPMENT AND CARE 23

chapter 3
DENTAL RADIOLOGY 93

chapter 4
DENTAL PROPHYLAXIS 105

chapter 5
PERIODONTAL THERAPY 137

chapter 6
EXODONTICS 173

chapter 7
ENDODONTICS 207

chapter 8
RESTORATIVE DENTISTRY 267

chapter 9
ORTHODONTICS 339

chapter 10
DENTAL ORTHOPEDICS 389

appendix 409

index 419

chapter 1

DENTAL RECORDS

General Comments

- Written records are necessary to identify the patient; to record the patient's status before, during, and after treatment procedures; to document client/owner acceptance or rejection of the treatment plan; to record therapy sequence, prognosis, results, and sequelae; to measure progress at successive appointments; to document consultations and referrals; and to provide ease of transfer to another practitioner.[1]

TOOTH IDENTIFICATION SYSTEMS

General Comments

- A number of tooth identification systems can be used in a dental record.
- In some systems a specific number is given to each tooth, whereas other systems use symbols and numbers to designate an individual tooth. The systems that use numbers without symbols are more readily adapted for use with computers.
- In this work we will use the terms "type" to refer to primary (deciduous) or permanent dentition and "function" to refer to the four common functional groups, i.e., incisor, canine, premolar, and molar.

PALMER NOTATION SYSTEM

General Comments

- Teeth are given letters corresponding to their function.
- Capital letters are used for permanent teeth and lower-case letters for primary teeth.
- The teeth are numbered consecutively within their functional group and a cross symbol is used to denote the quadrant. Note that right and left are as viewed and do not indicate the patient's right or left.

  P $\lfloor$ 2 = upper left second permanent premolar.
  P $\lceil$ 1 = lower left first permanent premolar.
  C1 $\rceil$ = lower right first permanent canine.

Advantages

- Identifies tooth function and type.
- Easy identification of quadrant.

Disadvantages

- Not easily used with a computer.
- Difficult to use to describe tooth verbally.

TRIADAN SYSTEM

General Comments

- Each tooth has a three-digit number.
- The first number represents the quadrant, with the upper right quadrant being 1, going counterclockwise to the lower right quadrant.
- The upper right quadrant is 1, the upper left quadrant is 2, the lower left quadrant is 3, and the lower right quadrant is 4 for the permanent teeth. Quadrants for primary teeth are represented by the numbers 5, 6, 7, and 8. The individual teeth are represented by two digits, with 01 being the first tooth from the midline and continuing distally around the arch to the last tooth. In the dog the last number is 10 for the upper arches and 11 for the lower arch. The number 309 in the dog would represent the permanent lower left first molar. The number 504 in the dog would represent the primary upper right canine tooth.

Advantages

- Is adaptable for computer use if computer is nonalphanumeric.
- Each tooth has an individual number.
- Easy to use in dealing with a single species or when records with anatomic charts printed on them are used.

Disadvantages

- Difficulty in learning and remembering if not used frequently.
- Same tooth in different species may have different numbers because of the variance of dental formulas among species.
- Tooth function is not identified by this system.

Palmer	$3\rfloor$	$2\rfloor$	$1\rfloor$	$\lfloor1$	$\lfloor2$	$\lfloor3$
Tridan	101	102	101	301	203	201
Anatomic	I^3	I^2	I^1	^1I	^2I	^3I
Universal	13	12	11	10	9	8
Haderup	3+	2+	3+	+1	+2	+3
Zsigmondy	$3\rfloor$	$2\rfloor$	$1\rfloor$	$\lfloor1$	$\lfloor2$	$\lfloor3$
Federali	1,3	1,2	1,1	2,1	2,2	2,3

Right

Left

Palmer	Tridan	Anatomic	Universal	Haderup	Zsigmondy	Federali		Federali	Zsigmondy	Haderup	Universal	Anatomic	Tridan	Palmer
$C1\rfloor$	104	C^1	14	4+	$4\rfloor$	1,4		2,4	$\lfloor4$	+4	7	^1C	204	$C\lfloor1$
$P1\rfloor$	105	P^1	15	5+	$5\rfloor$	1,5		2,5	$\lfloor5$	+5	6	^1P	205	$P\lfloor1$
$P2\rfloor$	106	P^2	16	6+	$6\rfloor$	1,6		2,6	$\lfloor6$	+6	5	^2P	206	$P\lfloor2$
$P3\rfloor$	107	P^3	17	7+	$7\rfloor$	1,7		2,7	$\lfloor7$	+7	4	^3P	207	$P\lfloor3$
$P4\rfloor$	108	P^4	18	8+	$8\rfloor$	1,8		2,8	$\lfloor8$	+8	3	^4P	208	$P\lfloor4$
$M1\rfloor$	109	M^1	19	9+	$9\rfloor$	1,9		2,9	$\lfloor9$	+9	2	^1M	209	$M\lfloor1$
$M2\rfloor$	110	M^2	20	10+	$10\rfloor$	1,10		2,10	$\lfloor10$	+10	1	^2M	210	$M\lfloor2$
$\overline{M3}\rfloor$	411	M_3	42	11−	$\overline{11}\rfloor$	4,11		3,11	$\lfloor\overline{11}$	−11	21	$_3M$	311	$M\lfloor\overline{3}$
$\overline{M2}\rfloor$	410	M_1	41	10−	$\overline{10}\rfloor$	4,10		3,10	$\lfloor\overline{10}$	−10	22	$_2M$	310	$M\lfloor\overline{2}$
$\overline{M1}\rfloor$	409	M_1	40	9−	$\overline{9}\rfloor$	4,9		3,9	$\lfloor\overline{9}$	−9	23	$_1M$	309	$M\lfloor\overline{1}$
$\overline{P4}\rfloor$	405	P_4	39	8−	$\overline{8}\rfloor$	4,8		3,8	$\lfloor\overline{8}$	−8	24	$_4P$	308	$P\lfloor\overline{4}$
$\overline{P3}\rfloor$	407	P_3	38	7−	$\overline{7}\rfloor$	4,7		3,7	$\lfloor\overline{7}$	−7	25	$_3P$	307	$P\lfloor\overline{3}$
$\overline{P2}\rfloor$	406	P_2	37	6−	$\overline{6}\rfloor$	4,6		3,6	$\lfloor\overline{6}$	−6	26	$_2P$	306	$P\lfloor\overline{2}$
$\overline{P1}\rfloor$	405	P	36	5−	$\overline{5}\rfloor$	4,5		3,5	$\lfloor\overline{5}$	−5	27	$_1P$	305	$P\lfloor\overline{1}$
$\overline{C1}\rfloor$	404	C_1	35	4−	$\overline{4}\rfloor$	4,4		3,4	$\lfloor\overline{4}$	−4	28	$_1C$	304	$C\lfloor\overline{1}$

Federali	4,3	4,2	4,1	3,1	3,2	3,3
Zsigmondy	$\overline{3}\rfloor$	$\overline{2}\rfloor$	$\overline{1}\rfloor$	$\lfloor\overline{1}$	$\lfloor\overline{2}$	$\lfloor\overline{3}$
Haderup	3−	2−	3−	−1	−2	−3
Universal	34	33	32	31	30	29
Anatomic	I_3	I_2	I_1	$_1I$	$_2I$	$_3I$
Tridan	403	402	401	301	302	304
Palmer	$\overline{3}\rfloor$	$\overline{2}\rfloor$	$\overline{1}\rfloor$	$\lfloor\overline{1}$	$\lfloor\overline{2}$	$\lfloor\overline{3}$

DENTAL SHORTHAND/ ANATOMIC IDENTIFICATION SYSTEM

General Comments

- Each tooth is given a letter corresponding to tooth function and type.
- Upper-case letters are used for permanent teeth and lower-case for primary teeth.

  I = incisor   i = primary incisor
  C = canine   c = primary canine
  P = premolar   p = primary premolar
  M = molar

- Each quadrant of the mouth corresponds to a corner around the letter.
- Upper or maxillary teeth are indicated by superscript numbers, and lower or mandibular teeth are indicated by subscript numbers
- Teeth on the patient's right are indicated to the right side of the letter, and teeth on the patient's left are indicated to the left side of the letter.
- The teeth are numbered consecutively, for each functional group of teeth, starting from the midline. This number is placed in the appropriate corner around the letter. For example:

  The permanent upper right central incisor is represented by the number 1 placed as a superscript on the right side of the letter $I = I^1$.

  Second and third permanent lower left premolars are represented by the numbers 2 and 3 placed as a subscript on the left side of the letter $P = {}_{2-3}P$.

  The primary upper left canine is represented by the number 1 placed as a superscript on the left side of the letter $c = {}^1c$.

Advantages

- Easy to learn as it is more self explanatory.
- The same tooth number is used on the same corresponding tooth in different species.
- May be used with alphanumeric systems by placing "U" or "L" or "+" or "−" before or after the tooth number.

The permanent upper right central incisor = IU1 or I + 1.
Second permanent lower left premolar = L2P or − 2P.
Primary upper left canine = U1c or +1c.

Disadvantages

- May not be used with all computer systems without the above modifications.
- May be confusing to a noninformed reader as to whether reference is to animal's or observer's right or left.
- Is easier to use in written than oral form.

NUMERICAL ORDER (UNIVERSAL TOOTH NUMBERING SYSTEM)

General Comments

- Each permanent tooth is given a number 1 to 30 in the cat, 1 to 42 in the dog. Primary teeth are lettered (a to z in the cat; a to z, A to B in the dog).
- The teeth are numbered starting in the upper left quadrant with the last tooth and continuing with consecutive numbers around the arch to the opposite last upper tooth. The lower arch is numbered starting from the last lower left tooth continuing around the arch to the last lower right tooth.

Advantages

- Easy communication if both parties know the numbers and the system.
- Easily used with computers.

Disadvantages

- The same tooth from species to species will have a different number because of the differences in dental formulas.
- Difficult to memorize all the numbers, especially if numerous species are treated or if used infrequently.
- Does not identify tooth function.

HADERUP SYSTEM

General Comments

- This system numbers each tooth in a quadrant consecutively, starting at the midline.
- The upper or lower arch is indicated by a + or − next to the number, with + corresponding to the upper jaw and − to the lower jaw.
- The right or left is indicated by which side of the tooth number the symbol is placed; +2 = left upper second incisor, 6 − = lower, right second premolar.

Advantages

- The system is readily used in computerized records.
- Easier to use in oral communication than the anatomic system. All parties involved must still know the system well.

Disadvantages

- The practitioner must memorize the numbering for each species worked with. This becomes cumbersome.
- Does not identify tooth function.

ZSIGMONDY SYSTEM

General Comments

- This tooth identification system uses the arms of a cross to identify the quadrant. Looking at the patient head on, visualize a horizontal line between the upper and lower jaws and a vertical line separating the right side from the left.
- The intersecting arms of this cross are used as the symbol to denote the corresponding quadrant. These are written as viewed, not corresponding to the patient's right or left.
- The permanent teeth are numbered consecutively in each quadrant, starting from the midline. The primary teeth are lettered consecutively, starting with the letter A for the first tooth from the midline.

  $\underline{5|}$ = permanent upper right first premolar in the dog.

  $\overline{|4}$ = permanent lower left canine in the dog.

  $\underline{|B}$ = primary upper left second incisor in the cat or dog.

Advantage

- Clearly defines maxillary vs mandibular and right vs left quadrant.

Disadvantage

- Inconsistent with other systems in that with this system the tooth is identified by how the observer sees the tooth, rather than by where the tooth is in the patient's mouth.

FÉDÉRATION DENTAIRE INTERNATIONALE SYSTEM

General Comments

- In this system each quadrant is identified by a number 1 to 4 for permanent, 5 to 8 for primary teeth. 1/5 = upper right, 2/6 = upper left, 3/7 = lower left and 4/8 = lower right.
- The teeth are numbered consecutively in each quadrant from the midline, with the corresponding quadrant number for the permanent or primary tooth in front of it. In the dog 1,1 = upper right permanent central incisor.
- In the cat 6,4 = upper left primary canine.

Advantages

- Easy identification of quadrant (upper or lower, left or right).
- Can be used readily in computer record systems.

Disadvantages

- Difficult to learn.
- Does not identify tooth function.
- Not good for multiple species use.

VETERINARY MEDICAL RECORDS

General Comments

- Written records must be dated, accurate, and readable and should be signed if many people are making entries.
- Recording dental findings and procedures performed is necessary to provide a legal record if that treatment is ever questioned and provides continuity of treatment for various dental disorders.
- The medical record should have the owner's name, address, and telephone numbers along with name, breed, age, and sex of the patient.
- Having a telephone number where the owner can be reached during a patient's dental procedure can be beneficial if additional abnormalities are found after the patient is anesthetized.

Client number _____

Pet Clinic
Initial Oral Exam

Owner _____ Patient _____ Date _____

Species _____ Breed _____ Sex _____ Date of Birth _____

Chief complaint _____

Past dental history _____

General medical history _____

Diet _____

Home oral hygiene _____

Other _____

Medical Alert

Skull type:

- ☐ Brachycephalic
- ☐ Mesiocephalic
- ☐ Dolichocephalic
- ☐ _____

Oral Hygiene

- ☐ Plaque   N S M H
- ☐ Calculus   N S M H

Normal Slight Moderate Heavy

Periodontal Exam

- ☐ Inflammation   I C P M
- ☐ Gingival Edema   I C P M
- ☐ Pockets >3mm   I C P M
- ☐ Pockets >5mm   I C P M
- ☐ Recession   I C P M
- ☐ Hyperplasia   I C P M
- ☐ Mucogingival loss I C P M
- ☐ Tooth Mobility   I C P M
- ☐ Further evaluation I C P M

Incisor Canine Premolar Molar

Occlusion:

- ☐ Scissors
- ☐ Brachygnathic
- ☐ Prognathic
- ☐ Wry
- ☐ Level
- ☐ Crossbite
- ☐ Occlusal wear   I C P M

Tooth Abnormalities

- ☐ Ret. Primary   I C P
- ☐ Missing   I C P M
- ☐ Supernumerary I C P M
- ☐ Caries   I C P M
- ☐ Resorptive   I C P M
- ☐ Injured   I C P M

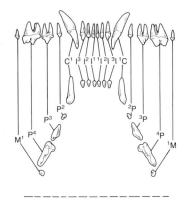
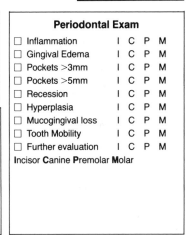
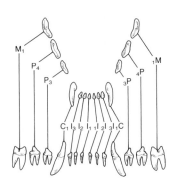
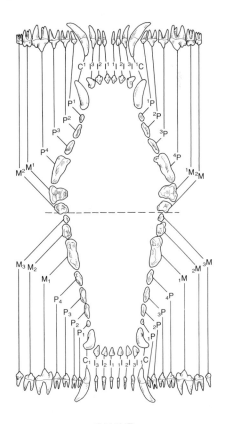

FELINE

CANINE

DENTAL RECORDS

General Comments

- Dental records can be designed to record information by fill-in or check-off formats, dental anatomic charts, or a combination of these to provide easy recording in a short period of time.
- Dental anatomic charts are important because we are describing three-dimensional objects that are often difficult to discuss in written terms. This allows an ongoing record.
- The type of record used will vary with each practice but should include: patient/client identification; chief complaint; a general health history; dental history; tooth identification system, either numerical or illustrated; recording of specific findings, treatment plan, procedures done, and follow-up care; radiographic interpretation; documentation of discussions and consultations, missed appointments, or deviation from recommended follow-up; and documented informed consent.

INITIAL ORAL EXAMINATION

General Client/Patient Information

- The client number (if used), owner, patient, date of examination, species, breed, sex, and date of birth (or age) is recorded.

Chief Complaint

- Listing the chief complaint ensures that this problem is dealt with even though additional dental problems may be found on examination.

General Health History

- The general health of the patient is extremely important because the treatment of most dental diseases requires a general anesthetic.

Past Dental History

- This includes past dental problems and their treatment and any complications.

Diet

- The patient's current diet and amounts fed, whether moist, dry, or table scraps, should be recorded. Other treats fed and chewing habits (fence, bones, rocks, etc.) are listed.

Home Oral Hygiene

- Home oral hygiene performed is noted.

Recording Specific Findings

- In a systematic way the oral cavity is examined and initial findings and abnormalities are recorded.
- The skull type (dolichocephalic, brachycephalic, mesocephalic, or variation) is noted.
- The occlusion is noted as well as occlusal wear.
- The amount of plaque and calculus present in general is recorded.
- Tooth abnormalities, including retained primary teeth, missing teeth, and supernumerary teeth, should be noted. Other

dental findings such as carious lesions, resorptive lesions, dental trauma, or any other abnormalities are noted by indicating the tooth involved and the location on the tooth.

- The periodontal status is recorded by noting gingival inflammation, gingival edema, periodontal pocket depth if significant, gingival recession, gingival hyperplasia, mucogingival junction loss, and tooth mobility or by noting that further diagnostic evaluation is necessary.
- Other oral disease is noted in the dental chart.
- A permanent initial record of dental findings can be kept for future reference.

ANATOMIC CHARTING

- Pretreatment and subsequent findings can be recorded in pencil on the anatomic chart on the left. This side is updated as the patient's condition changes. (See the canine dental chart on the opposite page.)
- Treatment performed is recorded in ink on the anatomic chart on the right. This becomes the continuing record of the patient's dental status.
- Symbols or letters to indicate a variety of abnormalities can be used on a dental anatomic chart to speed recording and allow a quick reference to all the abnormalities and treatment performed.
- Many symbols are in common usage in dentistry, or the practitioner may develop his or her own.
- A key for symbols and letter abbreviations used should be available to eliminate confusion for others reading the record. (See pp. 13 and 14.)
- The additional box rows (2 and 3) can be used for additional probings, footnoting to

the record, and for other descriptive abbreviations.

Remarks

- Miscellaneous remarks may be entered.

Diagnostics/Treatment Plan/Treatment Completed

- A date is recorded, the tooth or teeth involved are indicated, and treatment, plan, or options are entered. A "P" is placed in the column to denote a plan or a "T" is placed to denote a treatment. The date may be written alongside the "P" to indicate a plan that has been followed up with a treatment.
- Complications and follow-up may be recorded in this area.
- Radiographic findings, discussions, and consultations may also be recorded in this section.

Pet Clinic
Canine Dental Chart

Diagnosed and Untreated Conditions/Abnormalities

Fill in this side with pencil, transfer to "Treatments Performed"
when treatment completed and erase this side.

Treatments Performed

Write this side in ink, use color to
indicate different treatment dates

M2	M1	P4	P3	P2	P1	C1	3	2	1	I	I	1	2	3	1C	1P	2P	3P	4P	IM	2M

Buccal

Occlusal

Palatal

Lingual

Occlusal

Buccal

M3	M2	M1	P4	P3	P2	P1	C1	3	2	1	I	I	1	2	3	1C	1P	2P	3P	4P	1M	2M	3M

M2	M1	P4	P3	P2	P1	C1	3	2	1	I	I	1	2	3	1C	1P	2P	3P	4P	IM	2M

M3	M2	M1	P4	P3	P2	P1	C1	3	2	1	I	I	1	2	3	1C	1P	2P	3P	4P	1M	2M	3M

Remarks:

Diagnosis/Treatment Plan/Treatment Completed

Date	Tooth		Plan	Treatment

PERIODONTAL CHARTING

- Periodontal charting is a more specialized record of the periodontal status of each tooth. (See the feline dental chart.) It can include evaluation of the various indices to quantitate gingival health, such as: gingival bleeding and edema (gingival index); amount of plaque and calculus (plaque index or calculus index); probing depths; mobility; and attachment levels. These measurements are important in quantitating the degree of periodontitis present in general and the involvement of individual teeth and allows for greater assessment of treatment and home-care procedures needed.

Periodontal Indices

- Changes in the periodontium in response to disease can be quantitated by the use of various indices. This helps to assess the severity of the pathologic process and can be used to evaluate success of treatment.
- Epidemiologic studies use indices in order to have a consistent evaluation of disease and to be able to compare the data statistically.
- A number of indices have been developed to evaluate the presence of plaque, calculus, gingival changes, probing depth, attachment loss, and mobility.

Plaque Index (Silness and Loe[2])

Grade
0   No plaque.
1   Thin film of plaque at gingival margin visible when checked with explorer.
2   Moderate amount of plaque along gingival margin. Interdental space is free of plaque. Plaque is visible to the naked eye.
3   Heavy plaque accumulation at the gingival margin. Interdental space filled with plaque.

Gingival Index (Loe and Silness[2])

Grade
0   Normal gingiva, no inflammation, discoloration, or bleeding.
1   Mild inflammation, slight color change, mild alteration of gingival surface, no bleeding on probing.
2   Moderate inflammation, erythema, swelling bleeding on probing or when pressure applied.
3   Severe inflammation, severe erythema and swelling, tendency toward spontaneous hemorrhage, some ulceration.

Mobility

Grade I, slight mobility—Represents the first detectable sign of movement greater than normal.

Grade II, moderate mobility—Movement of 1 mm.

Grade III, marked mobility—Movement of more than 1 mm in any direction and/or intrusive movement.

Furcation Exposure

Class I—The periodontal probe can barely detect the entrance to the furcation.

Class II—The periodontal probe can enter the furcation, but does not extend to the other side. Early radiographic changes may be seen.

Class III—The periodontal probe can pass through the furcation to the other side.

Pet Clinic
Feline Dental Chart

Diagnosed and Untreated Conditions/Abnormalities

Fill in this side with pencil, transfer to "Treatments Performed"
when treatment completed and erase this side.

Treatments Performed

Write this side in ink, use color to
indicate different treatment dates

M1	P4	P3	P2	C1	3	2	1	1	2	3	1C	2P	3P	4P	1M

Buccal

Occlusal

Palatal

Lingual

Occlusal

Buccal

M1	P4	P3	C1	3	2	1	1	2	3	1C	3P	4P	1M

Remarks:

_____
_____
_____
_____
_____
_____
_____

Diagnosis/Treatment Plan/Treatment Completed

Date	Tooth	Plan	Treatment

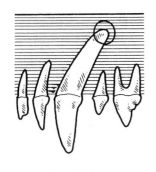

Periapical
pathology

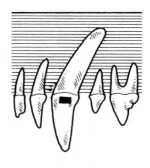

Restoration

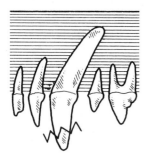

Root canal
treatment

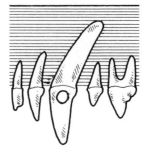

Caries

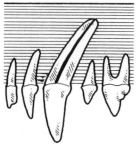

Fractured
crown

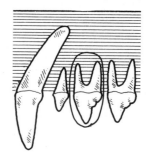

Missing
tooth

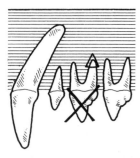

Retained
root

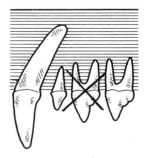

Extracted
tooth

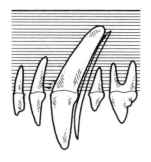

Retained
primary
tooth

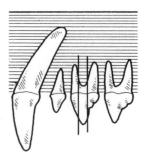

Planned
extracted
tooth

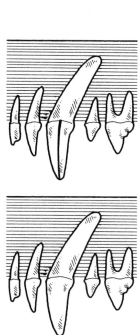

Posts

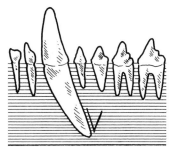

Frenula
problem

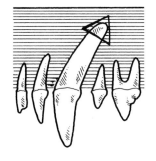

Malpositioned
tooth

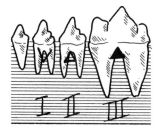

Furcation

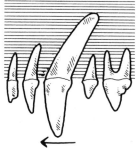

Apicoectomy

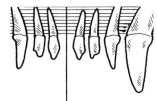

Bridge

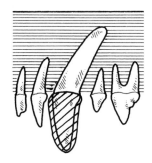

Crown

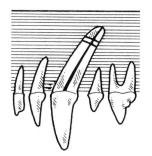

Implant

SAMPLE DENTAL CHART WITH DISEASE

Various standard marks can be used to record conditions of the teeth and gums. The sample chart on the opposite page shows many of these marks; numbers in the text refer to points on the chart.

1. Periapical disease is indicated by a circle around the root tip in the buccal view.

2. Fractured crown is indicated by a jagged line over the crown in all three views, with an attempt made to show the missing area.

3. Retained root is indicated by an "X" over the crown in the buccal, occlusal, or palatal (lingual) view and by drawing in the root portion retained in the buccal view.

4. Retained primary tooth is indicated by drawing in the tooth on the buccal view, including the root.

5. Cavities are indicated by an irregular circle on the appropriate views in the area of the lesion (do not fill in because this would indicate a restoration).

6. Missing teeth are indicated by a circle around the tooth in all three views.

7. Planned extractions are indicated by parallel lines over all three views.

8. Malpositioned teeth are indicated by an arrow in the direction of malposition in the appropriate views.

9. A need for a frenectomy is indicated by a "V"-shaped figure in the buccal view at the involved area.

10. An exposed furcation (Class 1) is indicated by a "V."

11. An open triangle denotes a Class 2 furcation.

12. A filled-in triangle denotes a Class 3 furcation.

13. A hatched line over the "V" indicates that a frenectomy has been performed.

14. Probing depth measurements can be recorded in the first row of boxes.

15. A line is drawn on the buccal view to show the level of the gingival margin. Combining the charted gingival margin line with the charted probing depth allows the practitioner to determine the level of the gingival attachment. See periodontal charting in this chapter for more specifics.

16. Root canal treatment is indicated by a solid line in the root canal (not in pulp chamber) in the buccal view.

17. A restoration is indicated by blacking in the area of restoration on appropriate views.

18. Extracted teeth or roots are indicated by an "X" over the tooth/root extracted in all three views.

19. Posts are indicated by a line in the pulp chamber (not root canal, which would indicate root canal therapy).

20. Apicoectomy is indicated by an open triangle around the apex.

21. A crown/cap is indicated by a circle around the coronal views. If porcelain, it is left clear; if metal, it is filled in with hatch lines.

22. A bridge is indicated by parallel lines connecting the involved crowns in the occlusal view.

23. An implant is indicated by a line in the root area, with perpendicular lines on the buccal view.

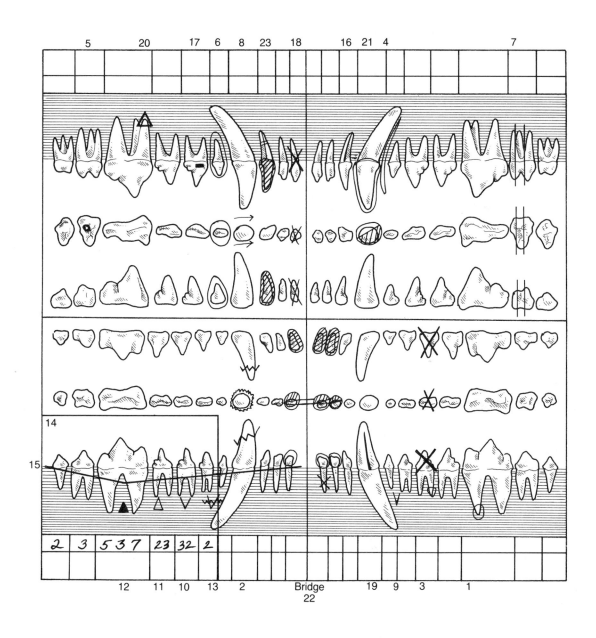

| 5 | 20 | 17 | 6 | 8 | 23 | 18 | 16 | 21 | 4 | 7 |

14

15

| 2 | 3 | 5 | 3 | 7 | 23 | 32 | 2 |

| 12 | 11 | 10 | 13 | 2 | Bridge 22 | 19 | 9 | 3 | 1 |

DENTAL TERMINOLOGY

- An understanding of dental terminology is important in understanding a technique, in discussing a case with another veterinarian, dentist, or student, and in reporting a finding or procedure in a record, to eliminate confusion and misunderstandings. A list of common dental and anatomic terms is included.

GLOSSARY

Anatomic Terms

Alveolar bone – Cancellous bone directly surrounding the tooth roots.

Alveolar crest – The ridge of bone between two adjacent teeth or between the roots of a tooth.

Alveolar mucosa – Less densely keratinized gingival tissue covering the bone.

Alveolus – The cavity or socket in either jaw bone that surrounds and supports the root of the tooth.

Anterior teeth – The canine and incisor teeth.

Apex – Terminal portion of the root.

Apical delta – The diverging branches of the root canal at the apical end of the tooth root.

Apical foramen – The opening(s) in the apex of the root through which nerves and vessels pass into the root canal.

Attached gingiva – The gingiva that extends from the free gingival groove to the mucogingival line.

Attachment apparatus – The periodontal ligament, cementum, and alveolar bone that hold the tooth in place.

Canine tooth – Large, single-root tooth designed for tearing and grasping.

Carnassial tooth – Shearing tooth. Upper P4 and lower M1 in the dog and cat.

Cementoenamel junction – Found at the neck of the tooth where the enamel and the cementum meet.

Cementum – Bony layer covering the root surface.

Cingulum – The cervical third of the palatal surface of the anterior teeth.

Crown – The portion of the tooth covered with enamel.

Cusp – Tip or pointed prominence on the occlusal surface of the crown.

Deciduous teeth – Teeth of the primary dentition ("baby teeth").

Dental arch – Formed by the curve of the crowns of the teeth in their normal position or by the residual ridge if the teeth are missing.

Dental Quadrant – Half of each dental arch when divided at the midline.

Dentin – The main component of the tooth. It consists of multiple tubules that extend from the pulp to its outer surface. The tubules contain sensory nerve fibers that register various degrees of pain. Harder than bone, dentin is covered by enamel on the crown and by cementum on the root.

Diastema – The space between two adjacent teeth that are not in contact with each other in an arch.

Enamel – The hard, shiny outer layer of the crown composed of hydroxyapatite crystalline components.

Epithelial attachment – Tissue attaching the gingiva to the tooth.

Free gingiva – Portion of the gingiva not directly attached to the tooth that forms the gingival wall of the sulcus.

Free gingival groove – On the surface of the gingiva a slight concavity or line separating free from attached gingiva.

Free gingival margin – The free edge of the gingiva on the tooth surface.

Furcation – The space between tooth roots where they join the crown.

Gingiva – Soft tissue surrounding the teeth.

Gingival sulcus – The normal space created by the free gingiva and the tooth.

Gnathic – Referring to the jaw.

Halitosis – Foul, offensive, or unpleasant breath.

Incisal edge – The cutting edge of the incisors.

Incisor – Small anterior tooth with a single root.

Infrabony pocket – A periodontal pocket in the alveolar bone.

Interdental – The area between the proximal surfaces of adjacent teeth in the same arch.

Interproximal – Between adjoining surfaces of teeth in the same arch.

Interradicular – Between roots of multi-rooted teeth.

Juga – The depressions between the ridges of bone formed by roots in the alveolar process on the mandible or the premaxilla and maxilla.

Lamina dura – The dense cortical bone forming the wall of the alveolus next to the tooth. It appears on a radiograph as a white line next to the dark line of the periodontal ligament.

Lateral or accessory canal – Small canal leading from the root canal to the outer surface of the root.

Line angle – The imaginary intersection of two tooth walls.

Mental foramen – Openings in the mandible through which nerves and vessels pass.

Molar – Large, multicusp teeth designed for grinding. Upper (two) molars have three roots and lower (three) molars have two roots in dogs.

Mucogingival line – Definite line of demarcation where the attached gingiva and alveolar mucosa meet.

Neck (cervical line) – The junction of the crown and root.

Odontoblast – The cells in the pulp that produce dentin.

Palate – The structure that separates the oral and nasal cavities.

Periodontal ligament – A network of fibers connecting the tooth to the bone.

Periodontium – The supporting structures of the teeth including the periodontal ligament, gingiva, cementum, and alveolar and supporting bone.

Posterior teeth – The premolar and molar teeth.

Premolar – The teeth distal to the canine and mesial to the molars with one to three roots.

Primary teeth – The first teeth to erupt; they are replaced by adult teeth.

Proximal – The surface of a tooth that is adjacent to another tooth.

Pulp – Soft tissue component of the tooth consisting of blood and lymphatic vessels, nerve tissue, and loose connective tissue.

Pulp chamber – Portion of the crown containing the pulp.

Radicular – Pertaining to the root.

Root – The portion of the tooth normally covered by cementum.

Root canal – Portion of the root containing the pulp.

Ruga palatina – The irregular ridge in the mucous membrane covering the anterior part of the hard palate.

Dental Positioning/Surfaces

Apical – Towards the apex.

Buccal – Surface of the tooth nearest the cheek (posterior teeth).

Coronal – Towards the crown.

Distal – Away from the midline in the dental arches.

Facial – Surface of the tooth nearest the face. This term is awkward to use in most veterinary patients because there is little delineation of face and cheek. Buccal and labial are more accurate.

Incisal – Biting surface of anterior teeth.

Interproximal – Between adjoining surfaces of teeth.

Labial – Surface of the tooth nearest the lips (anterior teeth).

Line angle – Imaginary line formed by the junction of two adjacent surfaces/walls of a tooth.

Lingual – Surface of the tooth nearest the tongue.

Mandible – The bone that forms the lower jaw.

Maxilla – The bone that forms most of the upper jaw.
Mesial – Toward the midline of the dental arch.

Occlusal – The chewing surfaces of the caudal teeth.

Palatal – Surface of the tooth towards the hard palate.

Sublingual – The structures and surfaces beneath the tongue.

Dental Fields

Endodontics – The diagnosis and treatment of diseases inside the tooth that affect the tooth pulp and apical periodontal tissues.
Exodontics – Branch of dentistry that deals with extraction of teeth.

Oral surgery – Pertaining to surgery of the oral cavity.
Orthodontics – Branch of dentistry that deals with the prevention and correction of irregularities of the teeth and malocclusion.

Periodontics – Branch of dentistry dealing with the study and treatment of periodontal diseases.
Prosthodontics – Branch of dentistry that deals with the construction of appliances designed to replace missing teeth and/or other oral structures.

Restorative/operative dentistry – Branch of dentistry dealing with restoring the form and function of teeth.

Oral Diseases/Conditions

Abrasion – The wearing away of teeth due to abnormal contact with structures other than teeth.
Acquired Pellicle – The thin film composed mostly of protein that forms on the surface of teeth. It forms with or without bacteria and can be removed by abrasive action.
Anodontia – The absence of teeth
Anterior crossbite – An orthodontic condition in which canine, premolar, and molar occlusion is normal but one or more mandibular incisors are anterior to the maxillary incisors.
Attrition – The wearing away of teeth by tooth-against-tooth contact during mastication.
Avulsion – The separation of the tooth from its alveolus.

Brachygnathia – The lower jaw is markedly shorter than the upper jaw.

Calculus – Hard, mineralized plaque on the tooth surface.
Caries – A demineralization and loss of tooth structure due to action of microorganisms on carbohydrates.

Edentulous – Without teeth.
Embedded tooth – A tooth that has not erupted into the oral cavity and is not likely to erupt.

Erosion – Loss of tooth structure by chemical means not involving bacteria.

Facet – A flattened or worn spot on the surface of a tooth.
Freeway space – The space between the opposing mandibular and maxillary premolar cusps when the mouth is closed.
Fused teeth – The joining of two teeth in development where they have developed from different tooth buds.

Gemini tooth – The partial division of a tooth bud attempting to form two teeth.
Gingival hyperplasia – A pathological increase in the amount of normal gingival tissue in a normal arrangement.

Horizontal bone loss – Loss of crestal alveolar bone along an arch secondary to periodontal disease.

Impacted tooth – An unerupted or partially erupted tooth that is prevented from erupting further by any structure.

Level bite – Occlusion where the upper and lower incisors meet incisal edge to incisal edge.
Luxation – The displacement or partial displacement of a tooth from its alveolus.

Odontalgia – Pain in a tooth.
Oligodontia – Reduced number of teeth.
Open bite – The failure of the upper and lower incisors to contact each other when the mouth is closed.
Oronasal fistula – An abnormal opening between the oral and nasal cavity.
Overbite – Layman's term for the upper jaw overlapping the lower jaw.

Periapical abscess (or apical abscess) – An abscess at the apex of the root, involving the pulp and surrounding apical tissues.
Periodontal abscess – An abscess involving the periodontium.
Periodontal pocket – Pathologic increase in the depth of the gingival sulcus with loss of epithelial and periodontal ligament attachments.
Plaque – A thin film covering the teeth, composed of bacteria, saliva, food particles, and sloughed epithelial cells.
Posterior cross bite – An abnormal occlusion where one or more mandibular premolars or molars occlude buccal to their occlusal partner.

Pulpitis – Inflammation of the pulp.
Pyorrhea – A discharge of pus from the peridontium.

Resorption – The loss of substance by a physiologic or pathologic process.
Reverse scissor bite – Occlusion where all the lower incisors occlude anterior to the upper incisors.
Root fenestration – A window-like opening of bone and gingiva over the root.

Stomatitis – Inflammation of the soft tissues of the mouth.
Supernumerary teeth – Teeth in excess of the normal number.

Vertical bone loss – Bone loss at an acute angle to the root surface, forming an infrabony pocket.

Wry bite – A malocclusion in which the midline of the lower jaw does not oppose the midline of the upper jaw.

Dental Devices

Abutment – A tooth or implant that is used for the support or anchorage of a prosthesis or appliance.
Anchorage – Used orthodontically, it is the resistance to unwanted tooth movement.

Bite impression – Used to align casts to the occlusion of the patient.

Cast – A replication of the teeth and tissues made from an impression.
Crown or Cap – A cast metal covering of the crown of the tooth.

Impression – A negative replication of the teeth and tissues used to make a cast.

Orthodontic appliance – A device used to apply force to the teeth for tooth movement or to maintain tooth position.

Prosthesis – An artificial part that replaces part of the body.

Splint – An apparatus designed to prevent motion or displacement.

References

1. Cohen S, Burns RC. Pathways of the Pulp. St Louis: C.V. Mosby Co., 1984:302.

2. Rateitschak KH, et al. Periodontology. Stu Hgart: George Thieme Medical Publishers, 1989:35–37.

chapter 2

DENTAL EQUIPMENT AND CARE

SELECTING DENTAL EQUIPMENT

A variety of equipment is available and this leads to a frequently asked question: "What type of dental equipment should I buy?" The question has several factors to consider, depending on the practice situation. How much and what type of dentistry will be performed? How much space is available? How much capital is available to purchase the equipment?

When purchasing dental equipment, frequency of use, type of use, space available for equipment, and the cost should be evaluated before making a decision. For example, if the intent is to perform endodontic therapy, more than a casual interest should be exhibited and the purchase of an air-driven unit is almost a necessity. Other advanced dental procedures also require specialized equipment.

After reviewing the practice situation and goals, one hopes that the choice suited for the practice will become easier to make. The purchase of dental equipment provides an excellent return on investment.[1]

POWER EQUIPMENT

When purchasing power equipment, the practitioner should consider the cost of the unit, locations available for the compressor and dental consoles, noise levels at the location, track record at the clinic for equipment maintenance, and present and future dental caseload.

Features to Look for When Purchasing

Feature: Foot Pedal

Advantage

- Allows hands to concentrate on work rather than switching on and off.

Feature: Variable Speed

Advantage

- Allows for a broader range of work with more control.

Feature: Reverse Direction

Advantages

- Can use with caution to back out of wrapped hair.
- Can use with diamond disk to cut in direction you would like to cut.

Disadvantage

- A mandrel or screw-in prophy cup may become unscrewed if turned in the direction opposite to its design.

Accessories

- Prophy angles are used for polishing during prophylaxis, restorations, and other times where abrasives are used.
- Contra angles are used to change the angle of rotation of the device used on the teeth.
- Reduction contra angles are used to reduce speed at an angle.
- Acceleration contra angles will increase speed at which the device used on the teeth spins.
- Handpieces are instruments used to create force and to hold contra angles, prophy angles, burs, or other devices.

Uses

- Prophylaxis.
- Endodontics.
- Restorations.
- Exodontics.
- Orthodontics.
- Orthodontic laboratory.
- Oral surgery.

Electric-Motor-Driven Bands

Description

- The electric motor driving a steel or nylon band is one of the oldest types of power equipment used in human dentistry (A).
- They are still used mostly in dental labs.
- They are best suited for a new practice or a practice with a small dental load or limited procedures and are available on the used dental equipment market for low cost.
- Speed range of 3000 to 30,000 rpm.

Advantages

- Lower cost.
- Portability.
- Small size.

Disadvantages

- Slow speed.
- Breaking the band and difficulty in replacing parts.
- No water for cooling.
- Catching hair in the mechanism.

Maintenance

- Replacement of band.
- Lubrication according to manufacturer.

Handpieces Connected to Cable Driven by Electric Motor

Description

- Cable mechanisms that are hooked to electric motors come in several types.
- They are fairly inexpensive and are suited to a practice with a low volume and limited load, or as a secondary unit to handle additional patients when the primary unit is in use.
- Speed range is usually less than 3000 rpm.

Advantages

- Lower cost.
- Low maintenance.
- Portability.
- Small size.

Disadvantages

- Cable breakage, no water for cooling.
- Slow speed.
- Inability to do dental procedures other than polishing.

Maintenance

- Lubrication as directed by manufacturer.

Electric Motor Handpieces

Description

- Handpieces with electric motors built in *(B)*.
- A control box serves to connect the handpiece electrically.
- Speed range 3000 to 20,000 rpm; with accelerating contra angles speed can be increased to 125,000 rpm. (These contra angles are expensive.)

Advantages

- Most cost less than air units.
- Low maintenance.
- Portability.
- Small size.

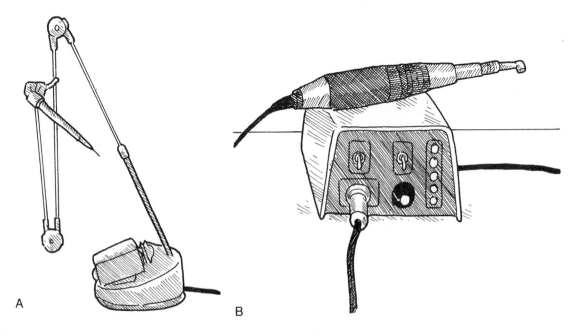

A   B

Disadvantages

- Handpiece and motor breakdown with heavy use.
- Except for models with accessories, inability to run water through the handpiece as a coolant for dental tissue.
- Slow cutting speed, cumbersome to use.
- Heavier handpiece may lead to more operator fatigue.

Air-Driven Power Equipment

Description

The air-driven systems have three components: the compressor, the "plumbing," and the handpieces. Compressors are rated by horsepower (hp) and the ability to deliver a flow of air. Most dental handpieces require the compressor to maintain 30 to 40 pounds per square inch (psi) at a flow of 3 cubic feet per minute. The control section is an array of air and water switches, regulators (valves), and hoses that control the flow of air and water into the air and water hoses and, in turn, into the handpieces. The control section can be mobile stands, carts, wall-mounted extension arms, or small countertop units.

Advantages

- Air acts as a coolant to the handpiece.
- Water passing through the handpiece and acting as a coolant/irrigant of dental tissues.
- Longer life of the compressor and handpiece.
- Ability to run at higher speeds for rapid performance.
- Air compressor units are easy to use.

Disadvantages

- Larger size.
- Noise from some types of compressors.
- Greater expense.

- Aerosol formed by spray mist.
- Accumulation of water in the oral cavity.
- Handpiece's noise may cause hearing loss.

Variable Features

- These are features the practitioner should consider when purchasing these units.

Electric Foot Switches

Comment

- The electric foot switch compressors operate with an electrical circuit to turn the compressor on and off, and air is delivered directly to the handpiece without storage.

Advantage

- Require less horsepower and thus can be smaller units at tableside.

Disadvantage

- Their disadvantage is the handpiece is either on full speed or off; there is no intermediate speed.

Air Rheostat Controls

Comments

The compressor is turned on and off by a preset pressure switch and runs only to fill the storage tank. Compressors of less than 3/4 hp are running more than they are off. This leads to overheating and temporary shutdown. If the practitioner's intent is infrequent use, the smaller, chairside units will work well. If frequent use or the use of multiple dental stations is anticipated, a larger, remote compressor with a storage tank is the best selection.

Advantage

- Wide variability in speeds.

Disadvantage

- Greater expense.

Remote Compressors

Comments

Compressors can be located away from the dental area. This removes another item from occupying space in the dental area and allows for multiple station use.

Advantages

- Can be used to power multiple stations.
- Many smaller, tableside compressor control units without compressors are compact and can be moved around and used at different locations, or stored out of the way.
- Remove compressor noise from dental area.

Disadvantages

- Require space with ventilation for cooling.
- Require a location where compressor noise will not interfere with practice routine.

Tableside Compressors

Comments

Primary considerations for selection of a tableside compressor are: space in the dental area, if the unit has enough power for current and future use, and noise tolerance of staff using the facility.

Advantages

- Can be stored in a different location when not in use.
- Can be moved easily.

Disadvantages

- Low power with some units that translates into a low volume of air flow and low air pressure.
- Excessive noise with some units.

Oil-Free/Oil-Containing Compressors

Comments

- Air heats up as it is compressed, and this heat is transmitted to the compressor.
- Compressors are cooled either by air or oil.
- Air-cooled, oil-free compressors do not have oil to check or change.
- As a general rule, "oil-free" compressors are noisier and more expensive than the equivalent oil-containing variety.
- To overcome the problem of monitoring oil level with a dipstick, several oil-containing models have level view ports for observation of the oil level.
- In-line filters to separate oil and water are recommended with all types of compressors.

"Whisper-Quiet" Compressors

Comments

- Traditional air compressors are fairly noisy.
- Very quiet refrigerator compressors have been converted from pumping refrigerator coolant to pumping air.
- These units are available in portable carts, portable cabinets, and countertop units.
- The single-unit compressor rates around 1/2 hp. If multistation use or a sonic scaler handpiece is being considered, a double-unit, 1-hp compressor should be considered.
- Because converted refrigerator compressors contain oil, the oil level must be monitored and changed on the manufacturer's recommendation.

Advantages

- Quiet compressor.
- Tabletop models are available.

Disadvantages

- Contain oil.
- Expensive.
- If used for long periods of time without stopping, some models may overheat and shut down until cool.

Three-Way Syringes

Comments

The three-way syringe (A) is used for:

- Flushing the oral cavity for better visualization.
- Rinsing chemicals off dental structures.
- Air drying tooth structures during restorations and other procedures.
- Air drying teeth to visualize calculus deposits that turn chalky when dry.[2]

Automatic Switches/Mechanical Switching

Comments

- Some units have switches that turn air on/off when the handpieces are placed in or taken from their holders.
- Others require mechanical switching on the part of the operator.

Automatic Drain Valves

Comment

- When pressure is released from air storage tank, condensed water is released.

Advantages

- Automatic drainage of water requires less maintenance because water is automatically drained.
- The compressor tank will last longer (decreases rust).

Disadvantages

- One more piece of equipment that may break down.
- Does not always work.

Oil-Level Indicators

Comment

- A view port is located at the same level as the oil stored inside the compressor (B).

Advantages

- Checking the oil level may be performed without the mess of a dipstick.
- The color of oil may be periodically inspected.

Do-It-Yourself Experimentation versus Plug-in "Turnkey" Units

Comments

- Components purchased at a department or hardware store can be used to assemble a dental unit.
- A minimum of 1 hp, and preferably a 2-hp compressor, is desirable.
- The control panels, regulators, and foot pedals can be purchased from dental suppliers.

Advantage

- No doubt there is a financial savings by putting together your own dental unit. However, we are veterinarians, not fluid engineers and mechanics!

Disadvantages

- This approach requires experimentation and time to manufacture a functional unit.
- In most cases, if the time to research and assemble a dental station were spent in

practice, you would have money ahead to purchase a "turnkey" unit.

- The turnkey units have been tested, the "bugs" worked out, and they are warranteed and serviceable.
- The practitioner will find, in most cases, the return on investment in a dental compressor will justify the purchase of a turnkey unit.

Compressor Maintenance

- All compressors with air storage tanks require periodic drainage of condensation from the tank (C).

- The last stage regulator should be set between 30 and 40 psi (D).
- The pressure in the tank may be 80 to 120 psi, depending on the brand.

Compressor Accessories

- Filters to filter out oil and water from the compressed air.
- Dryers to dry the air.
- Water filters to filter the water before entering the handpiece.

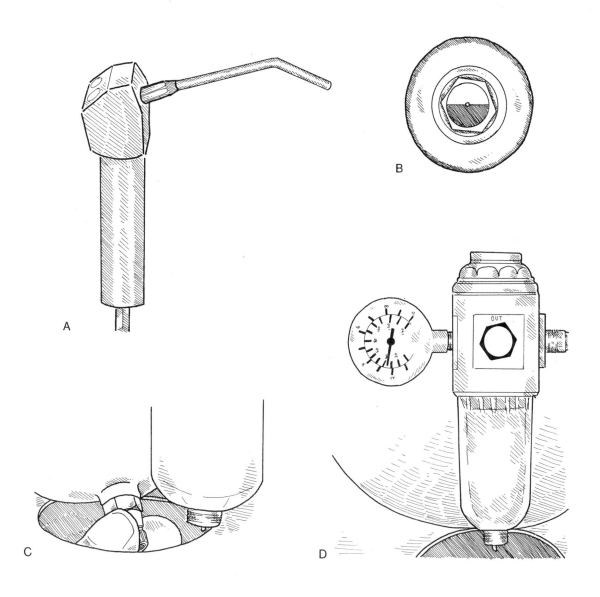

A

B

C

D

Handpieces

- Handpieces are instruments that enable the operator to work on teeth.
- Many types of handpieces are available, and they can be categorized into three basic types: slow-speed, high-speed, and sonic scalers.

General Maintenance

- A handpiece should never be turned on without a bur or "blank" inserted into the chuck to prevent damage.
- In addition, be sure to follow the manufacturer's recommendations on handpiece lubrication and air pressure.
- Lubricant should be placed in the smaller of the two large holes (A).

Slow-Speed Handpieces

Description

- Slow-speed handpieces produce a range of 5000 to 20,000 rpm, with high torque.

Uses

- Polishing with prophy angles.
- Contra angles can be attached to allow use of burs, endodontic files, polishing discs, and other specialized instruments requiring slower speeds and higher torques.

Advantages

- High torque, less likely to "stall out."
- Slower speed for cutting bone.

Disadvantages

- Slow speed is a disadvantage when cutting teeth; increases working time.
- May shatter tooth if the bur binds while cutting the tooth.
- May create thermal injury because of the slow speed and pressure between the bur and tooth surface (drilling pressure).
- Slow-speed handpieces usually do not have water as a coolant and irrigant.

Autoclavable Option

Comment

- Many of the newer slow-speed handpieces can be autoclaved.

Advantage

- Increase in rust resistance.

Maintenance

- Lubricate according to manufacturer's instructions.
- If a heavy oil is used, spraying with a light oil* once every 2 weeks may help to dissolve oil accumulations.
- Run the handpiece for 20 to 30 seconds after lubrication.
- Exterior should be wiped with a gauze sponge lightly soaked with alcohol between patients.

Accessories: Prophy Angles

Comments

- Prophy angles are used to polish teeth.
- There are two types of prophy angle rubber cup attachments, snap on and screw on. Which to use is an individual preference.

Circular Prophy Angles

Description

- These prophy angles rotate 360°.
- Metal styles are manufactured both to be disposed of when they break and to be repaired.
- Disposable styles are designed for single use and are made of plastic.

Advantages

- Circular prophy angles tend to be less expensive.
- The less-expensive styles are replaced rather than repaired.

Disadvantages

- Require taking apart and lubricating.
- May "spit" oil, contaminating the prepared dental surface.

Oscillating Prophy Angles

Description

- The oscillating prophy angle oscillates back and forth 90°.
- This style is a sealed unit.

Advantages

- Does not require lubrication.
- Prophy paste is not thrown because the cup is not spinning.

---

*WD-40.

• Hair does not become trapped in a spinning cup.

Disadvantages

• Greater expense to purchase.
• Repairs, if possible, may cost more than prophy angle.

Maintenance of Nonsealed Prophy Angles

• The prophy angle can be unscrewed and lubricated. There are usually two locations where the instrument can be opened for cleaning; by removal of the head or removal of the cap. With most prophy angles, only one method needs to be used.

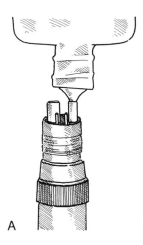

A

Removal of Head

Step 1—The head is unscrewed by turning it counterclockwise *(A)*.

Step 2—The gears are cleaned with WD–40 or other solvent *(B)*.

Step 3—The gears are lubricated with Prophy Lube* or other appropriate lubricant *(C)*.

Step 4—The head is replaced by screwing it on clockwise.

Removal of Cap

Step 1—The cap is unscrewed by turning it clockwise *(D)*.

_____

*Young Dental Mfg, 13705 Shoreline Ct., Earth City, MO 63045.

Step 2—The gears are cleaned with WD–40 *(E)*.

Step 3—The gears are lubricated with Prophy Lube *(F)*.

Step 4—The cap is replaced by screwing it on counterclockwise.

Accessories: Contra Angles

- Contra angles can increase or decrease the rpm's at the working end, change angulation, or provide 90° rotation.
- Contra angles use right angle (RA) or latch-type burs, which have larger-diameter shanks than high-speed burs.

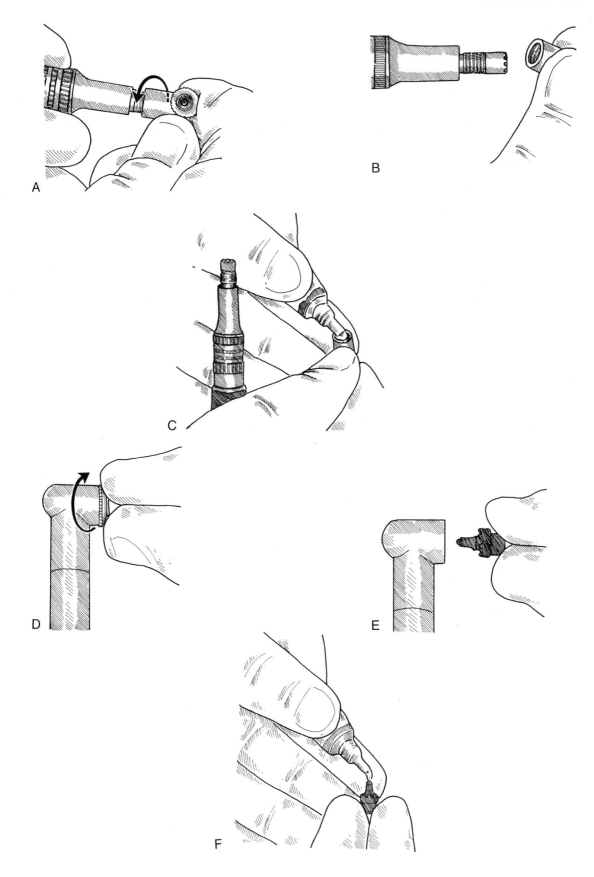

Slow-Speed Burs

- Burs are held by handpieces in three ways: "straight," "latch," and "friction grip."
- The straight-type bur fits directly into the slow-speed handpiece (A).

Changing Straight-Type Burs

Step 1—Twist the collar to open the chuck (B). Proper position is usually noted by dots on the handpiece.

Step 2—Remove straight bur and replace with new bur (C).

Step 3—Twist chuck latch collar to close, as noted by dots on the handpiece (D).

- The latch or RA type fits into a contra angle that holds the bur in place (E).

Changing Latch-Type Burs

Step 1—Holding the contra angle with the working side away from the operator, slide handle to the right (F).

Step 2—Remove old bur (G).

Step 3—Replace with new bur, lining up the flat portion of the bur to slide all the way in (H).

Step 4—Slide handle to left (I).

- The friction grip or FG is usually used in high-speed handpieces and will be discussed under high-speed handpieces.

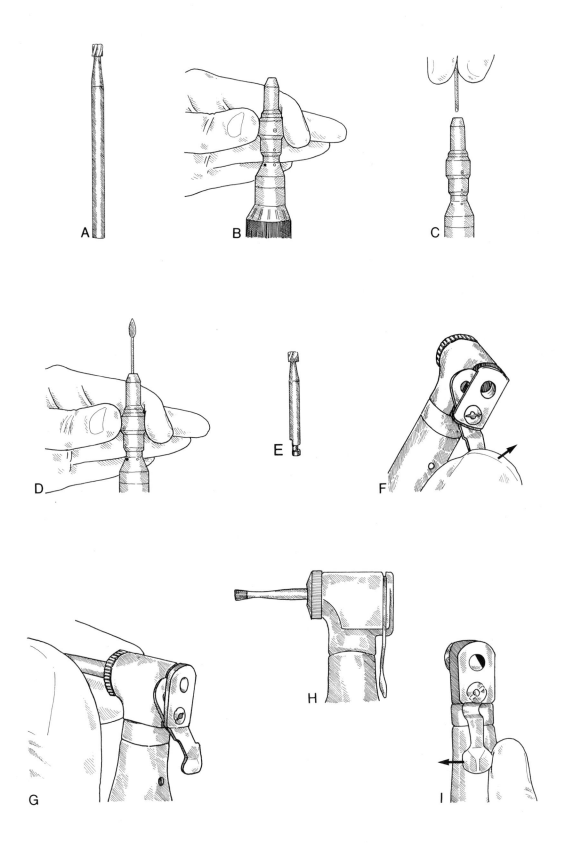

Types of Burs/Drills

- Many types of slow-speed burs are similar to high-speed burs.
- Some types of burs and drills are available for slow speed only.

Gates Glidden Drills

Description

- The Gates Glidden drills have relatively long, narrow shafts with a flame-shaped boring head *(A)*.
- The size of the Gates Glidden drill is marked by bands on the shaft.

Uses

- The Gates Glidden drill is used to expand the opening into the endodontic system for easier instrumentation and filling of the canal proper during root canal therapy.
- The Gates Glidden drill tends to follow the path of a pre-existing hole.

Cautions

- If bound in the canal or bent, the drill will break, usually at the latch end of the shaft.
- Use with slow-speed handpiece only.

Peeso Reamers

Description

- The Peeso reamer has a longer, torpedo-shaped head and shorter shaft than the Gates Glidden drill *(B)*.
- The Peeso reamers have bands to indicate the size on the shank.

Uses

- The Peeso reamer is used to widen the diameter of a prepared root canal in preparation for a post *(C)*.
- The Peeso reamer may cut its own path, not necessarily following the canal *(D)*.

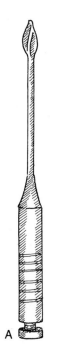

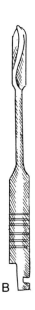

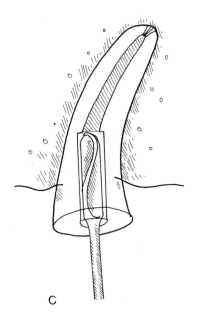

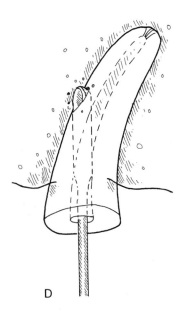

A

B

C

D

Green Stones

Description

- Green stones are silicon carbide abrasive stones in carefully controlled grits of various shapes and sizes.

Uses

- Green stones are used for finishing restorations and to produce a moderately rough surface.
- Green stones are used for the bulk removal of restorative material prior to the final finish.

White Stones

Description

- White stones are dense aluminum oxide abrasives of fine texture *(A)*.

Use

- White stones are used for final restoration to produce a smooth surface.

Discs

Description

- Discs are flexible, molded or cut paper, plastic, rubber, stone, or metal *(B)*.
- Discs may have their own shafts or may be held by a mandrel.

Use

- Discs are used for finishing restorations, occlusion adjustment, and cutting tooth and material.

Wheels

Description

- Wheels, composed of molded abrasive materials of phenolic resins or rubber with an abrasive, come in various shapes and sizes *(C)*.

Uses

- Wheels are used primarily for laboratory procedures, finishing, and polishing.
- Shofu polishing disc* *(D)*.

---

*Shofu Dental Corp., 4025 Bohannon Drive, Menlo Park, CA 94025.

Mandrels

Description

- Mandrels attach to the slow-speed handpiece with latch-type, straight-shaft, or FG-type grips.
- Mandrels hold discs or wheels by pop-on, screw-on, or rod-type screw.
  - Pop-on mandrel *(E)*.
  - Screw-on mandrel *(F)*.
  - Rod-type screw-on mandrel *(G)*.

Use

- Mandrels are used to hold finishing materials.

Paste Fillers

Comments

- Paste fillers are attached to the reduction gear contra angle of the slow-speed handpiece *(H)*.
- When rotated they will spin paste root canal filling material down into the canal.
- Because of their reverse spiral, they work in the forward (clockwise) rotation.
- Paste fillers are manufactured in various sizes and lengths.

Advantage

- Paste fillers auger root canal pastes or sealers apically into the canal, eliminating air bubbles.

Disadvantages

- May not fit into canal.
- Must use 10:1 reduction gear contra angles or risk breaking spiral filler.
- Must have adequate-diameter access to prevent binding and breakage.

Slow-Speed Bur–High-Speed Handpiece Adapter

Description

- The adapter holds high-speed burs in latch-type contra angles *(I)*.

Advantage

- Allows slower speed use of FG bur.

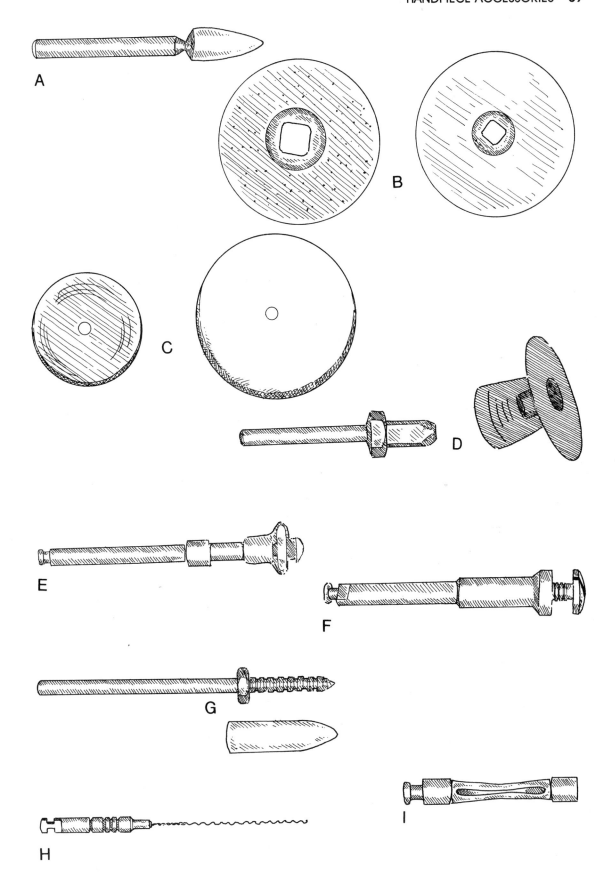

A

B

C

D

E

F

G

H

I

High-Speed Handpieces

Description

- High-speed handpieces rotate in the range of 200,000 to 400,000 rpm.

Use

- Cutting teeth, endodontic access, cavity preparation, and restorations.

Advantages

- High speed allows for rapid cutting of teeth.
- Water cooling protects dental tissue.
- Low torque, "stalling" protects dental tissue from shattering.

Disadvantages

- Stalling may slow down work.
- May create excessive heat or burning if not using adequate water cooling or too much drilling pressure.
- Moisture or oil blown through the handpiece may destroy the turbine bearings.

Options

Wrenchless Handpieces

Comment

- This feature allows bur exchange without using a chuck key.

Advantage

- Speed in changing burs.

Disadvantage

- The wrenchless type is more prone to breakdown.

Fiberoptics

Comments

- Light is directed at the operating field.
- A light source provides light that is transferred by fiberoptics to the head of the handpiece.

Advantage

- Greater visualization of working area.

Disadvantages

- One more thing to break down.
- Additional expense.

High-Speed Handpiece Maintenance

- Lubricant must be used on a regular basis. Follow the recommendations of the handpiece manufacturer for which spray or liquid lubricant to use. Oils are not recommended for most high-speed handpieces.
- The lubricant should be placed in the smaller of the two large holes (A).

Changing Friction Grip Burs

Overhead Chuck-Key Type

Step 1—Place chuck key over the head of the handpiece (B).

Step 2—Rotate the chuck-key knob counterclockwise (C).

Step 3—Remove old bur (D); if resistance is initially encountered, it may help to first gently push in on bur to loosen the chuck grip and then pull the bur out.

Step 4—Push new bur in until completely seated (E). Caution must be exercised here. If the bur is not completely seated, the turbine bearings may be damaged.

Step 5—Rotate chuck-key knob clockwise just until snug (F). Do not overtighten.

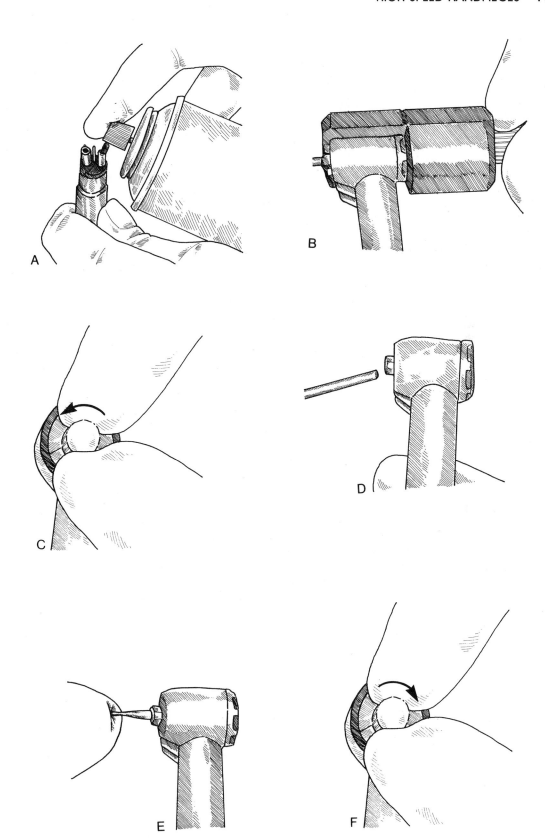

Replacement of Turbine Cartridge

Signs of defective turbine cartridge:

- Chuck will not tighten around the bur.
- Increased noise or vibration.
- Roughness felt when spinning bur by hand, with turbine in or out of handpiece.
- Handpiece intermittently stops.
- Handpiece will not work.

Cap-Style Handpiece Back

Step 1—Place "blank" bur in handpiece (A). If bur that is in handpiece cannot be removed, proceed with caution to avoid cutting hands on bur.

Step 2—Place small metal ring (wrench) supplied with handpiece on cap of handpiece (B).

Step 3—By rotating wrench counterclockwise, unscrew the handpiece cap and remove (C).

Step 4—Press on blank or bur to remove turbine cartridge from handpiece head (D).

Step 5—The new turbine cartridge is placed into the handpiece head (E).

Step 6—The new turbine cartridge is aligned with pin side up (F). If the pin is not lined up with the slot, the turbine cartridge will not slide completely into the handpiece head (G).

Step 7—Slide cartridge all the way into handpiece head (H).

Step 8—Replace handpiece cap by twisting wrench clockwise (I).

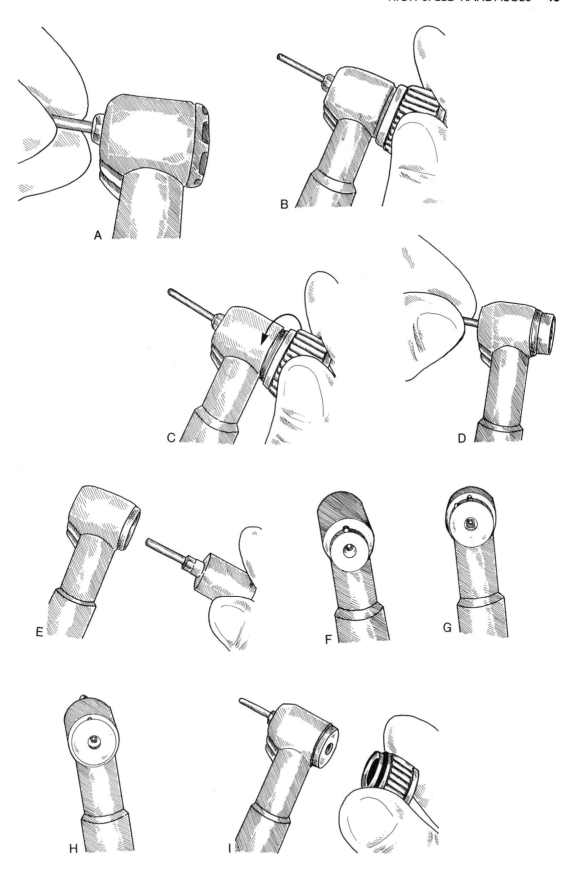

Handpiece Burs

- High-speed handpieces use friction grip burs.
- Only high-speed burs should be used with high-speed handpieces.
- There are three parts to burs: shank, the portion that attaches to the handpiece; shaft, the portion from the shank to the head; and head, the working portion.
- Different length heads may be denoted as S (short) or L (long); if no letter it is the standard length.

    Longer shanks are denoted as surgical length (A).

    Flutes can be cut plain, without notches (B) or crosscut, with notches (C).
- Most cutting burs are 6 fluted. Finishing burs have 10 or more flutes.
- When discussing bur types, we are discussing the shape of the head of the bur. Most shapes come in plain or cross cut. Common shapes are round, cylinder (fissure), taper fissure, pear, flame, inverted cone, and wheel.
- The tips of the bur can be cutting, noncutting, rounded, or square. The noncutting tip is used to cut straight sides without cutting the floor of the cavity preparation. The cutting tip may cut into the cavity floor. The square tip creates a 90° angle at the interface between the floor and the wall. This may be difficult to fill with restorative material and creates a "break on angle" line. The round tip creates a rounded transition between the floor and wall. This interface is easier to fill and is less fragile.

Round Burs (1/4, 1/2, 1, 2, 3, 4, 6, 8)

Uses

- The smaller burs (1/4, 1/2) can be used to create retentive grooves in tooth structure or mark locations for larger slow-speed bur placement (D).
- The medium-sized burs (1, 2) can be used for initial cavity preparation and outline.
- The larger burs are used for bulk removal of dental tissue.
- Some round burs are designed to be placed parallel to the tooth with the shank as a limit to marking cutting depth in crown preparation.

Fissure Burs (556, 557, 558)

Description

- The sides of the head of the fissure bur are parallel (E).

Use

- The fissure bur has straight, parallel sides that create parallel cavity sides.

Tapered-Fissure Burs (plain 168, 169, 169L, 170, 170L, 171, 171L, 172, 172L, 173; crosscut 699, 700, 701, 701L, 702, 702L, 703, 703L)

Description

- The head of a tapered-fissure bur is narrower at the tip than toward the shank (F).

Uses

- The tapered-fissure bur is a general-purpose bur that can be used for bulk removal of dental tissue, in sectioning teeth for extraction, or endodontic access.
- When held perpendicular to a cavity preparation, it can be used to prevent an undercut.

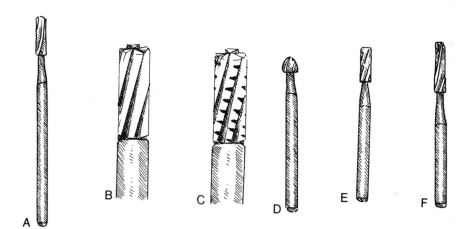

A B C D E F

Pear-Shaped Burs (330, 331, 332)

Uses

- The pear-shaped bur is a general-purpose bur that can be used for root canal access or undercutting dentin in cavity preparation (A).
- The pear-shaped bur creates smoothly rounded internal line angles.

Flame Burs

- The flame bur head has a pointed tip and wider body that rounds toward the shank.
- One of the commonly used Rotopro burs is the flame shape.

Inverted-Cone Burs (33½, 34, 35, 37, 38, 39)

Description

- The inverted-cone bur has a head that is wider toward the tip than toward the shaft (B).

Uses

- Smaller inverted-cone burs are used to penetrate into root canals.
- Larger inverted-cone burs are used to undercut cavity preparations to create a mechanical interlock.

Special-Use Burs

Rotopro Bur

- Used for scaling teeth (C).
- Frequency is 30,000 kHz at the working tip, depending on speed of air turbine and air pressure.
- See periodontics section for information.

Multifluted Finishing Burs

- Come in a variety of shapes.
- Have an increasing number of flutes; the more flutes, the smoother the finish.

Diamond Burs (Many Sizes and Shapes Available)

- Diamond burs cut by grinding and can be used for cutting (D) or finishing (E).
- Are manufactured by electroplating diamond grit onto a one-piece bur blank by either a nickel or chromium bonding material.
- Either natural or artificial diamonds are used.
- Different grits of diamonds are used. Commonly used are extrafine, fine, medium, and coarse.

Bur Accessories

Bur-Cleaning Brush

- Bur-cleaning brushes clean the flutes of the bur, but will not sharpen the flutes (F).
- The brush is used by brushing the bur, without running the handpiece.

Diamond-Bur Cleaning Stone

- The diamond-bur cleaning stone removes debris from the surface of the diamond bur (G).
- The bur is run over a wet stone using the high-speed handpiece.

Bur Block

- The bur block is used to store burs (H).

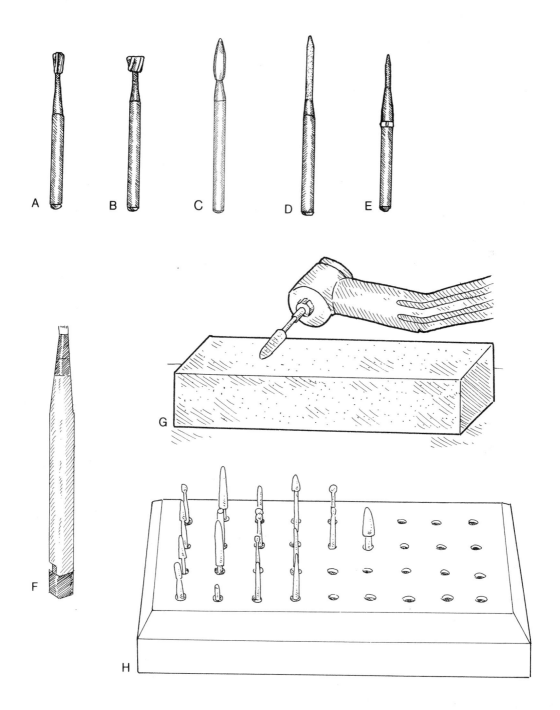

A   B   C   D   E

F

G

H

DENTAL RADIOLOGY EQUIPMENT

Veterinary Medical Units

Description

- 100-ma to 500-ma veterinary medical units may be used to expose dental film.

Advantage

- No additional expense required when using standard veterinary medical machines.

Disadvantages

- The patient must be moved between the dental area and radiology area during procedures.
- The flexibility of most veterinary medical units does not allow the radiographic head to move for optimum positioning. Thus, the patient must be positioned; that is more time consuming and difficult than moving the radiographic head.

Dental Radiographic Units

Description

- Used or new dental units are available.
- They are usually low-milliamperage units suited for dental film exposure.

Advantages

- Dental radiology may be carried out in the normal dental area.
- The regular veterinary radiographic unit is available for use by the rest of the hospital while the dental procedure is performed.
- A higher-quality image is generated.

Film-Processing Systems

- Film may be processed either manually or with an automatic processor.

Manual Processing

- There are three types of manual developing solutions: standard veterinary dip-tank solutions, one-step rapid process solutions, and two-step rapid processing.

Standard Veterinary Medical Solutions

Description

- The regular developer and fixing solutions that are normally used in manual processing of veterinary radiographic film may be used to develop dental film.

Advantage

- If the hospital is already using this system, these solutions are available at no additional cost.

Disadvantages

- Loss of detail.
- Longer processing time.

One-Step Rapid Processing

Description

- A single developing solution that contains both developer and fixer to process the film in approximately 1 minute.

Advantage

- Single-step processing.

Disadvantages

- There is a loss of detail when using the single-step technique.
- "Greening" of processed film may occur several days after developing.

Rapid Two-Step Processing

Description

- A developing solution and a separate fixing solution designed to process film in approximately 1 minute.

Advantages

- The rapid two-step processing solutions provide high-quality developing and rapid processing.
- If properly used, these solutions create films that may be stored without loss of quality.

Mechanical Processing

- There are two types of mechanical processing systems: the large-film automatic processors and the smaller dental processors.

Large-Film Processors

Description

- Large-film automatic processors are commonly found in veterinary hospitals.
- Dental radiographic film may be taped to larger radiographic film and sent through the processor.

Advantage

- None; in most practices, manual systems are best.

Disadvantages

- Risk loss of film into the processor.
- Must use leader film to attach the smaller film.
- Possible damage to processor if improper tape is used.

Small-Film Processors

Description

- Small-film processors are designed to transport dental films through the processing solutions and the dryer.

Advantages

- Greater quality control.
- No need to use leader films.

Disadvantages

- Expense.
- Usually require greater time to process than manual rapid process methods.

Location of Processing
Dip Tanks for Darkrooms

Description

- Tanks or containers may be used in the darkroom with rapid processing solutions to process the radiographs.

Advantage

- Less expense.

Disadvantages

- Personnel must leave the dental area to go to darkroom to process the film.
- May create additional mess in the darkroom due to inadvertent spillage.

Chairside Darkrooms

Description

- Chairside darkrooms are small, portable lightproof boxes that have hooded hand ports to process the film in darkness. Because this process is manual, a special see-through plastic cover allows the operator to see the film and dip tanks. The cover does not allow exposing light to affect the film.

Advantages

- Rapid (usually less than 1 minute) process.
- Avoids tying up a darkroom.

Disadvantages

- Use caution to avoid opening the lid accidentally and exposing the film during processing.
- The amber filter will protect the film for a limited time and intensity of light.
- Must have space at tableside or in the dental area.

Maintenance

- The frequency of chemical change depends on the number of radiographs processed, the amount of exposure to air, and the age of the chemicals.
- Close lids to unused chemicals.
- Replace damaged hand porthole covers.
- Clean box with mild detergent and water.
- Do not damage the porthole sleeves with jewelry.
- Chairside darkrooms need to be used in subdued-light areas. To test the location, place the chairside darkroom where you plan to use it. Open a film packet in the "darkroom." Lay the film on top of one of the jars and cover all but one strip of it. At 15- to 30-second intervals uncover another strip of the film until the last strip has been exposed for the set time interval. Develop the film in the normal fashion. After fixing, examine the film for fogging. If there is no fogging, it is safe to develop film at that location under the same light-intensity conditions. If there is fogging, determine the length of time it took to cause fogging and whether you can process films in less time at that location and light intensity. If the fogging occurred in a short time, the location or the amount of light needs to be changed.

EQUIPMENT FOR PERIODONTICS

Sonic Scalers

Description

- Sonic scalers are used for gross calculus removal from teeth (A).
- Inside most sonic scalers is a shaft that is connected to the air supply and tip.
- The vibration at the tip of the scaler is caused by air passing out of a hole in the shaft that spins a ring that encircles the shaft.
- There is little difference between the action of the ultrasonic scaler and the sonic scaler on the surface of the tooth.
- Frequency is 16,000 kHz at the working tip.

Use

- Gross calculus removal.

Advantages

- Very little heat is created at the working tip compared to the ultrasonic scaler.
- There is less chance of injuring the tooth with pulp hyperthermia.
- Do not have to sharpen the instrument.
- Performs a lavage function by irrigating and flushing while effecting calculus removal.

Disadvantages

- Conflicting reports regarding the relative strengths of the sonic and ultrasonic scaler. One study showed that some models of subsonic scalers have been shown to be as effective at calculus removal as ultrasonic scalers set at maximum power.[3] However, another study claimed that the ultrasonic scaler cleared hard deposits of calculus faster.[4]
- Some units must be cleaned and lubricated periodically.
- Higher rate of breakdown than ultrasonic scalers.

Ultrasonic Scalers

Description

- The ultrasonic scaler has long been the mainstay of veterinary dentistry.

- Vibration frequency at the working tip with pot/stack is 25,000 kHz, with piezoelectric 40,000 kHz. We have seen little advantage or disadvantage between the piezoelectric and pot/stack models.

Uses

- Removes gross calculus from the teeth.
- Removes orthodontic bonding materials.

Advantages

- Durability.
- No need to sharpen instrument.
- Performs a lavage function by irrigating and flushing while effecting calculus removal.

Disadvantages

- Heat production and possible injury to tooth.
- Expense of replacement tips.
- With improper use, can damage enamel.

Tip-Only Replacement

Comment

- Some models are available in which only the tip needs to be replaced (B).

Advantage

- Tips are a lot less expensive than the whole stack arrangement.

Disadvantage

- May require entire handpiece to be repaired or replaced.

Pot/Stack Model Maintenance

- The "leaves" should be periodically inspected for fracture and replaced if fractures are found (C).

Calculus-Removal Forceps

Description

- Calculus-removal forceps are specially designed forceps used for the removal of gross calculus (D).

Use

- Periodontics, gross calculus removal.

Advantage

- This instrument is for the quick removal of large pieces of gross calculus.

Disadvantages

- They remove only gross supragingival calculus (and are only one of the first steps of a complete and thorough prophylaxis).
- Can damage the crown, enamel, or gum tissue if improperly used.

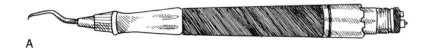

A

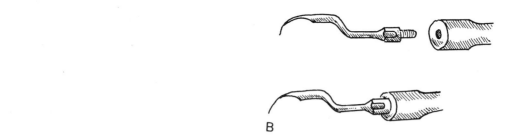

B

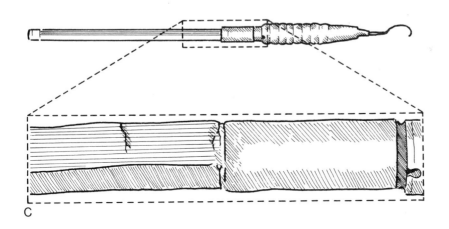

C

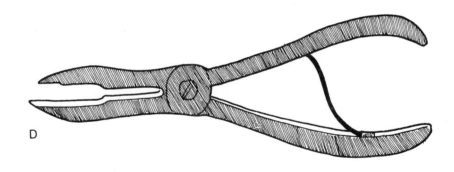

D

Large Hand Instruments

Dental Hoe (Chisel)

Description

- The working tip is a wide, chisel-like blade (A).

Use

- Supragingival gross calculus removal only.

Advantage

- Strong instrument.

Disadvantage

- It is for removal of large deposits only, not for removal of subgingival or small calculus and plaque.

Dental Claw

Description

- The dental hoe and claw were once the mainstay hand instruments of veterinary dentistry.
- The claw is a large, thick, sickle-shaped scaler (B).

Use

- Used only to break off large pieces of supragingival gross calculus.

Advantage

- Removal of gross calculus in absence of sonic or ultrasonic scalers or calculus-removing forceps.

Disadvantages

- Slow speed.
- Some mechanical hand strength required.
- Potential damage to the tooth and gingival structures.

Fine Hand Instruments

- The selection of a curette or scaler is a matter of personal preference.
- If you do not like a particular instrument, do not replace it with the same one.
- If properly used and sharpened, these instruments will need to be replaced on a periodic basis.
- When properly performed, hand scaling is preferable to ultrasonic scaling. It causes less damage to the tooth structure and is more efficient.[2]

- Use of fine scalers lets the operator remove calculus and plaque from above and below the gumline.[5]

Options

Comments

- Both curettes and scalers are made of carbon steel or stainless steel.
- Dry storage of dental instruments is an accepted procedure in human dentistry.

Carbon Steel

Advantage

- Carbon steel instruments will maintain a sharper edge than stainless steel, provided they are kept rust free.

Disadvantage

- Carbon steel instruments rust and become brittle if left in water containing cold disinfecting solutions for extended periods of time or if steam autoclaved without a rust inhibitor.

Stainless Steel

Advantage

- Stainless steel instruments are resistant to rusting.

Disadvantage

- Stainless steel instruments will still dull if left in disinfecting solutions and do not maintain as sharp an edge as carbon steel.

Replaceable Tips

Comment

- Some manufacturers make hand instruments that have a cone socket handle and removable tips (C).

Advantages

- The tips rather than the entire instrument are replaced when the tip is worn down or broken.
- The operator can select different tips for each end of the instrument and customize the instrument.

Disadvantage

- The replaceable tip instruments generally are expensive to purchase initially.

Scalers

Description

- The blade of a scaler is triangular and tapers to a pointed tip, with two parallel cutting edges *(D)*.

Use

- Scalers are used for supragingival scaling.

Advantages

- The angulation of a scaler is convenient for supragingival scaling.
- The pointed tip may be used to remove calculus from pits and fissures and interproximal areas *(E)*.

Disadvantage

- Because of the shape and sharp tip, the scaler should not be used below the gumline. It can distend and lacerate soft tissues.

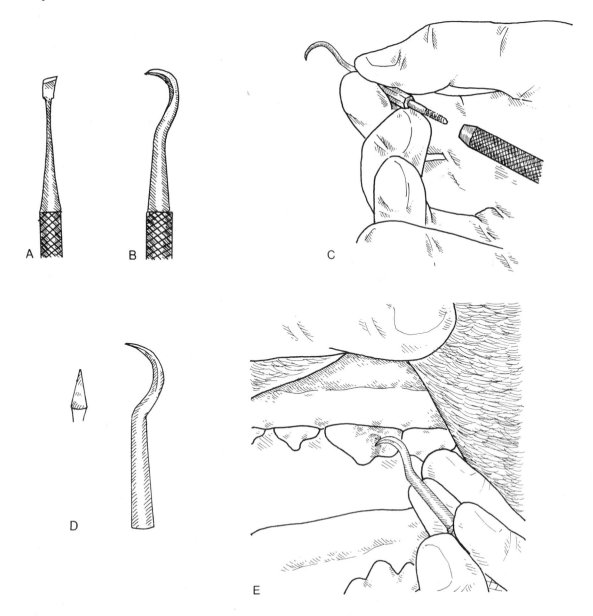

Types

Jacquette 2Y-3Y Scaler *(A)*

- Has medium blade, acute round angle at the blade, and no shaft; the blade is slightly longer than the Morse 0–00.

N135 Scaler

- Has a medium shaft, thin blade, with sharp curve, good for supragingival interproximal work, between incisors or between maxillary fourth premolar and first molar *(B)*.

H6-H7 or N6-N7 Scaler

- Long, sickle-shaped blade of medium thickness *(C)*.

Morse 0–00 Scaler

- Has no angle, very thin, short blade, acute 90° angulation *(D)*.

Maintenance

- To remain functional, a scaler must be kept sharp. Sharp scalers fracture, cleave, and remove calculus; dull scalers ineffectively crush and burnish it.
- Ideally, hand instruments should be sharpened between each use.

Curettes

Description

- Curettes have two sharp working edges, a flat face, and a rounded back *(E)*.
- Looking end on, they have a half-moon shape.

Uses

- Curettes are used for removing calculus and plaque above and below the gumline.
- Curettes are used for subgingival curettage and root planing.

Advantage

- The rounded tip and back are less traumatic to soft tissue and adapt easily to root surfaces.

Disadvantages

- The rounded tip may not be able to get into all crevices.
- If used improperly may break or cause tissue damage.

Types

Universal Curettes

- Universal curettes are adaptable throughout the mouth, hence the "universal" title. Although the anatomy varies from humans to animals, this general concept is still valid.

Columbia 13/14 Curette

- Has a short shank, medium to thin blade, and medium curve *(F)*.

Barnhart 5/6 Curette

- Has a short shank, medium blade, and small to medium curve *(G)*.

Columbia 3/4

- Has a medium shank, medium blade, and small to medium curve *(H)*.

Posterior Curettes

- Posterior curettes have a longer terminal shank for interproximal access.

4R-4L Curette

- Has a medium shank, medium blade, with medium curve, primarily for posterior teeth.

2R-2L Curette

- Has a long shaft, medium blade, with medium curve; fits shape of canine patients' teeth, primarily for anterior teeth.

Barnhart 1/2 Curette

- Has a long shaft, thin blade, medium curve; good for root planing in tight fits.

Maintenance of Scalers and Curettes

Cleaning and Care of Scalers and Curettes

Step 1—The instrument should be washed with a disinfectant soap* to remove all debris.

Step 2—The instrument should be dried.

Step 3—The instrument is sharpened (see sharpening techniques).

Step 4—The instrument is soaked in a disinfectant solution, autoclaved, dry sterilized, or gas sterilized.

---

*Nolvasan scrub, Fort Dodge Laboratories, 800 Fifth Street NW, Fort Dodge, IA 50510.

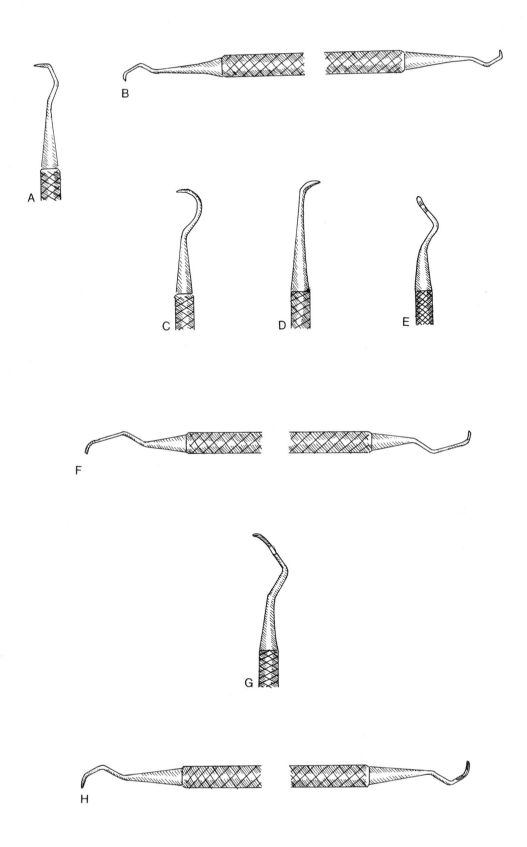

Sharpening Curettes and Scalers

Objectives

- Remove as little of the instrument as possible.
- Obtain sharp edge.
- Retain original design of the instrument.

Materials: Sharpening Stones

- Sharpening stones are used to restore the cutting edge on a dull instrument without changing the original design of that instrument.[6]
- The coarser the stone, the faster the sharpening, and the rougher the edge.
- Fine stones are used for sharpening only slightly dull instruments and to finish sharpening to remove rough edges or flash.
- Coarse stones are used for dull instruments, or for reshaping.

Arkansas Stones

Description

- Arkansas stones are fine stones, used for routine sharpening and finishing.
- Arkansas stones are used with oil.

Advantages

- Give a fine finish.
- Relatively little of the instrument is reduced.

Disadvantage

- May be slow if used to recontour the instrument.

Maintenance

- After use, should be wiped clean.
- May be cleaned with routine soaps or detergents.
- May be autoclaved.

India Stones

Description

- India stones are either fine or medium in coarseness.
- India stones are used with oil.

Advantage

- Good for use to sharpen excessively dull instruments.

Disadvantage

- May excessively wear away the instrument if used for routine sharpening.

Maintenance

- After use, should be wiped clean.
- May be cleaned with routine soaps or detergents.
- May be autoclaved.

Ceramic Stones

Description

- Stones are made from compressed glass.
- They are used with water or dry.
- They are fine to medium grit.

Advantages

- Do not create mess, as does oil.
- Are found in kits.*

Disadvantage

- Additional expense of the stone.

Moving Flat Stone Technique

Advantages

- Easiest technique to learn.
- Good visibility of sharpening surface.
- Sharpens side of instrument, maintaining strength (A).

Disadvantage

- Some operators like stationary stone technique better.

Materials

- Stone oil.
- Sharpening stone.

Technique

Step 1—A drop of oil is placed on an India or Arkansas sharpening stone (B).

Step 2—The oil is distributed over the face of the stone by wiping with a tissue (C).

Step 3—The instrument is held vertically over the side of a table with the edge to be sharpened down (D).

Step 4—The stone is placed so that the open angle between the face and stone is 110° (E). This creates a 70° angle between the face and side of the blade. The stone is drawn

---

*Sharpen-Rite, P.O. Box 03371, Portland, OR 97203.

up and down to sharpen the blade while maintaining this angle.

Step 5—The sharpening sequence *ends on the down stroke.*

Step 6—The other side blade and the blades of the opposite tip are sharpened in a similar manner.

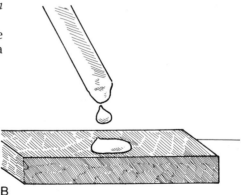

B

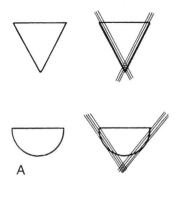

A

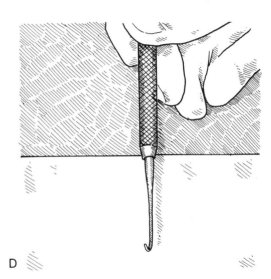

D

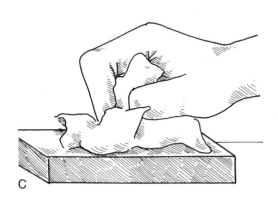

C

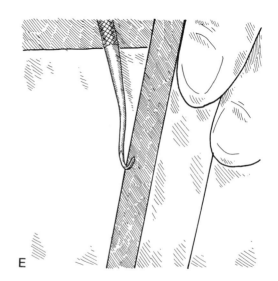

E

Moving Flat Stone—Sharpen-Rite Technique

Advantages

- Guides the inexperienced sharpener effectively.
- Helps achieve a sharp instrument.

Disadvantages

- Cumbersome and slower to use.
- Requires time to read instructions and figure out.

Materials

- Sharpen-Rite Kit.*
- Does not require stone oil.

---

*Sharpen-Rite, P.O. Box 03371, Portland, OR 97203.

Technique

Step 1—The Sharpen-Rite Guide is taped to the edge of a counter *(A)*.

Step 2—The operator is sitting directly in front of the counter top *(B)*.

Step 3—The stone is placed parallel to one of the two black lines marked "stone" *(C)*.

Step 4—The instrument is held with the toe pointing directly toward the operator with the hand resting firmly on the counter top *(D)*.

Step 5—The instrument is lined up in the area corresponding to the marking for that type of instrument *(E)*.

Step 6— Keeping the stone parallel to the stone line, the stone is moved up and down to sharpen the instrument.

Step 7—The toe of the instrument is sharpened by repositioning the instrument at a 45° angle between the stone and face of the blade.

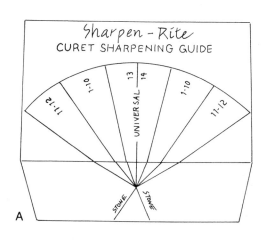

A

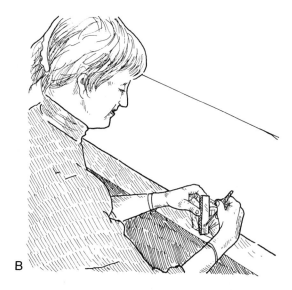

B

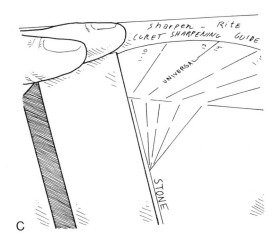

C

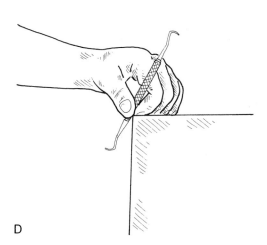

D

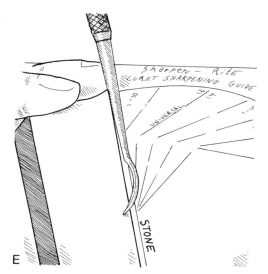

E

Stationary Flat Stone Technique

Advantage

- Once learned, may be the fastest technique to perform.

Disadvantage

- Takes time and practice to use this technique effectively.

Technique

Step 1—The stone is oiled as with other techniques.

Step 2—The stone is placed flat on a table and is held by hand *(A)*.

Step 3—The instrument is held in the opposite hand with a modified pencil grip *(B)*. The index and thumb hold the instrument while the middle, ring, and little fingers act as a guide and slide along the table. The blade to be sharpened is positioned with the face of the instrument opened at a 110° angle to the stone. The cutting edge is formed between the face and side of the blade, and that angle should be between 70° and 80°. The instrument is moved back and forth on the stone while keeping the blade at this constant angle.

Conical Stone Technique

Advantage

- Less skill is involved in using a conical stone.

Disadvantages

- Decreases the strength of the instrument by taking away the body of the blade where previous techniques remove sides but keep the thickness *(C)*.
- Changes the angle between the face and side of the blade of a curette.

Materials

- Stone oil.
- Conical stone.

Technique

Step 1—A small amount of stone oil is placed on the stone *(D)*.

Step 2—The stone is wiped with a tissue *(E)*.

Step 3—The stone is placed on the face of the instrument and is rotated and, at the same time, rubbed along the face toward the tip *(F)*. One to three rotations over the face of the blade are made to remove excess flash or uneven edges.

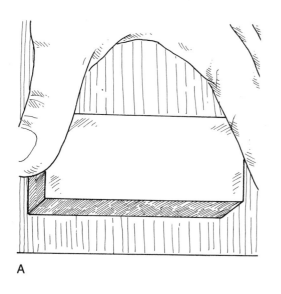

A

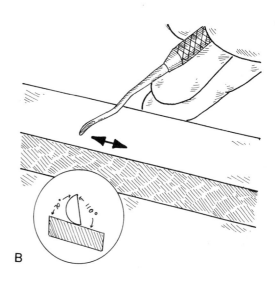

B

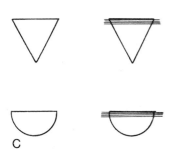

C

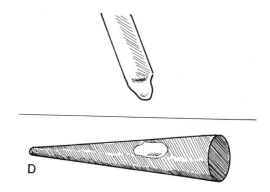

D

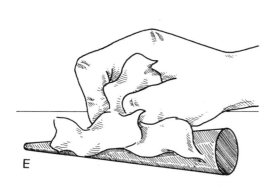

E

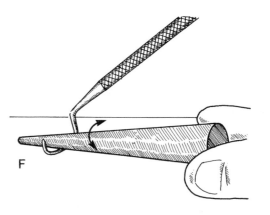

F

Instruments for Periodontal Diagnosis

Periodontal Probes

Description

- Periodontal probes are either notched or color coded and may be single ended or double ended in combination with another type of probe or explorer.
- Periodontal probes may be contra-angled for more accurate reading on the distal side of teeth.

Use

- Periodontal probes are used to measure the gingival recession and periodontal pocket depth, allowing the evaluator to estimate epithelial attachment level.[5, 7]

Advantage

- Probes can be used to measure the degree of periodontal disease.

Disadvantage

- If used improperly, probes can damage epithelial attachment.

Types

Notched Probes

Description

- The notched types are generally notched in millimeters.
- The notched types are either flat or round. The flat probes are easier to fit into a thin sulcus, whereas the rounded ones are easier to see at different angles.
- The Goldman Fox and Williams probes have notches at 1-2-3-(skips 4)-5-(skips 6)-7-8-9-10 mm (A).

Advantage

- The notch is a clear indication of depth.

Disadvantage

- May not be as easy to read as color-coded probes.

Color-Coded Probes

Comments

- The color-coded probes have color-coded bands.

- The probes come in 10-, 11-, and 12-mm lengths.
- The 3-6-9-12-mm readings are popular markings (B).

Advantages

- The longer probes may record deeper depths.
- The probes are longer and easier to see at different angles than are the flat probes.

Disadvantage

- The color coding may wear off with time or in ultrasonic cleaners; however, some manufacturers will recoat probes for a reasonable cost.

Periodontal Explorers

Description

- Explorers are used to examine the tooth and detect abnormalities through the senses of touch and sound.[8]
- Of the several types of explorers available, the most common is the Shepherd's hook (no. 23) (C).
- The number 17 explorer is shown in (D).
- The finer tips allow greater sensitivity.
- "Springier" steel helps tactility.

Use

- Explorers are used subgingivally to detect calculus and supra- and subgingival irregularities, to assess tooth mobility, to evaluate root smoothness,[9] and to probe for soundness.

Advantage

- Ability to detect soft dental areas, open pulp chambers, subgingival calculus, and surface irregularities easily with minimal equipment.

Disadvantage

- May damage tissue.

Mirrors

Description

- Dental mirrors are usually attached to handles for easier access and extension.
- Some mirrors come with light sources attached to them.

Uses

- Mirrors are used to provide direct vision, retraction of lips and cheeks, and illumination of dark areas.
- Mirrors may be used for transillumination for caries detection.

- Large mirrors are used for intraoral photography.
- Saliva or warming the mirror may prevent fogging.

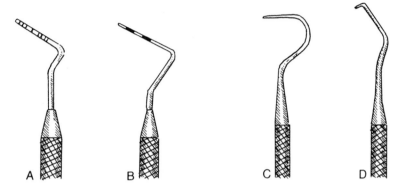

Instruments for Periodontal Surgery

- With a few additional instruments, the general veterinary surgical pack can be adapted for periodontal surgery.
- Necessary instruments are periodontal knives, periosteal elevators, curettes, and chisels.
- These instruments should be as fine as possible to allow delicate manipulation of the tissues.

Scalpel Blades

Description

- Generally, smaller blades are more useful for periodontal surgery.
- A number 2 scalpel handle is used with these blades.

Types

Number 11

Description

- The number 11 blade has a sharp, triangular point (A).

Uses

- The number 11 blade is used for stab-type incisions.
- Used for delicate sulcular incisions, especially in extractions.

Advantage

- Sharp, pointed tip.

Disadvantage

- Pointed tip may not give as much control as other blades.

Numbers 12 and 12B "Hawk-Billed"

Description

- Both numbers 12 and 12B have hooked-type tips; the 12 has a cutting surface only on the inner side, and the 12B has a cutting surface on both sides (B).

Uses

- Both may be used with a lifting (pulling) motion that places tension on the tissue, giving increased stability.

- The number 12B may be used for pulling or pushing.
- Numbers 12 and 12B may be used for flap, mucogingival, and graft operations; gingivoplasty; and gingivectomy.

Advantage

- Getting to distal surfaces that may not be reachable with a number 11 or 15C.

Disadvantage

- Locking in bone, breaking the tip in osseous bone.

Number 15

Comment

- Thin blade (C).

Advantage

- Finer blade than the standard-use small animal veterinary blade (no. 10).

Disadvantage

- May break if used for heavy-duty work.

Number 15C

Comment

- Thinner blade than the number 15 (D).

Advantage

- Allows for finer work.

Disadvantage

- May break if used for heavy-duty work.

Surgical Knives

Description

- Various angles and shapes are available.

Use

- Periodontal surgery.

Advantages

- The angulation of the surgical knives gives greater flexibility and ease of cutting soft tissue.
- Thicker; can be used for reflection as well.

Disadvantage

- The blades must be kept sharp, a skilled process that takes practice.

Types

Orban Knife

Advantage

- Good for interproximal removal of tissue (E).

Kirkland Knife

Advantage

- Good for the removal of a lot of firm, fibrous tissue (F).

Disadvantage

- Must be kept sharp, and cannot be used for fine, delicate procedures.

Maintenance: Sharpening Technique

Step 1—The sharpening stone is placed flat on a table and oiled as described under curette and scaler sharpening.

Step 2—The edge of the blade is held at a 15 to 25° angle to the stone (G). The wrist is rotated so the blade edge moves along the stone to sharpen the tip.

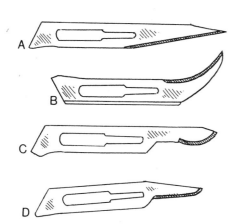

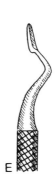

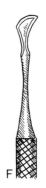

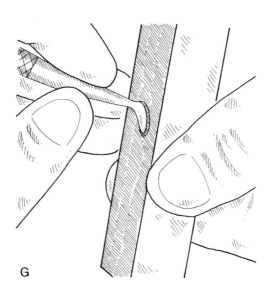

Periosteal Elevators

Description

- The blade shapes of periosteal elevator blades include rounded, straight, and sharp points.

Uses

- Periosteal elevators are used to reflect and retract mucoperiosteum after the initial incision of gingival tissue.
- The blade portion is used with the convex side against the soft tissue, thus reducing the chance for tearing or puncturing the gingiva.

Types

Molt Number 9 *(A)*
B55B Number 7 Wax Spatula *(B)*
B55A Pritchard Periosteal Elevator *(C)*

Maintenance

- Sharpening as with other sharp instruments.

Surgical Curettes

Description

- Surgical curettes are thicker and wider than other curettes, with a less flexible shank.

Use

- Removal of hard deposits, granulation tissue, necrotic cementum, and fibrous interdental tissue.

Advantage

- Stronger, less likely to break.

Disadvantage

- Bulkier; may not allow access into all areas.

Surgical Scissors

Goldman Fox Number 15

Description

- Goldman Fox scissors are sharp-sharp scissors that have slightly curved blades *(D)*.

Use

- Surgical scissors are used for enlarging initial incisions, trimming tissues, and incising muscle attachments.

LaGrange Scissors

Comment

- Are sharp-sharp scissors that have "S"-shaped blade and handle *(E)*.

Advantage

- Better accessibility to the osseous side of the flap.

Minnesota Retractor

Comment

- Used for retraction of gingival tissue *(F)*.

INSTRUMENTS FOR EXTRACTIONS

Dental Elevator

Description

- Dental elevators are available in various sizes and shapes to fit different tooth sizes.

Use

- As different types of levers or gouges to stretch and break the periodontal ligament.

Disadvantage

- Because of mechanical advantage, careful use of these instruments is needed to avoid fracturing the crown, root, or alveolar bone.

Types

Manufacturers vary the appearance of each instrument, even though they may use the same number. The armamentarium should consist of a small (number 301) *(G)*, a medium (number 34) *(H)*, and a large (number 3) *(I)* elevator.

Maintenance

- The working edges of elevators should be kept sharp. A conical stone is used to sharpen inside edges of rounded elevators.

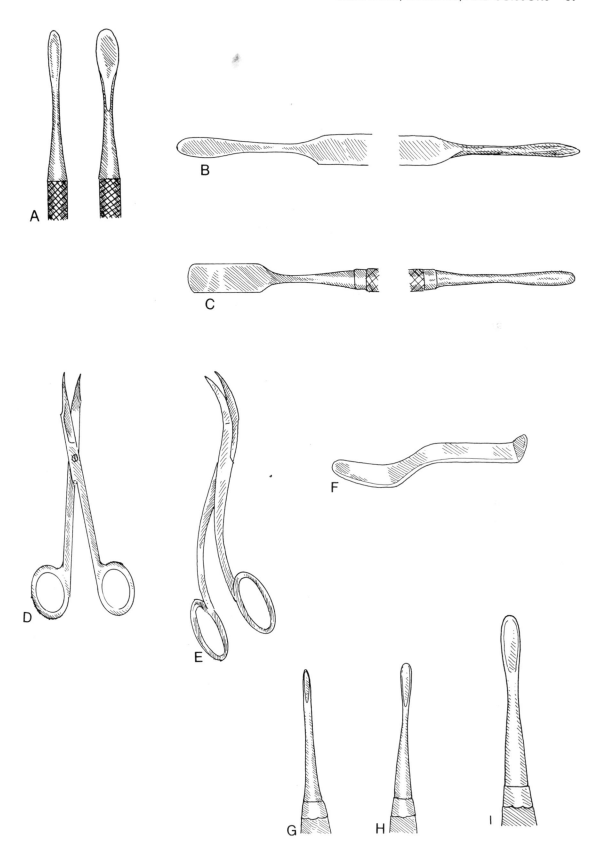

Heidbrink Root Tip Pick

Description

- Heidbrink root tip picks have narrow, sharp points *(A)*.

Uses

- Stretching and breaking the periodontal ligament.
- Retrieving fractured root tips.

Advantage

- Small size to retrieve broken root tips.

Disadvantages

- Use light touch to avoid alveolar perforation.
- May break the tip of the instrument if too much force is applied.

ED10-11 Root Tip Pick

Description

- A double-ended root tip pick *(B)*.

Uses

- Stretching and breaking the periodontal ligament.
- Extraction of retained root tips.

Advantage

- Small size.

Disadvantage

- Use light touch to avoid alveolus perforation /instrument fracture.

Extraction Forceps

Description

- Many different varieties are available.
- Human dental extraction forceps can be used, but available veterinary models fit the conical teeth better and have less rocking when gripping the tooth.

Uses

- Extraction forceps are used for gripping the tooth.
- They can be used with caution to remove gross calculus.

Advantage

- Allow gripping the tooth to lift it out of alveolus.

Disadvantage

- Because of mechanical advantage, careful use of these instruments is needed to avoid fracturing the crown, root, or alveolar bone.

Types
Veterinary "Cat Forceps"*

Comments

- The beaks are parallel to better adapt to the conical teeth *(C)*.
- Smaller forceps.

Advantages

- Smaller size, fits most hands comfortably.
- Is shaped to contour most small animal teeth.

Veterinary "Dog Forceps"*

Comments

- The beaks are parallel to better adapt to the conical teeth *(D)*.
- Larger forceps.

Advantage

- May fit larger teeth better than human or cat extraction forceps.

Disadvantage

- May cause operator to "overpower" and fracture crown or root tip.

Human Extraction Forceps

Description

- The grasping surfaces are concave to accommodate the bulge of the crown of human teeth and to grasp the crown down at the neck.

Disadvantage

- The concavity makes for poor contact with the conical teeth commonly encountered in veterinary dentistry.

---

*Depen Industries, San Mateo, CA.

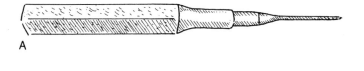

A

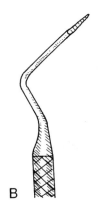

B

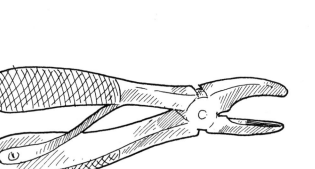

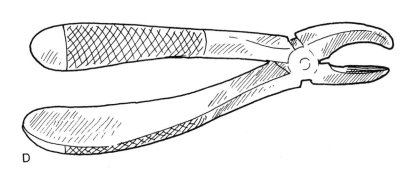

C

D

EQUIPMENT FOR ENDODONTICS

Cotton Pliers

Description

- Cotton pliers (forceps) have two beaks and a handle; some are locking.

Uses

- Cotton pliers are used to grasp materials to transfer them into and out of the oral cavity.
- They have use in all phases of dentistry, including endodontics, orthodontics, and periodontics.
- Cotton pliers are not intended to handle tissue.

Endodontic Broaches

Description

- Broaches are manufactured by notching the walls of a round blank (A).

Uses

- Broaches are used for the bulk removal of pulp tissue or other debris from the pulp chamber and root canal.
- Broaches should not be used to prepare the canal.
- Broaches are for one time use only; however, they may be cleaned intraoperatively by passing through rubber glove material.

Endodontic Files and Reamers

Description

- The files and reamers have two dimensions, length and diameter.
- The length is indicated by a millimeter (mm) notation.
- Typical lengths are 19, 22, 25, 28, 31, 40, 49, 55, and 60 mm.
- In general, the shorter files can be used for the incisors, premolars, and molars, whereas the longer lengths are necessary for the canines.
- The other dimension is the diameter. The diameter is indicated by a number only.

- The number represents the diameter of the file at the working end.
- For example, a number 10 file is .1 mm, a number 50 file is .5 mm, and a number 100 file is 1 mm at the working end.

Use

- Endodontics.

Types

Reamers

Comments

- Reamers are manufactured by twisting tapered, faceted wire, to produce cutting edges or flutes (B).
- Reamers are used for either filing or reaming.
- Filing with a reamer is accomplished by pushing and pulling the instrument in and out of the tooth.
- When filing, flutes scrape against the wall, gouging and removing dentin.
- Reaming is twisting the file in a clockwise direction. With this movement, the flutes scrape the walls and widen the canal.

Advantage

- May be used for reaming or filing.

Disadvantages

- Do not have the cutting ability of most files.
- Should not be turned counterclockwise while filing.

K-Files

Comments

- K-type files are also manufactured in the same manner as reamers but are twisted to a greater degree (C).
- The resulting flutes are greater in number and more angulated than reamers.
- K-files may be used in reaming or filing.

Advantage

- K-files have a greater number of cutting edges than a reamer.

Disadvantage

- With continued twisting they can penetrate the tooth apex.

Hedström Files

Comment

- Hedström files are manufactured by cutting triangular pieces from tapered wire (D).

Advantage

- Sharp when new.

Disadvantages

- Hedström files are only used in filing and never should be used for reaming.
- Hedström files are more prone to breakage than K-files or reamers.
- Hedström files are less flexible.

Maintenance: Cleaning Files and Reamers

- Many manufacturers recommend single-use applications. These instruments should be disposed of in proper waste containers, according to regulations dealing with "sharps."
- Caution should be exercised when handling files and reamers not to stab oneself.

Step 1—Disinfect by soaking in chlorhexidine solution diluted as recommended on bottle.
Step 2—Surgically scrub.
Step 3—Disinfect by soaking in chlorhexidine solution.
Step 4—Rinse.
Step 5—Place in storage.

- An alternate approach would be to use a bead sterilizer in place of steps 3 and 4.

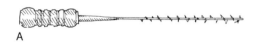

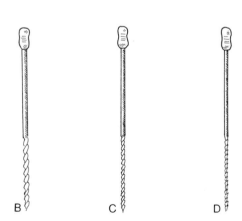

Accessories

File Organizers

Comments

- File organizers allow the orderly storage of endodontic files.
- Some organizers have containers for disinfectants *(A)*.
- Other models are autoclavable.

Advantage

- Allow an organized approach to file storage.

Disadvantages

- Vigilance must prevail to keep the organizer clean; it is difficult to keep sterile.
- The best system would be to place only new files in the organizer when the file packages are opened. Files are then destroyed after first use. This decreases the incidence of file breakage in the canal.

Endo-Ring*

Comment

- Endo-Rings are plastic rings with ruler and sponge for intraoperative storage of files *(B)*.

---

*Almore International, Inc., Portland, OR 97225.

Advantages

- Allows an orderly storage of files and reamers as well as pastes such as RC Prep† by placing on the sponge.
- The Endo-Ring allows the separation of files that have been used from those in the organizer.
- The sponge on the Endo-Ring can be used to clean files intraoperatively.

Disadvantage

- Care should be taken when placing file in the sponge not to stab the fingers.

Maintenance

- The foam is intended to be used once and destroyed.
- The Endo-Ring itself (exclusive of the foam insert) may be sterilized by steam, ethylene oxide, or cold sterilization.

---

†Premier/ESPE Dental Products, Box 111, Norristown, PA 19404.

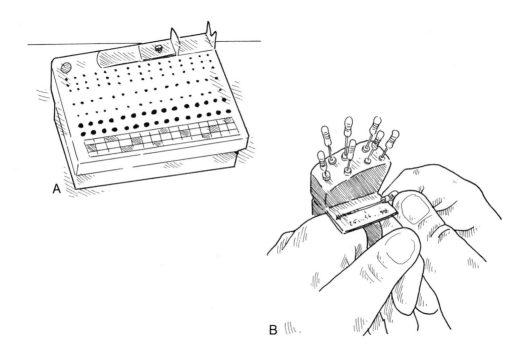

A

B

Bead Sterilizers

Comment

- Small sterilizer to place the tips of instruments for sterilization (A).

Advantage

- Allows relatively quick sterilization of instruments.

Disadvantage

- Only the tip of the instrument is sterilized.

Automated Files

Comments

- With the use of a special contra angle that oscillates at 90° and files that fit into these contra angles, the canal can be filed with the slow-speed handpiece.
- These instruments are best used in short canals.

Advantages

- Less physical strength required.
- May speed filing of canal.

Disadvantages

- Time to change files.
- Less tactile sense.
- Possible perforation of apex or "zipping" of canal.
- Greater risk of breaking files.

Instruments for Filling the Canal

High-Pressure Syringes*

Description

- A metal syringe with mechanical advantage to increase the pressure placed upon the filling material to extrude it through a small opening.
- The pressure may be placed by a lever at the back of the plunger (B).
- The pressure may be created by a screw at the back of the plunger (C).

---

*Centrix Inc., 30 Stran Road, Milford, CA 06460.

Advantage

- Material may be injected into small canals through a fine needle, as small as 30 gauge.

Disadvantages

- Special needles for these syringes have one-time use.
- Additional time must be taken to clean the syringe.

Maintenance

- E.L. Cor Solvent† Cleaning solution is used to clean the zinc-oxide-eugenol compounds.

Pluggers

Description

- A plugger has a blunt tip (D).

Use

- Pluggers are used to push gutta percha into the root canal in the vertical condensation technique.

Advantage

- Pluggers assist gutta percha to reach the apex of the root canal.

Disadvantage

- Pluggers will not laterally condense gutta percha.

Finger Pluggers or Finger Spreaders

Description

- A plugger or spreader with a handle similar to files or reamers (E).

Use

- Ability to reach into canals when intraoral space is limited.

Advantage

- Better tactile sense.

Disadvantage

- Shorter, sometimes harder to hold.

---

†Lang Dental Manufacturing, 2300 W. Wabansia Ave., Chicago, IL 60647.

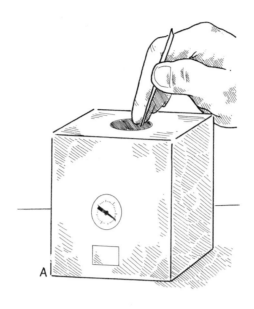

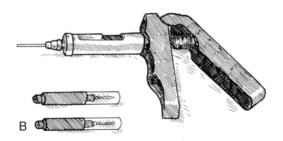

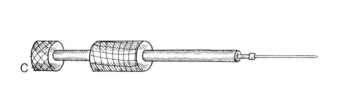

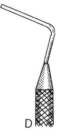

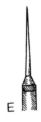

Spreaders

Description

- Spreaders are pointed and sized according to the original standardized sizes of gutta percha (A).

Use

- Spreaders are used to laterally condense gutta percha.

Advantage

- Spreaders will laterally condense gutta percha.

Disadvantage

- Will slide along side of gutta percha rather than pushing it deeper into canal toward apex.

Electrically Heated Spreaders*

Description

- An electrical current passed through the spreader causes it to heat up (B).

Uses

- Warming and further condensing gutta percha.
- Cutting gutta percha.

---

*Touch and Heat, Analytic Technologies, 3301 181st Place, Redwood, WA 98052.

Advantage

- Warming the gutta percha speeds up the process of placement, particularly in large canals.

Disadvantages

- The possibility of causing thermal damage to the tissue surrounding the tooth.
- Gutta percha expands when warm and shrinks when cold.

Warmed Gutta Percha Cannules

Description

- Cannules of gutta percha that are first warmed in a heating unit and are placed into a special syringe for injection into the canal (C).

Use

- Plasticized root canal filling.

Advantage

- Allows more rapid filling of canals.

Disadvantages

- Cost of unit and cannules.
- Canal must be filed to size 70.

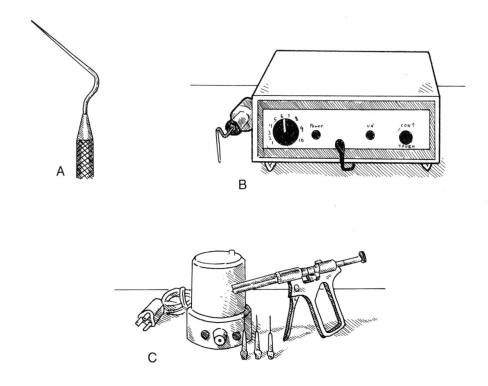

RESTORATIVE EQUIPMENT AND INSTRUMENTS

Chisels

Description

- The cutting edge of a chisel forms a right angle with the long axis of the handle.
- When double ended, one cutting edge is distal to the handle and termed "reverse bevel."
- The other end is termed "standard bevel" (A).
- The reverse bevel is indicated on the instrument shaft by an indented ring (B).
- Chisels have:
    Straight (C),
    Monangle (D),
    Biangle (E), or
    Triple angles (F).

Use

- Chisels are used to reshape or smooth dental tissue.

Hatchets

Description

- The cutting edge of a hatchet is parallel to the angle of the handle (G).

Use

- A hatchet is used for trimming and smoothing dental tissue.

Light-Cure Gun

Description

- A high-intensity light-cure gun is used to start the photochemical reaction which sets up the light-cure dental materials.

Uses

- Curing light-cure restorative materials.
- Curing light-cure periodontal packs.
- Curing light-cure orthodontic resins.
- Curing light-cure calcium hydroxide.
- Curing light-cure rubber dams.

Advantages

- Light curing allows easy shaping of the restoration and then rapid curing.
- Decreased polymerization shrinkage.

Disadvantages

- Cost of light-cure gun.
- Special eyeglasses or shields must be used to protect the eyes from the intense light.

Options
Continuous "On"

Comment

- Many guns will turn themselves off automatically, slowing the procedure down.

Advantage

- A gun with continuous "on" will allow long curing times.

Disadvantage

- May cause breakdown of light filter if used frequently for long periods of time.

High Energy Output

Comment

- Light-curing guns are manufactured with different light intensities.

Advantage

- Brighter lights penetrate for a greater depth of cure.

Disadvantage

- Greater risk of eye damage.

Fiberoptic Cord versus Pistol

Comment

- Some light-cure guns have their light source in the control box and transmit the light via a long fiberoptic cord.

Advantage

- Having the light source in a box allows for larger fans than can be hand held. This decreases the chance of bulb burnout caused by overheating with long exposures.

Disadvantages

- Fiberoptic cords are very delicate; small breaks in the fibers may occur and decrease the output.
- Fiberoptic cords are thicker and harder to handle.

Accessories
Multiple Tips

Comment

- Some units come with a variety of tips with different sizes and shapes.

Advantage

- Multiple tips allow greater range of uses (restorative, light-cure orthodontic materials, light-cure periopacks, light-cure rubber dams, etc.)

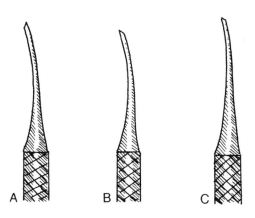

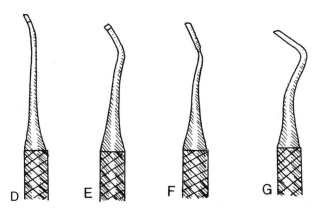

Maintenance

- Inspect filter (with light turned off!) on a regular basis (*A*).
- It should look like a blue-purple mirror (*B*).
- Holes in filter indicate that dangerous wavelengths of light may be escaping (*C*).
- Inspect light bulb—black, discolored bulbs may need to be replaced.

Shield Tip

Comment

- Small plastic light shields fit over the fiber-optic tip (*D*).

Advantage

- The shield is always with the light-curing gun.

Disadvantage

- Usually will not completely conform to shape of tooth; therefore, light shines out around the edges.

Light Analysis Tool

Comment

- For checking intensity of the light output.

Advantage

- Periodic (yearly) monitoring of light ensures optimum curing.

Disadvantages

- Expense.
- Physical inspection usually is enough.

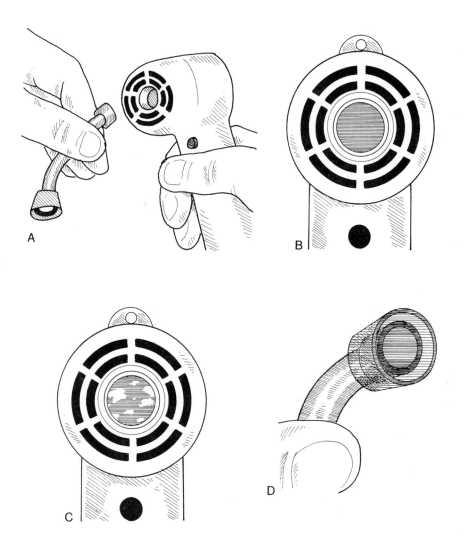

Amalgamators

Description

- Amalgamators hold a capsule that contains amalgam or glass ionomer (A).

Use

- Rapid mixing of glass ionomers and amalgam restorative material.

Advantages

- Rapid mixing of restorative materials.
- Thorough mixing of material.
- Helps prevent improper mixing and environmental contamination.

Disadvantage

- As with all equipment, instruments, and material, instructions must be followed.

Amalgam Wells

Comment

- An amalgam well is a small metal bowl to hold the amalgam while waiting to be transferred to the cavity preparation.

Amalgam Carriers

Description

- Amalgam carriers are used to transfer amalgam from the amalgam well to the restoration site (B).

Use

- Amalgam restorations.

Advantage

- Amalgam carriers quickly transfer amalgam to the restoration.

Disadvantage

- Training is required; the operator and assistant must know not to compact the amalgam into the carrier. If this occurs, the carrier will jam and amalgam cannot be removed from the carrier.

Maintenance

- Periodic cleaning with paper points or cotton swabs.
- Replacement of plastic tips.

Retrograde Amalgam Carriers

Description

- Retrograde carriers carry a smaller amount of amalgam and fit into smaller spaces (C).

Use

- Retrograde carriers are used in surgical root canals.

Advantage

- Small tip for placement of amalgam into apical opening.

Disadvantage

- Limited to use in surgical root canals or very small fillings.

Amalgam Condensers (Pluggers)

Description

- Condensers are used to pack (condense) amalgam into the restoration (D).
- A variety of sizes are available for different size restorations.

Use

- Amalgam restoration.

Advantage

- By using different sizes and shapes, amalgam can be compacted into all sizes and shapes of cavity preparations.

Amalgam Carvers

Description

- Various sizes and shapes have been designed to trim and shape amalgam (*E*).
- If working with amalgam, the practitioner will accumulate a variety of carvers.

Advantage

- Rapid trimming of amalgam.

Amalgam Burnishers

Description

- Amalgam burnishers are used to smooth down the surface of the amalgam restoration (*F, G*).
- They are more beneficial when hand mixing amalgam.

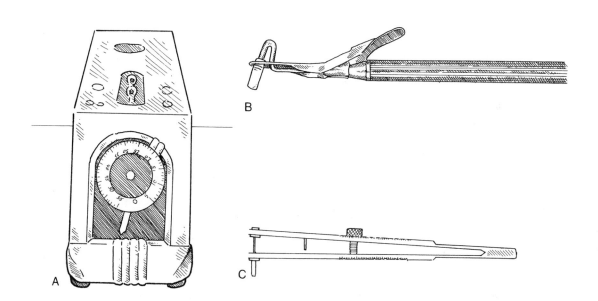

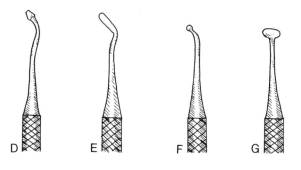

Plastic-Working (Filling) Instruments

Description

- Plastic-working instruments are either plastic or metal instruments used to shape plastic restorative material prior to curing.
- Plastic-working instruments come in several sizes and shapes and are double or single ended.

Advantage

- Plastic-working instruments do not leave a metal stain or discolor the restoration.

Mixing Spatula

Description

- The thin-blade metal spatula.

Use

- Mixing filling and restorative materials.

Mixing Pads

Description

- Glass or waxed paper slabs are used for mixing dental materials.

Uses

- Orthodontics.
- Restorations.
- Periodontics.
- Endodontics.

Types
Glass

Comments

- Glass slabs come in varying thicknesses and sizes.
- They may be cooled prior to use to provide longer working time for materials.
- Storing in refrigerator and using while cold may add working time to materials. This technique should not be performed in areas of high humidity.

Advantage

- Provides a smooth, sturdy working surface.

Disadvantages

- Must clean up slab immediately after each mixing.
- Chemical residues may be present that could interfere with the mixing of the next chemical.

Paper

Comment

- Pads of wax-coated paper are available.

Advantage

- Ease of cleaning; simply tear off contaminated paper and a new sheet is present.

Disadvantage

- Some types of materials (glass ionomers) may pick up the wax coating on the paper pad.

Jiffy Tubes

Description

- A jiffy tube is open at one end and drawn down to a fine point at the other.
- The dental material is introduced into the open end, which is then pinched closed, forcing the material out of the fine point.

Use

- Restorative materials such as glass ionomers, liners.

Advantages

- Easy to use.
- Disposable, no clean up.

Disadvantages

- Small size.
- A little messy in use.
- Less control and pressure than with other restorative placement methods.

Curved-Tip Syringes*

Description

- Syringes with curved tips and rubber pluggers.

---

*Centrix, Stratford, CT 06497.

- The restorative material is pushed into the barrel of the curved tip.
- The rubber plugger is inserted.
- The syringe has a plunger on the shaft that advances the rubber plunger into the curved tip, forcing the material out of the tapered end.

Use

- Placement of restorative.

Advantages

- The plastic tips and rubber pluggers are disposable.
- Can inject under a fair amount of pressure.
- A very fine and controlled flow of restorative material is created.

Disadvantage

- Small volume of material that can be accommodated by the tip.

Options
Plastic

Advantage

- Less expensive than metal.

Disadvantage

- May be stained by materials.

Metal

Advantages

- More resistant to staining.
- Easier to clean.

Disadvantage

- Slightly greater initial cost.

Maintenance

- Cleaning with alcohol or other solvent.

EQUIPMENT AND INSTRUMENTS FOR ORTHODONTICS

Impression Trays

Description

- Because of the variety of sizes of veterinary patients, a number of different-sized impression trays are necessary (A).
- Impression trays can be custom made by the practitioner or purchased as preformed trays.
- Several veterinary dental impression trays are manufactured.
- Styrofoam or paper cups should not be used. They do not provide enough stability.

Uses

- Orthodontics.
- Restorative dentistry (crowns and bridges).

Options
Custom Trays

Comment

- The practitioner may need to make custom trays to fit an individual patient because of variations in width and length of the mouth.

Advantage

- The tray can be varied according to the shape of the patient's mouth.

Disadvantages

- It takes time to mix, shape, and cure the tray.
- For precision work (crowns and bridges) a tray should be manufactured and allowed to cure 24 hours prior to use to avoid distortion of the impression from polymerization (curing) of the impression tray.

Veterinary Manufactured Trays

Comment

- Several companies have begun to manufacture trays that are shaped to fit dog and cat mouths.

Advantages

- Will fit most patients.
- Fairly inexpensive.

Disadvantage

- Will not fit all patients; still need to have the ability to manufacture custom trays.

Maintenance

- Cleaning and disinfecting.

Trays Manufactured for Human Dentistry

Comment

- Various sized and shaped trays are available for human dentistry.

Advantages

- Less expensive.
- Good when relatively small impression or an impression of only one tooth is required.

Disadvantage

- Will not fit the entire arch of most patients.

Accessories
Tray Adhesive

- Improves the ability of the material to stick to the tray.

Rubber Bowls

Description

- Soft rubber bowls allow easy mixing and spatulation of alginate and plaster dental materials (B).

Advantages

- The slight flexing of the bowl is easier to grasp and position material for mixing.
- The alginate is easy to clean up because it peels off the bowl once set up and plaster breaks free of rubber once dried.

Large Mixing Spatulas ("Buffalo" Spatulas)

Description

- Larger mixing spatulas are made of plastic, nylon, or metal (C).

Advantage

- Rapid mixing of a large volume of material is performed with the use of a large spatula and rubber bowl.

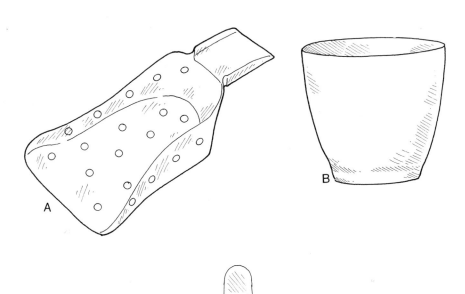

Vibrators

Description

- Vibrators aid in working with dental plaster and stone by removing bubbles and facilitate the flow of the plaster or stone into the impression (A).

Uses

- Formation of dental models for orthodontics.
- Formation of cast for crown and bridge restoration.

Advantage

- Without a vibrator, air bubbles will be trapped in the dental stone, particularly in the long, narrow canine teeth; these air bubbles may cause fracture or distortion.

Maintenance

- The vibrator should be covered with a plastic bag or paper towel to prevent stone and plaster from getting inside the unit.

Accessories
Model Trimmer

Description

- An electric motor drives a circular grinding disc; water is circulated to remove ground plaster (B).

Use

- Trimming models for orthodontics and restorations.

Advantages

- Allows mounting of the model.
- Much more cosmetic appearance for client education.

Disadvantages

- Operation is very messy.
- Steps must be taken to prevent clogging of hospital plumbing.
- Expense.

Articulators

Description

- Articulators are made of metal and plastic with two flanges hinged together.

Use

- Articulators are used to hold casts of jaws in proper alignment during various stages of prosthodontics or orthodontics.

Welders

Description

- Small, compact miniature arc welders that weld or solder by electrical current.

Use

- Orthodontic welders allow the veterinarian to custom make orthodontic appliances in the office.

Advantages

- Increased control over the quality and style of the appliance.
- Ability to do tableside adjustments (not on the patient!).

Disadvantage

- Expense and time it takes to learn to use this equipment.

Maintenance

- Replacement of carbon electrodes.

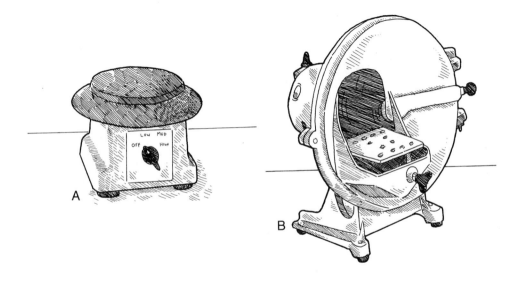

Pliers

Description

- Orthodontic pliers are used for bending wire for the manufacture of orthodontic appliances.

Uses

- Orthodontics.
- Oral orthopedic surgery.

Types
How Pliers

Description

- How pliers are used for holding wire and for free-form bending (A).

Uses

- How pliers are general-use orthodontic pliers; they may be used for gripping wire during placement or removal, seating bands, making adjustments to appliances, etc.

Bird Beak (Loop Forming) Pliers

Description

- Bird beak pliers have one round tip for round wire bends and one flat tip for sharp, angular bends (B).

Uses

- Bird beak pliers are used for bending wire.
- Either a sharp or gradual curve may be created.

Three-Prong (or Triple-Beaked) Pliers

Description

- Triple-beaked pliers have two prongs on one side and one on the other (C). The single prong is centered to move between the paired prongs.

Uses

- Three-prong pliers bend by placing the pliers on the wire and squeezing.
- Three-prong pliers are useful in adjusting wire, bending heavier orthodontic wire, and activating appliances.

Tweed Arch-Adjusting Pliers

Description

- Tweed arch-adjusting pliers have heavy, nonslip beaks (D).
- Their size limits use in the oral cavity, and are mainly used for laboratory work.

Use

- Tweed pliers are used for holding and adjusting arch wires.

Tweed Loop-Forming Pliers

Description

- Tweed loop-forming pliers have various diameters at the tip (E).

Use

- Forming loops.

Band/Bracket-Removing Pliers

Description

- Band-removing pliers have a protective nylon cap over the longer beak that is placed on the crown of the tooth (F).
- The shorter beak is placed along the bracket or band to be removed.
- The pliers may also be used to shear the remnants of the bonding cement off the tooth.

Maintenance

- The shorter beak may require sharpening to grasp fine bands.

Wire Cutters

- Wire cutters can be purchased from dental suppliers or local hardware stores (G).

Accessories
Storage Trays

- Storage trays are for organization and visualization of instrumentation.

Boley Gauge

Description

- A caliper that is calibrated in millimeters.

Use

- Measurement of the size of teeth.

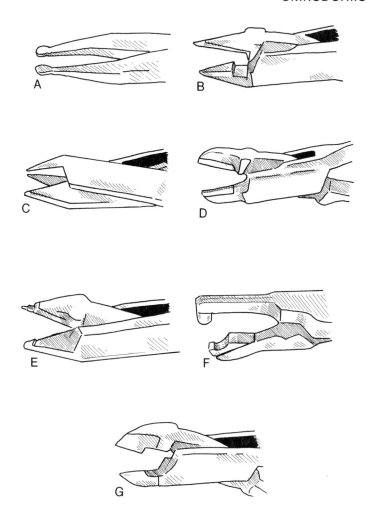

References

1. Williams CA. Dental Equipment Needs. Las Vegas: Western Veterinary Conference, 1988:6–12.
2. Grove K. Periodontal Therapy. Compendium on Continuing Education 1983;5(8):660–664.
3. Clinical Research Associates: Sonic and Ultrasonic Scalers. Provo, Utah, 1982; 6(7):1.
4. Loose B, Kiger R. An evaluation of basic periodontal therapy using sonic and ultrasonic scalers. J Clin Periodont Res 1987;14:29–33.
5. Parr RW, Pipe P, Watts T. Periodontal Maintenance Therapy. Berkeley: Praxis Publishing Co, 1974:87.
6. Hu-Friedy. Smarten Up, Sharpen Up. Chicago: Hu-Friedy, 1982.
7. Tholen MA. Concepts in Veterinary Dentistry. Edwardsville, KS: Veterinary Medicine Publishing Co., 1983:164.
8. Finkbeiner BL. Periodontal instruments. In: Carter LM, Yaman P, eds. Dental Instruments. St Louis: C.V. Mosby Co., 1981:4.
9. Hawkins BJ. Periodontal Disease Therapy and Prevention. Philadelphia: W.B. Saunders Co., 1986:835–849.

chapter 3

DENTAL RADIOLOGY

GENERAL COMMENTS

- Dental radiology using intraoral film can be used by all practitioners.

INDICATIONS

- In young patients to evaluate the presence of unerupted or impacted teeth.
- During prophylactic or therapeutic teeth cleaning to evaluate the extent of periodontal disease by measuring bone loss and assist in treatment planning (A and B).
- In patients with oral stomas (fistulas), as a diagnostic tool (C).
- In patients undergoing endodontic therapy, to allow the practitioner to evaluate therapy and to study radicular health and size prior to, during, and after endodontic therapy (D).
- In patients with missing teeth, to ascertain the status of potentially impacted or resorbed roots or teeth (E).
- In all types of dental/oral disease, to document and study the progress of therapeutic programs.
- In cases where neoplasia or metabolic disease is suspected, to evaluate the involvement of teeth and bone.
- In oral trauma, to evaluate the mandible and/or maxilla.
- Prior to or during extractions, to evaluate the complete removal of root tips or the location of retained root tips (F).

CONTRAINDICATIONS

- Critically ill patients who may have difficulty undergoing anesthesia, which is necessary to position the patient properly.

OBJECTIVE

- To obtain a radiograph with fine detail that represents the patient's condition (G).

MATERIALS—FILM

- Intraoral radiographic film is inexpensive, small, and flexible, fitting well into the oral cavity and conforming to the area placed (see table). Intraoral film is nonscreen film, which provides greater detail than the screen films used in most veterinary situations. Intraoral film can be processed in 1 to 2 minutes with rapid developer and fixer solutions with minimal loss of detail. Using this film, small areas of interest can be isolated.

FILM SIZES

Size Periapical	Measurement	Ektaspeed	Ultraspeed
0	$\frac{7}{8}" \times 1\frac{3}{8}"$	EP-01	DF-54
1	$\frac{15}{16}" \times 1\frac{9}{16}"$	EP-11	DF-56
2	$1\frac{1}{4}" \times 1\frac{5}{8}"$	EP-21	DF-58
Occlusal			
4	$2\frac{1}{4}" \times 3"$	EO-41	DF-50

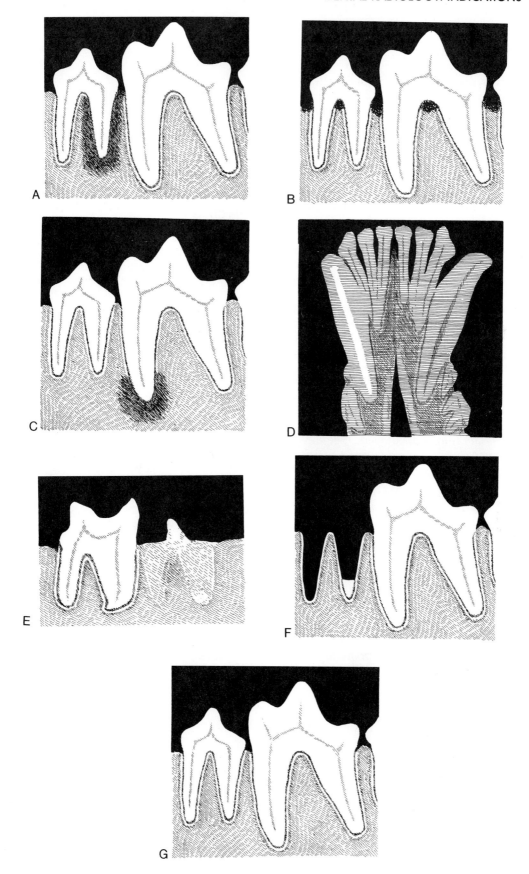

TECHNIQUE: TAKING AN INTRAORAL FILM

- Keep the distance from the patient to the film as short as possible.
- Use a fine-grain or high-detail nonscreen film.
- Use as small a focal spot on the x-ray tube as possible.
- Collimate to the area of the subject needed.
- Process film carefully after exposure.

Step 1—The patient is positioned appropriately for the radiograph to be taken.

Step 2—The intraoral film is placed in the proper position. As an aid in positioning the film, a mouth gag, film wedge, gauze sponge, or other object can be placed behind the film.

Step 3—The head of the x-ray machine is placed as close as possible to the structure being evaluated and positioned for the study.

Step 4—The appropriate milliamperage, kilovolt peak, and time are selected. (As a reference, 50 ma, 65 kVp, and 1/4 second comprise a good starting point. The technique should be adjusted to the situation.)

Step 5—The film is exposed.

Step 6—The film is developed. (See developing, later.)

Caution: Personnel should be protected by aprons, screens, and/or safe distance.

SPECIFIC INTRAORAL RADIOGRAPHIC TECHNIQUES

Parallel Technique

Indications

- Radiographs to evaluate the posterior mandibular teeth (A).
- Evaluation of portions of the mandible (B).
- Evaluation of the facial maxillary complex and nasal cavity (C).

Contraindications

- Any location where the film cannot be placed parallel to the structure being radiographed.
- Any area where other structures would be superimposed onto the film.

Objective

- To take a radiograph with the structure to be studied and the radiographic film parallel to each other, without interference by other structures being superimposed.

Technique

Note: In the drawings in this text, older-style cones are used to illustrate x-ray technique more clearly; tubular collimator cones with filter are preferable and in some states are the only equipment allowed by law.

- The film packet is placed parallel to the structure being radiographed. The plane of the film should be parallel to the plane through the structure (D).
- The head of the machine is placed as close to the film as is reasonable, and the x-ray beam should be perpendicular to the structure being radiographed.

Complication

- In many areas of the mouth it is not possible to place a film parallel because other structures interfere.

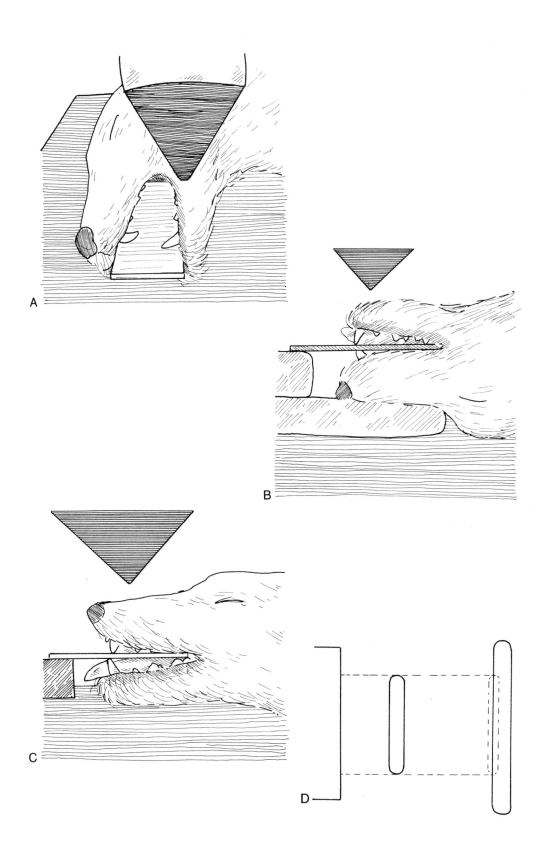

Bisecting Angle Technique

General Comments

- Ideally all film would be exposed using the parallel technique. However, in the mouth, few areas can be radiographed with this technique.
- The bisecting angle technique is an application of the geometric principle of equilateral triangles: In equilateral triangles we know that if two triangles share a side and both have an equal angle at their apex, then the opposite sides are the same length.

Indications

- The bisecting angle technique is used when parallel projections cannot be made.

- Posterior portion of the maxilla (*A*).
- Anterior portion of the maxilla including canines (*B*).
- Maxillary incisors and canines (*C*).
- Mandibular incisors and canines (*D*).
- Anterior portion of the mandible including canines (*E*).
- The posterior portion of the mandible may be taken with the bisecting angle technique if the parallel technique cannot be used.

Contraindications

- If parallel projections can be made they are easier to produce and have less error.

Objective

- To obtain an accurate representation of the tooth.

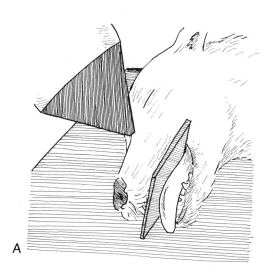

A

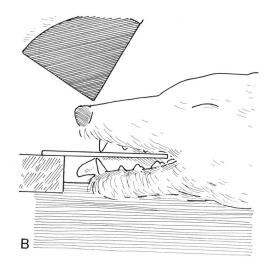

B

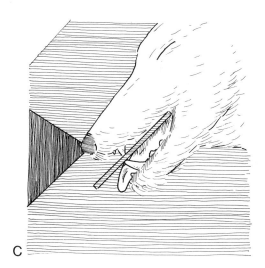

C

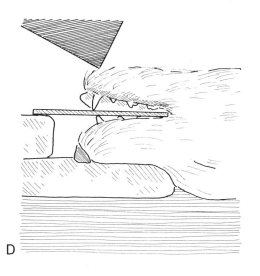

D

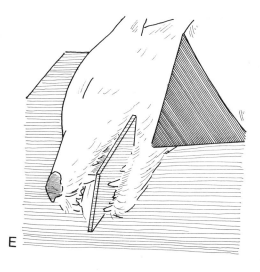

E

Technique

- The angle formed by the x-ray film and the structure is visualized and an imaginary line bisecting this angle is visualized (*A* and *B*).
- The head of the x-ray machine is positioned so the beam of x-rays will be perpendicular to the imaginary line.
- When first learning this technique it is often helpful to use props, such as sticks (cotton-tip applicators), to help visualize the angle and the bisected angle.
- As a rule of thumb aim the x-ray beam at a 45° angle lateral from the hard palate on maxillary projections.

Complications: Bisecting Angle

- The most common problems are not achieving a true bisecting angle and not having the x-ray beam perpendicular to the bisected angle.
- This may create foreshortening (*C* and *D*).
- Or it may cause elongation (*E* and *F*).

Complications: Radiographic Technique

- Improper exposure settings on the x-ray machine.
- Limitations imposed by the x-ray machine.
- Inability to determine which structure is which, particularly when evaluating maxillary fourth premolar palatal and mesial buccal roots. A second film is taken, with the x-ray beam moved either anterior or posterior; the structure that is more lingual (palatal root) will be shadowed on the film in the same direction as the x-ray beam. The structure that is more buccal (mesial buccal root) will be shadowed in the direction opposite to that of the x-ray beam. This phenomenon can be remembered by the acronym "SLOB rule." SLOB stands for Same Lingual Opposite Buccal.

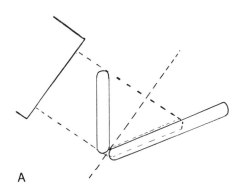

A

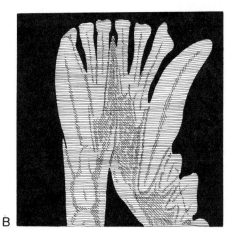

B

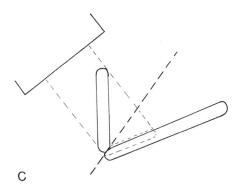

C

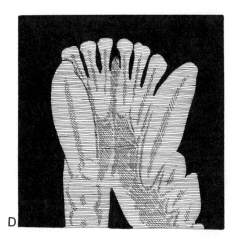

D

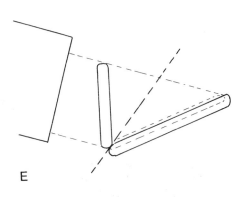

E

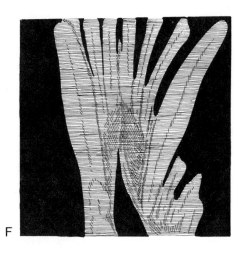

F

RADIOGRAPHIC DEVELOPING

There are four methods of developing the exposed film: standard hand-tank developing, rapid-processor developing, one-step rapid processing, and two-step rapid processing.

Standard Hand-Tank Developing

Description

- The procedure is the same as with other x-ray film.
- Specialized racks or holders may be used to hold the film(s) during the developing process (*A*).

Advantage

- Additional equipment and materials are not required.

Disadvantage

- The biggest disadvantage of this technique is the slow developing time.

Rapid-Processor Developing

Description

- An automatic processor is used to develop, fix, and dry the film.

Advantages

- Automatic processors establish constant developing and fixing, eliminating human error.
- Decreases operator time.

Disadvantages

- Unless the processor is designed to transport small films, there will be difficulty with this method. Some veterinary medical automatic processors will process occlusal-sized dental radiographic film.
- Automatic dental film processors are slower than the rapid-process developing systems.
- Automatic dental film processors are expensive.
- Standard veterinary x-ray film can be used as a "leader" by taping the smaller dental film to it. The large film is used to transport the dental film through the processors normally used in veterinary practices. This technique is discouraged because it is impractical and potentially damaging to the film processor.

One-Step Rapid Processing

Description

- A special combination developing/fixing solution is used for this procedure.

Disadvantages

- Because developing and fixing are done by the same solution, detail is compromised with this process.
- This process is not recommended because of the compromised quality of the processed film.

Two-Step Rapid Processing

- This is the recommended processing technique.

Description

- Solutions are designed for rapid developing and fixing of intraoral film.
- Three or four small containers are used.
- Small dip tanks are arranged with one tank for the developer, one or two for water rinse, and one for fixer.
- Small dip tanks may either be bought for this purpose or empty, clean medicine jars may be used.
- The dip tanks (*C*) may be housed in a darkroom or in a "chairside darkroom" (see Chapter 2).

Technique

Step 1—The solutions are stirred to mix.

Step 2—In a dark environment the film packet is opened and the film is removed from the packet and attached to a film clip (*B*).

Step 3—The film is immersed in the water

rinse for at least 5 seconds to hydrate the emulsion on the film.

Step 4—The film is next immersed in the developer, agitated to remove bubbles, and then no longer agitated. The time is dependent upon the solution used and the temperature; the manufacturer's recommendations should be followed. The film is removed from the developer with minimal drip-back into the developing tank.

Step 5—The film is placed into the water rinse with continuous agitation for 30 seconds.

Step 6—The film is transferred to the fixer and intermittently agitated during its fixing. Generally, the fixing time is twice the developing time.

Step 7—After the time prescribed for fixing by the manufacturer, the film is transferred into the final rinse. The fixer is allowed to drip back into the fixing tank. The film may be read at any time; however, it should be returned for a minimum of 10 minutes in a freshwater rinse (longer rinse time gives more assurance of removing all fixer from the emulsion).

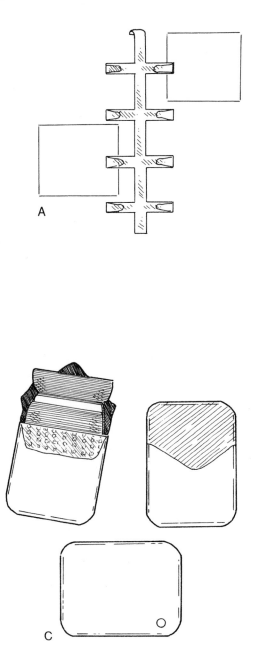

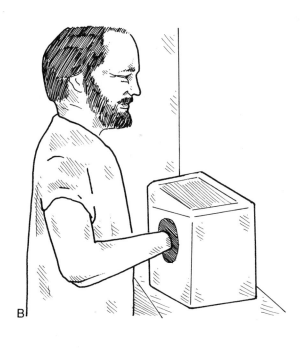

Complications

- Once the film is removed from the protective packet, processing should begin as soon as possible.
- Resist the temptation for prolonged viewing of the film between the developing and fixing stages.
- If Ektaspeed film (EP) is used, or if the unit is below a bright light source, a red filter should be placed over the amber filter.

- Old developer gives a "washed-out" background and fogs the film.
- If the films are not rinsed for a long enough time they will turn brown as the remaining fixer oxidizes with age.
- The film should be removed from the protective paper. If the paper is left attached to the film, the film will not develop properly.
- Silver jewelry should not come in contact with processing solutions!

chapter 4

DENTAL PROPHYLAXIS

General Discussion

- The deleterious effects of untreated dental disease on the rest of the body have long been recognized.
- The oral examination and prophylaxis are basic to good dentistry.

ORAL EXAMINATION

General Comments

- Perform the examination in a routine that is followed every time.[1]

Indications

- Cooperative patients receiving a physical examination.
- All patients undergoing general anesthesia.

Contraindications

- Unruly patients that will not allow examination without risk to the examiner.

Objective

- Thorough examination of all oral and dental structures for evidence of abnormality or disease.

Materials

- Periodontal probe/explorer.
- Mouth gag.

Technique

Step 1—Observe the head, muzzle, and nostrils.

Step 2—The lips are lifted, and starting rostrally, buccal and labial surfaces of the teeth and gingiva are examined.

Step 3—Working caudally, the mandibular and maxillary teeth, cheek tissues, and salivary gland ducts are evaluated.

Step 4—The opposite side of the mouth is scrutinized in a similar fashion.

Step 5—Once the entire buccal surface has been examined and you have gained familiarity with the patient, the mouth is opened.

Step 6—The lingual and palatal gingival tissues are examined. The lingual, palatal, interproximal, and occlusal surfaces of the teeth are evaluated. The examiner's thumb can be placed in the diastema behind the maxillary canine tooth so that it pushes on the hard palate as an aid in keeping the mouth open. However, in the awake patient, thorough visualization is limited.

Step 7—The tongue and floor of the mouth are examined. This area may be visualized more easily by pushing on the skin beneath the tongue on the ventral portion of the mandible posterior to the symphysis.

Step 8—The hard and soft palates are examined.

Step 9—The pharyngeal area and tonsils are examined. In tolerant animals a finger can be placed over the base of the tongue for better visualization of the caudal pharynx.

Complications

- May require general anesthesia if patient will not submit to examination.
- Mouth gag should be used only for a short time to prevent undue tension on the temporal mandibular joint.
- The practitioner should use caution to prevent being bitten intentionally or accidentally.

Aftercare—Follow-up

- Treatment is guided by the oral examination.

PERIODONTAL DISEASE

General Comments

Cause of Periodontal Disease

- The tissue degradation process appears to be driven by subgingivally advancing plaque, acute inflammation, and prostaglandin-induced bone resorption.[2]
- The host response, bacterial actions, and bacterial endotoxins destroy the periodontium.
- One authority has described it as similar to a battleground destroyed in the process of the battle.[3]

Stages of Periodontal Disease

- Stages of periodontal disease are recognizable both clinically and by the predominant cell types in the connective tissue of the marginal gingiva concomitant with increasing plaque and calculus formation.[4]
- The healthy gingiva has a knife-like margin (*A* and *B*).
- Radiographically, bone is seen close to the neck of the tooth.
- The *first stage* is described as the initial stage. A redness of the gingiva at the crest of the gingiva and a mild amount of plaque are noted (*C* and *D*).
- Radiographically, there is no change from healthy gingiva.
- The *second stage* is the early stage with an increase in inflammation including edema and subgingival plaque development. Amounts of supragingival plaque and calculus are increased (*E* and *F*).
- Radiographically, there is little change.

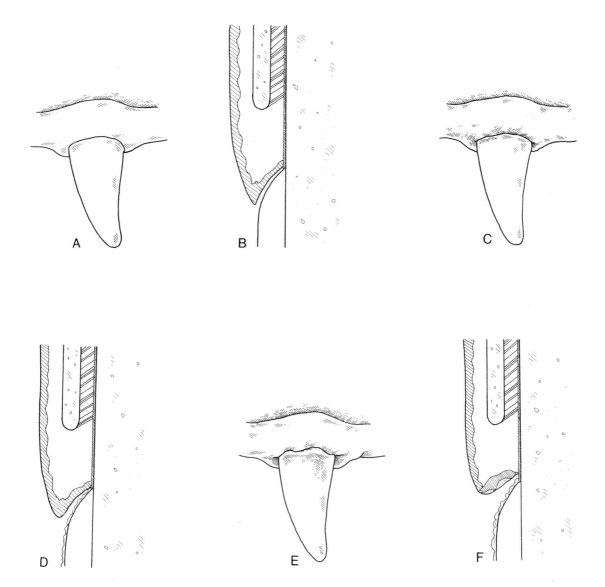

Stages of Periodontal Disease

(Continued)

- The *third stage* is the established stage, with gingivitis, edema, beginning pocket formation, and increasing amounts of plaque and calculus. The gingiva will bleed upon gentle probing at this stage (*A* and *B*).
- Radiographically, subgingival calculus may be noted.
- Some of the signs that may be associated with *stage 4*, or advanced periodontal disease, are the presence of severe inflammation, deep pocket formation, gingival recession, bone loss, pus, and mobility. The gingiva usually bleeds easily upon probing (*C* and *D*).
- Radiographically, subgingival calculus and bone loss are noted.

Prevention and Treatment of Periodontal Disease

- Patients with initial periodontal disease (stage 1) should receive home-care instruction and polishing supra- and subgingivally (above and below the gum line).

- A 1.64% stannous fluoride treatment administered by sulcular irrigation may be beneficial in causing a dramatic and sustained decrease of subgingival motile bacteria and spirochetes following irrigation.[5]
- Early periodontal disease (stage 2) should be treated with supra- and subgingival scaling, polishing the teeth, fluoride treatment, and regular home care.
- Established periodontal disease (stage 3) should receive thorough calculus removal supra- and subgingivally, polishing, fluoride treatment, and regular home care.
- Advanced periodontal disease (stage 4) should receive thorough scaling, subgingival curettage, root planing, flap surgery, polishing, fluoride treatment, and other periodontal procedures as indicated.
- Once periodontal disease reaches stage 3 (established) or stage 4 (advanced), a "simple dentistry," "dental," or "prophy" as commonly perceived in veterinary practice will not be enough to restore health.

TREATMENT AND PREVENTION PROTOCOLS FOR PERIODONTAL DISEASE

Procedure	Healthy	Stage 1	Stage 2	Stage 3	Stage 4
Home care	Yes	Yes	Yes	Yes	Yes
Scaling*	No	Possible	Yes	Yes	Yes
Polishing	Yes	Yes	Yes	Yes	Yes
Irrigation†	Yes	Yes	Yes	Yes	Yes
Subgingival Curettage	No	No	No	Yes	Yes
Root Planing	No	No	No	Yes	Yes
Flap Surgery	No	No	No	Rare	Yes
Splinting	No	No	No	No	Possible
Extraction‡	No	No	No	Possible	Yes

*Sub- and supragingival scaling.
†Chemical irrigation with chlorhexidine or fluoride.
‡Extraction for periodontal disease.

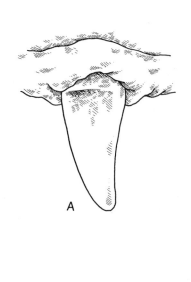

A

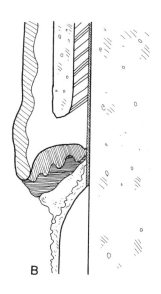

B

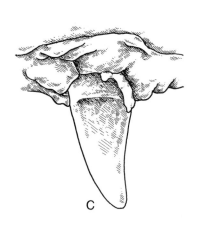

C

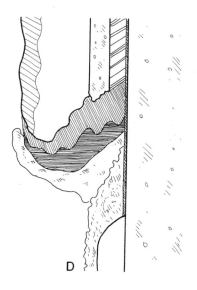

D

DENTAL PROPHYLAXIS

General Comments

- A complete and thorough prophylaxis consists of supra- and subgingival gross calculus removal, fine hand scaling, polishing, diagnostics, irrigation, and home-care instruction.
- The procedure must be performed with the patient under general anesthesia with a cuffed endotracheal tube.
- Steps for a complete and thorough prophylaxis are presented in order of use.
- Time needed for a thorough prophylaxis is 30 to 45 minutes with an uncomplicated case.

Step 1—Gross Calculus Removal

General Comments

- Gross calculus is removed by using scalers and curettes, calculus-removing forceps, ultrasonic scalers, sonic scalers, or rotary scalers.
- Larger particles of supragingival calculus are removed from the buccal, lingual, palatal, and interproximal surfaces of the teeth.
- Removal of gross calculus in itself is not a complete prophylactic dental procedure, and is of minimal therapeutic value.

Objective

- The gross removal of calculus from the tooth surface in preparation for other steps

to remove smaller particles of calculus and plaque.

Scalers and Curettes
Indications

- Removal of gross calculus above the gumline.
- Useful in areas that may be difficult to reach with power instrumentation.
- Hand instrumentation is necessary in all prophylactic procedures to remove all sizes of dental deposits.

Materials

- Scalers and curettes of choice.

Techniques

- The techniques to learn are instrument-holding techniques, use of finger rests, and proper working techniques.

Instrument-Holding Techniques

- Scalers are designed to be used with a modified pencil grasp for control (A).
- A pencil grasp should be avoided (B).
- The modified pencil grasp is achieved by first holding the instrument between the thumb and index finger, with the remaining fingers held straight (C).
- The remaining fingers are then moved over so that they are to the side and slightly on top of the index finger. The instrument remains in the front part of the hand (D).

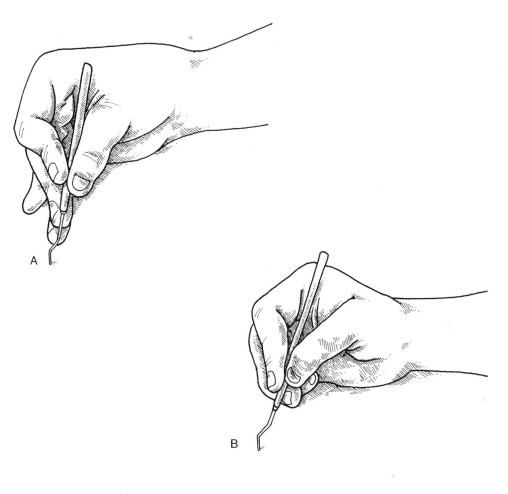

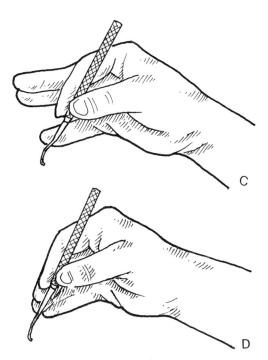

Finger Rests

- Accurate control is necessary to accomplish the task of cleaning the teeth and to prevent damage.
- A large variety of finger rests may be used in each situation.
- Hand size, position of operator to patient, and type of instrument all affect the selected finger rest.

Standard Position

- The second (middle) or third (ring) finger is placed against the tooth or proximal (adjacent) tooth. This finger becomes the fulcrum to effect power for the working stroke.
- The instrument is placed on the tooth to be scaled (A).
- The wrist is rotated while keeping the fingers straight, and as the blade of the instrument moves it is made to follow the contour of the tooth (B).

Cross-Arch Rest

- The fulcrum finger is placed on a tooth in the opposite arch (C).

Open or Extended Grasp

- The second (middle) and third (ring) fingers are allowed to separate (D).
- This technique is used when the finger rest (fulcrum) cannot be near the work area.

Long Reach

- The instrument is held further toward the middle of the handle (E).
- This technique decreases the amount of instrument control.
- A fulcrum is still used.

Secondary Rest

- The hand not holding the instrument is used as a rest for the fulcrum (F).

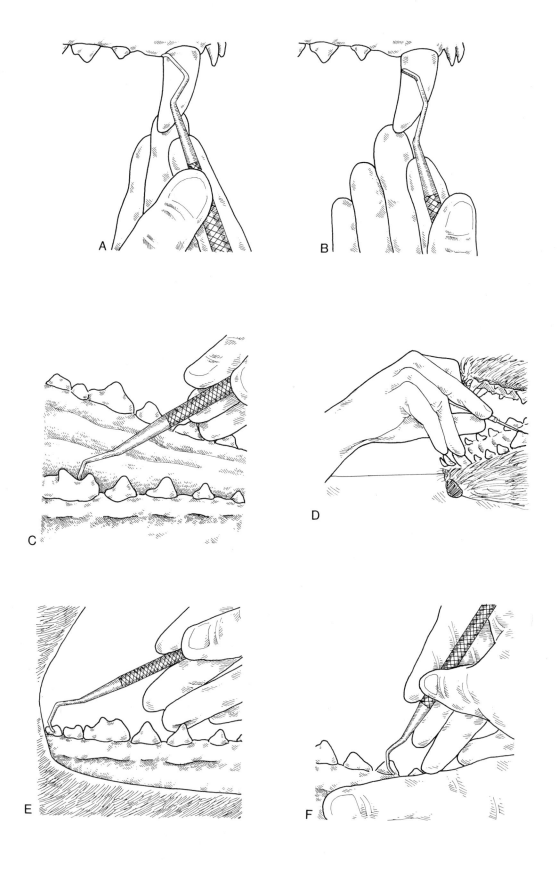

Working Techniques

- When one uses a scaler or curette, the blade of the instrument is placed at a 70 to 80° angle on the tooth surface (*A* and *B*).
- The instrument should follow the contour of the tooth and should maintain the 70 to 80° angle as the pull stroke is made away from the gingival margin over the tooth surface.
- The tip of the instrument may be used for the removal of calculus from pits and fissures; the maxillary fourth premolar is a site where this is often necessary.
- Scalers should not be used subgingivally because they distend and lacerate tissues.
- Curettes may be used supragingivally in a manner similar to that of the scaler.

Complications

- Scratching the enamel or dentin.
- Removal of restorative material from previously filled teeth.
- Gingival lacerations, abrasions, tears, and damage to the sulcus.

Calculus-Removing Forceps

Indication

- Removal of large pieces of calculus.

Contraindication

- Fractured teeth.

Basic Principle

- Rapid but uncontrolled removal of calculus.

Materials

- Calculus-removal forceps.*
- Needle holders.
- Extraction forceps.

Technique

- One jaw of the forceps is placed on the crown, the other below the calculus to be removed.
- The handle is squeezed and the calculus breaks free of the tooth.
- Extraction forceps may also be used in this technique (*C*).

---

*Deppen Industries, Inc., 111 St. Matthews Ave., San Mateo, CA 94401.

Complications

- Fracturing the crown.
- Tearing gingival tissue.
- Luxation or extraction of the tooth.
- Damage to enamel.

Power Instrumentation— Ultrasonic

General Comments

- If done properly, ultrasonic scaling is a safe method to remove large amounts of calculus rapidly.
- The "pot" should be inspected at regular intervals for fractures in the metal leaves (see Chapter 2, page 50).
- The correct angulation of the scaler is necessary for efficiency and safety.
- The side of the tip is most effective and least likely to cause damage if the handle is held parallel to the tooth surface (*D*), rather than perpendicular to it[6] (*E*).
- The pressure applied to the tooth surface should be no more than approximately the weight of two aspirin tablets.

Indication

- Removal of gross calculus from supragingival surfaces.

Materials

- Ultrasonic scaler with water source.
- Universal tip.

Technique

Substep 1—Handpiece is grasped with a modified pencil grip with fulcrum for control.

Substep 2—The terminal 1 to 2 mm on the side of the tip of the instrument is used (*F*).

Substep 3—Rapid, overlapping short strokes are made over the tooth surface. The strokes should start at the gingiva and move coronally.

Complications

- Overheating of the tooth causing pulpal damage.
- Etching the enamel with excessive pressure or using the instrument tip rather than the terminal side.

Aftercare—Follow-up

- Polish and use other techniques to ensure complete removal of plaque and calculus.

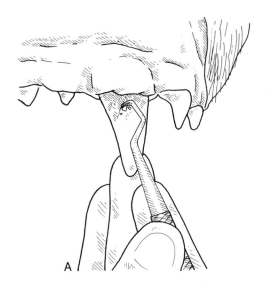

A

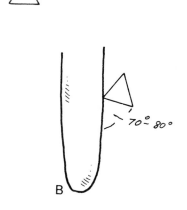

B

70°–80°

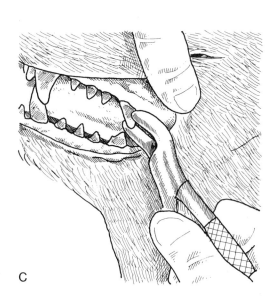

C

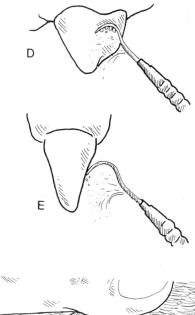

D

E

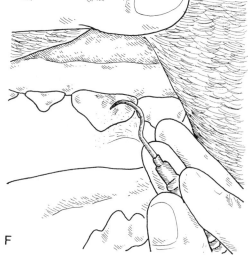

F

Power Instrumentation—Sonic

Basic Principles

- Less heat is created by sonic scalers than by ultrasonic scalers.
- Sonic scalers require compressed air to operate.
- The sonic scaler produces minimal heat, decreasing the chance of thermal damage to the pulp.
- Sonic scalers can be used subgingivally.

Indications

- Removal of gross calculus from supragingival and subgingival (with caution) surfaces.

Materials

- Dental station with compressed air.
- Sonic scaler.

Technique

- A systematic approach is recommended.
- The finger rest will vary from tooth to tooth and operator to operator.

Substep 1—The labial surface of the maxillary canine tooth is scaled with a sonic scaler and using extended-reach finger rests (*A*).

Substep 2—The buccal surface of the maxillary premolars is scaled using standard finger rests (*B*).

Substep 3—The palatal surface of the maxillary incisors is scaled using extended-reach finger rests (*C*).

Substep 4—The palatal surface of the maxillary canine is scaled using standard finger rests (*D*).

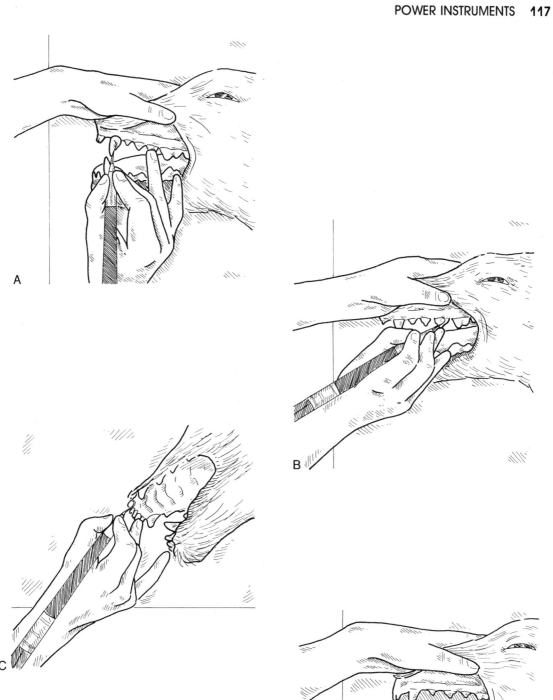

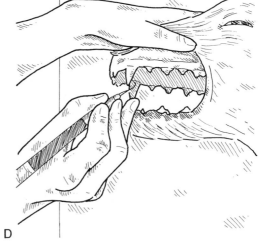

Technique *(Continued)*

Substep 5—The palatal surface of the maxillary premolars is scaled using cross-arch finger rests (*A*).

Substep 6—The labial surface of the mandibular canine is scaled using standard rests on the incisor (*B*).

Substep 7—The lingual surface of the mandibular incisor is scaled with standard rests (*C*).

Substep 8—The lingual surface of the mandibular molar is scaled with extended rests (*D*).

Complication

- Etching enamel.

Aftercare—Follow-up

- Same as with ultrasonic.

Power Instrumentation—Rotary Scaler (Rotosonic Scaling)

General Comments

- There is a limited place for this type of instrumentation in veterinary dentistry. However, it must be used cautiously in trained and skilled hands.

Indications

- Removal of gross calculus from supragingival surfaces.
- With care, the rotary scaler can be used for subgingival root planing.

Contraindication

- Inadequate training.

Basic Principle

- A high-speed bur is used to remove calculus.

Materials

- High-speed handpiece.
- Cleaning bur.*

Technique

- With *very light* pressure, the bur is moved over the surface of the tooth.

Complications

- Etching tooth enamel or dentin.
- Overheating tooth.
- Burning bone.
- Tends to remove calculus incompletely.
- If a burning smell is noted, the instrument is being used incorrectly.

---

*Rotopro, Ellman Dental Manufacturing Co., 1135 Railroad Ave., Hewlett, NY 11557.

RELATIVE SPEEDS OF POWER SCALING[7]

Pot/stack type	25,000 kHz
Piezoelectric type	40,000 kHz
Rotosonic	30,000 kHz
Subsonic	16,000 kHz

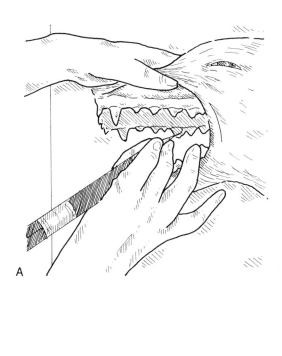

A

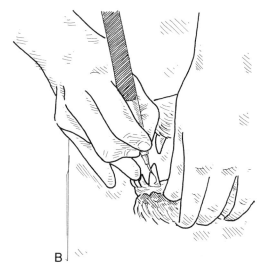

B

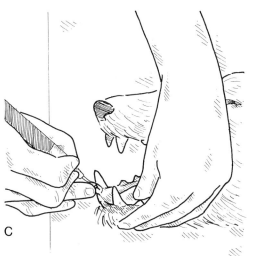

C

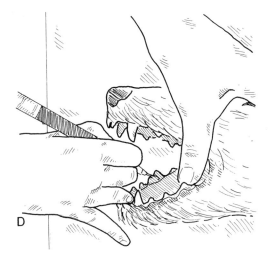

D

Step 2—Closed Subgingival Plaque and Calculus Removal

General Comments

- If subgingival calculus is left, only a cosmetic benefit and no health benefits have been accomplished.
- Sharp instruments are a must for this procedure.
- Pocket depth, pocket epithelium, rough tooth surface, and necrotic cementum may necessitate root planing, subgingival curettage, and/or periodontal surgery.

Indications

- Removal of calculus below the gingiva when pocket depth is less than 5 mm.
- If periodontal pocket depth is greater than 5 mm, surgical treatment may be indicated.

Contraindications

- Severe systemic disease.
- Increased bleeding time.

Objective

- The removal of all subgingival calculus and plaque.

Materials

- Curettes of operator's choice.

Technique

Substep 1—The angle of the face is near parallel to the tooth surface (closed position) (*A*). The curette is held with a modified pencil grip and gently introduced to the bottom of the sulcus/pocket (*B*).

Substep 2—The bottom of the sulcus or pocket is encountered and should feel soft and resilient versus the hard and firm feeling of calculus on the tooth surface (*C*).

Substep 3—Once the bottom is reached, the curette is rotated so the cutting edge is at a 70 to 80° angle with the tooth surface. Plaque and calculus are removed with a pulling stroke (*D*).

Substep 4—Repeated stokes are taken in different directions: vertical stoke (*E*), oblique stroke to distal (*F*), oblique stroke to mesial (*G*), and horizontal stroke (*H*), until the sulcus is clean.

- It may be necessary to start at an edge of the subgingival calculus and "chip away" at the calculus until the sulcus is clean.

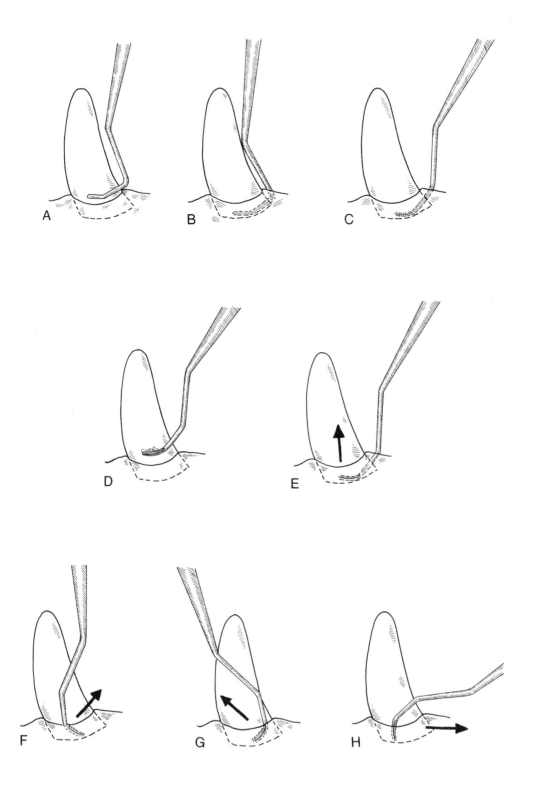

Complications

- The gingiva may be lacerated (*A*).
- The epithelial attachment may be torn (*B*).
- The tooth surface may be rippled or roughened (*C*).

Aftercare—Follow-up

- Routine home care, see pages 132 to 136.
- Re-examination in 14 to 21 days.
- Evaluation under general anesthetic in 3 to 6 months.

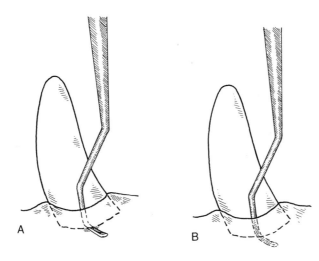

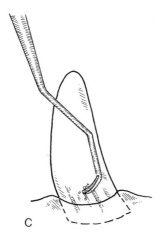

Step 3—Detection of Missed Calculus and Plaque

Objective

- To ensure removal of all calculus and plaque.

Techniques

- Techniques to detect calculus and plaque include air drying and the use of disclosing solutions, explorers, and periodontal probes.

Air

General Comments

- Calculus is more visible when dry.
- Calculus appears chalky on the dental surface after it is dried with air.
- This method is good to use during the prophylactic procedure on a tooth-by-tooth inspection after scaling. For examining the entire mouth, the staining techniques are preferable.

Indication

- Rapid detection of calculus and plaque that may not be visible to the eye.

Contraindication

- May not be as thorough as using a disclosing solution.

Materials

- Compressed air from a three-way syringe or other air source.

Technique

- Air is directed toward the gingival sulcus to gently lift the free gingival margin and to dry the tooth surface (*A*).

Disclosing Solutions

General Comments

- Plaque will retain the stain and clean teeth will not.

Indication

- Disclosing solution can help detect plaque that may otherwise be invisible to the eyes.

Contraindication

- White or light-haired dogs without their owners' consent because the haircoat may be temporarily discolored.

Materials

- One-stage disclosing solution, which stains plaque and calculus one color.
- Two-stage disclosing solution, which stains recently formed plaque a different color from long-standing plaque and calculus.
- Fluorescein stain, which may be observed in light or ultraviolet light.

Technique

Substep 1—A small amount of the disclosing solution is applied to a cotton-tipped applicator.

Substep 2—The disclosing solution is applied to the teeth (*B*).

Substep 3—The oral cavity is rinsed with water to remove nonadhering disclosing solution from enamel (*C*).

Substep 4—The disclosing solution stains the plaque and calculus. The stain does not absorb to normal enamel or dentin (*D*).

- Stained calculus and plaque are then visualized and removed using techniques described above.

Complications

- Staining gingiva and hairs. Because disclosing solutions are water soluble, they are washed away in several days by eating and drinking.

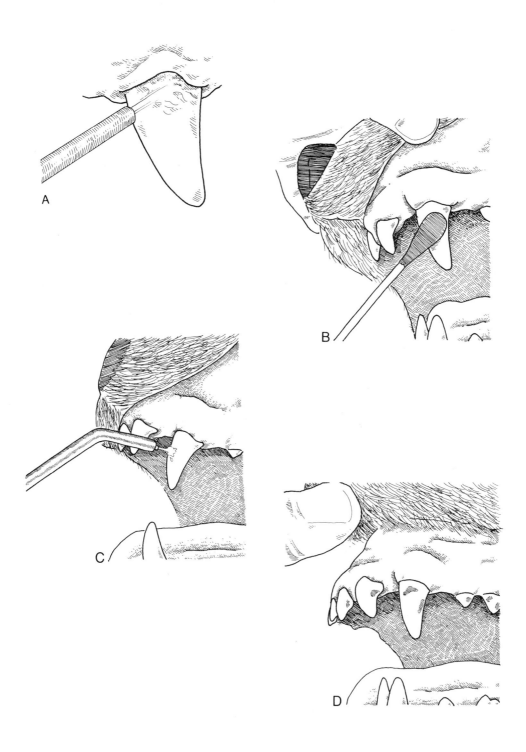

Step 4—Polishing

General Comments

- Slow speed should be used.
- The polisher should spend only a short time on each tooth to avoid overheating the tooth.
- Adequate prophy paste is used for lubrication and polishing.
- A light pressure minimizes thermal injury and tooth damage.
- If the teeth are not polished, the irregular or rough surface is perfect for bacterial plaque formation to recur promptly.

Indication

- After every tooth scaling.

Contraindications

- With some restorative materials alternative prophy pastes should be used.
- With some restorative materials, polishing should be avoided until curing is complete.

Objective

- Smoothing the tooth surface and removing residual plaque.

Materials

- Dental engine (electrical or air powered).
- Prophy angle.
- Prophy cup.
- Prophy paste.
- Prophy paste dish.

- The oscillating prophy angle (Prophy-matic*) creates less heat, does not tangle hair, and does not sling paste.

Technique

Substep 1—A small amount (1/2 teaspoon) of prophy paste is placed into a prophy paste dish (A).

Substep 2—The rubber prophy cup is dipped into the prophy paste dish (B).

Substep 3—The prophy paste is transferred to the surface of the teeth to be polished (C).

Substep 4—A liberal amount of prophy paste is used on each tooth surface because this acts as a lubricating as well as polishing compound (D).

Substep 5—The rubber prophy cup is lightly applied to the tooth surface and turned at a slow speed (2000 to 10,000 rpm) (E). The edge of the cup can be slightly flared to move subgingivally.

Substep 6—The tooth surface and sulcus are then thoroughly rinsed (F).

- Coarse or supercoarse ("stain-remover") prophy paste is available to assist in cleaning hard-to-clean enamel. When using coarse prophy paste, more enamel is removed. A fine prophy paste should be used after the coarse paste.

Complications

- Overheating the tooth surface.
- Wrapping patient's hair in the cup with the 360° prophy angle. Children's "banana" hair clips can be used to keep hair out of the operating field.

---

*Metadentia, 39–23 62nd Street, Woodside, NY 11377.

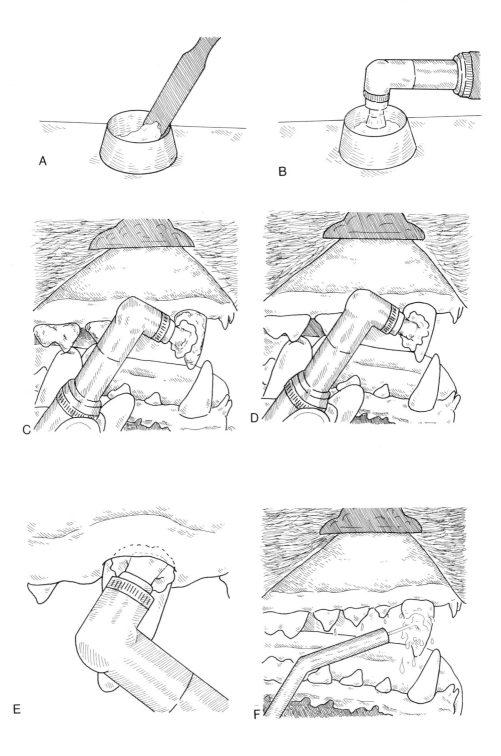

Step 5— Diagnostics

Periodontal Probing/Exploring
General Comments

- Periodontal probing and radiology are important diagnostic procedures.
- Proper treatment of any pocket over 5 mm in depth requires periodontal surgery.
- The periodontal probe/explorer is one of the most important diagnostic instruments for the veterinary dentist.
- The fine tip of an explorer may be moved along tooth surface at the gingival margin to detect tooth irregularities. It can be used to detect dentinal softening of carious lesions and to test the patency of pulp chambers in fractured or worn teeth.

Indications

- To examine dental structures.
- Detection of periodontal pockets and missed calculus.

Objective

- To assess periodontal health and monitor progress of therapy.

Materials

- Periodontal probe of operator's choice (see Chapter 2, pages 62 and 63).

Technique

Substep 1—The probe is gently inserted parallel to the long axis of the tooth to the bottom of the sulcus or pocket (*A*). Deep pockets are detected (*B*).

Substep 2—The probe is walked along the entire wall of the tooth, or at least six places around the tooth, measuring the depth of the sulcus or pocket (*C*).

Substep 3—The pocket depth is recorded in the dental record.

Complication

- Perforation of floor of gingival sulcus from too much pressure.

Dental Radiology
Indications

- Radiographs are taken to evaluate the dental and bony structure for loss due to periodontal disease.
- Intraoral dental radiology will enable the practitioner to find dental disease that may have been missed.

See Chapter 3 for further information.

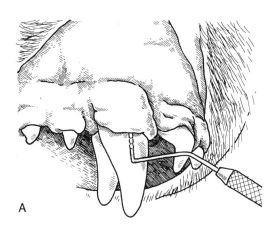

A

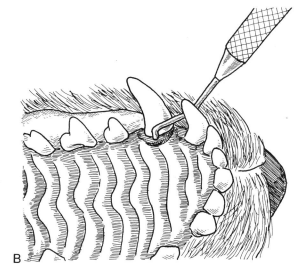

B

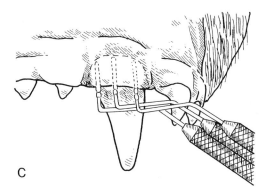

C

Step 6—Sulcus/Pocket Irrigation

General Comment

- Irrigation cleanses subgingival sulcus or pocket of loose calculus, prophy paste, and miscellaneous debris and decreases bacterial counts.[5]

Indication

- To remove debris after every scaling and polishing.

Contraindications

- Drug sensitivity.
- Mobile teeth.

Objective

- Flushing all debris from the sulcus or pocket and coating with antimicrobial substance.

Materials

- Blunted, 23-gauge needles with 6- or 12-ml syringe.
- Curved-tip syringes.
- Alternative rinsing solutions include water, 0.02% chlorhexidine, stannous fluoride gel, sodium fluoride foam.

Technique

Substep 1—The blunted tip is gently introduced into the pocket or sulcus and the irrigating solution is infused (A). Alternatively, a curved-tip syringe may be used (B).

Substep 2—Rinsing is continued until no debris is noted.

Substep 3—Depending on the material used, the irrigant is rinsed off the tooth structures.

Complications

- Tearing the gingival tissues caused by too great a pressure or mechanical action of tip.
- Failure to clean thoroughly.

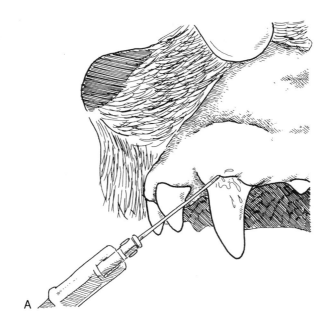

A

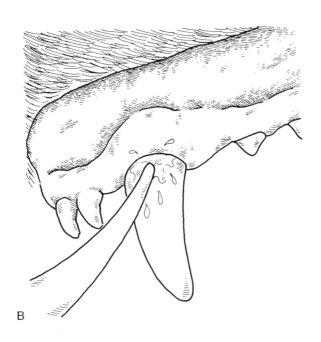

B

Step 7—Home-care Instruction

General Comments

- The veterinarian has assumed complete responsibility in the past for dental care, an impossible responsibility. The suggestion of home care to the client places more of the responsibility with the owner. At the time of the physical examination, a frank discussion to evaluate client willingness and patient cooperation in home-care procedure will help the practitioner create a proper treatment plan. If the client is unwilling, or if the patient will not allow dental home care, extraction of diseased teeth is indicated rather than advanced dental procedures. It is best to start home care as a pup or kitten, before dental disease starts.
- The client must be educated on how to perform proper home care to maintain clean teeth and a healthy mouth. After prophylaxis the teeth will stay clean only for a short time.
- Not all patients or clients are capable of providing home care; overexuberance in the presentation of the home-care procedure can "turn off" the client toward the clinic or hospital and can decrease the bonding between the owner and pet.
- Another equally important consideration is the animal's temperament. Clients and handlers should be warned of the potential risks involved in home care. The owner may be injured by the pet, and the veterinarian may be left open for possible litigation for advice given.
- It is important that a member of the staff spend some time reviewing brushing and home-care techniques with the client. Time spent in staff training will aid client rapport and increase the chances of successful therapy.
- The client should be educated in technique and product use, as well as recognition of oral disease. Clients should be encouraged to return for further instruction as often as necessary. Some clients may assume they are doing a great job, in reality giving them a false sense of security and causing unintentional damage.
- Client handouts are also beneficial in reinforcing the need for brushing and home care.
- After the dental procedure, the client should be informed of the extent of dental disease, the type of home care necessary, and the need for future professional follow-up. It is helpful to review the patient's dental chart and radiographs with the client at this time.

Indication

- To remove and prevent formation of plaque and prevent formation of calculus.

Contraindications

- Unruly or dangerous patient.
- Inability of client to perform.

Materials

- For demonstrations, the patient, a "demonstrator" dog/cat, or plastic/plaster models can be used to show brushing techniques.

Technique

- The two major methods of plaque control are mechanical and chemical.

Mechanical Devices

Toothbrush

- Preschool or child-size toothbrushes are generally the correct size for veterinary patients.

Advantages

- Readily available.
- A brush is the most effective method of removing plaque.

Disadvantage

- Some clients lack the manual dexterity required to brush effectively.

Mechanically Powered Toothbrush*

Advantage

- Easy to use.

Disadvantage

- Noise may scare the patient.

Gauze Sponge

- Pumice-impregnated gauze sponges.†

---

*Rotoplus; Interplaque, Rota-dent Professional Dental Technologies, P.O. Box 4129, Batesville, AR 72503.
†Cat-O-Dontic/Dog-O-Dontic, St. Jon Laboratories, Harbor City, CA 90710.

- These may be wrapped around a cotton-tip swab for ease of application.

Advantage

- Easy client use.

Disadvantages

- Greater risk to client of being bitten.
- Greater expense.
- May not be as thorough as a brush.

Water Pick

- The water pick should be used on low power.

Advantages

- Can be directed toward problem areas or areas that are hard to reach.
- May not be as painful as application of a brush or gauze after periodontal therapy or until gingival pain is decreased.

Disadvantages

- Messy.
- Patient may not tolerate it.
- Do not introduce directly into the sulcus. It can cause transient bacteremia.

Types of Compounds

- Various chemical agents have been proposed for the removal and prevention of plaque in humans and animals; unfortunately, a 100% effective agent has yet to be developed.

Powders

Advantages

- Powders have an abrasive quality that can vary with size, structure, and composition of the powder.
- Powders can be made into a paste.

Disadvantages

- Powders are messy.
- Particles may be accidentally inhaled.
- Particles can accidentally enter eyes and cause irritation.

Liquids

Advantages

- Have a variety of delivery systems ranging from spray to water-pick–type reservoirs.
- Can irrigate hard-to-reach areas.

Disadvantage

- Liquids are messy.

Sprays

Advantage

- Sprays are quick and easy to use.

Disadvantages

- The hissing noise may startle the patient.
- Sprays may accidentally enter eyes, causing irritation.

Pastes

Advantages

- Adhere well for application.
- Often flavored for better acceptance.

Disadvantage

- May stick to muzzle hairs or vibrissae.

Gels

Advantages

- Adhere well for application.
- Often flavored for better acceptance.

Disadvantage

- May stick to muzzle hairs or vibrissae.

Products

Na or K Pyrophosphate

- When present in dog biscuits, may inhibit plaque and supragingival calculus formation.

Saliva Substitutes*

- Helpful in patients with xerostomia.
- Has some fluoride in formulation.

Enzymatic†

- Marketed in pastes, spray, and impregnated pads.

Advantages

- Antiplaque; augments salivary peroxidase system.
- Flavored products available for pets.

Disadvantage

- Not as effective in plaque inhibition as chlorhexidine or fluoride.

Sanguinaria Based‡

- Marked as paste and rinse.

---

*Xero-Lube Scherer, GelKam International, P.O. Box 80004, Dallas, TX 75380.

†Enzydent, CET, St. Jon Laboratories, 1656 West 240th Street, Harbor City, CA 90710

‡Viadent, Viadent, Inc., 1625 Sharp Point Drive, Fort Collins, CO 80525.

Advantage

- Possible antiplaque agent.

Disadvantage

- Flavoring.

Chlorhexidine

- Marketed as a rinse* and gel.†
- Is for short-term use only.
- A premixed solution of chlorhexidine is recommended over dilution of a concentrated chlorhexidine.

Advantages

- True antimicrobial.
- Antiplaque.

Disadvantages

- Cost.
- Bad aftertaste.
- Hampers ability to taste after a short period of time.
- Black staining of protein pellicle may become noticeable after prolonged use.

Zinc Ascorbate‡

- Marketed as a spray, includes swab.

Advantages

- Supports collagen synthesis.
- Reduces odor.

Disadvantage

- Some patients object to spray.

Fluoride Based§

- Marketed as gel or liquid.

Advantages

- Antibacterial.
- Inhibits plaque formation.
- Reduces surface tension of tooth surfaces.
- Reduces dental hypersensitivity.

Disadvantages

- May be toxic in large doses.
- May combine with other fluoride sources to cause toxicity.

Types of Fluoride

- Stannous.
- Monofluorophosphate (MFP).
- Sodium fluoride.

Brushing Technique

Substep 1—Dentifrice is applied to the brush or sponge (A).
Substep 2—The brush is placed at a 45° angle to the tooth (B).
Substep 3—A circular, sweeping motion, with the emphasis on the coronal stroke away from the gingiva, is used to brush plaque away (C).

Wiping Techniques

Substep 1—The dentifrice may be placed on a cotton-tipped applicator (D).
Substep 2—The teeth may be wiped with a gauze sponge (E).
Substep 3–The teeth may be wiped with a gauze sponge wrapped around a cotton-tipped applicator (F).
Substep 4—To brush or wipe the lingual or palatal surface, a Nylabone is placed in the patient's mouth and the mouth is held closed on the Nylabone with the opposite hand while the teeth are brushed (G).

Complications

- The client should be warned of the dangers of being bitten or scratched.
- Iatrogenic oral trauma may occur because of poor technique.
- Failure to respond to conventional therapy may be a sign of: (1) a systemic disease such as diabetes; (2) hyperparathyroidism; (3) low calcium intake; (4) chronic nephritis; (5) leukemia; (6) leptospirosis; (7) deficiency of the vitamin B complex[8]; and (8) feline immunodeficiency virus (FIV) infection.
- Calculus left subgingivally may lead to periodontal abscess.

---

*Nolvadent, Peridex, Fort Dodge Laboratories, 800 Fifth Street N.W., Fort Dodge, IA 50501.
†CHX, St. Jon Laboratories, 1656 West 240th Street, Harbor City, CA 90710.
‡Maxiguard, Addison Laboratories, Route 3, Box 90-B, Fayette, MO 65248.
§GelKam International, P.O. Box 80004, Dallas, TX 75380.

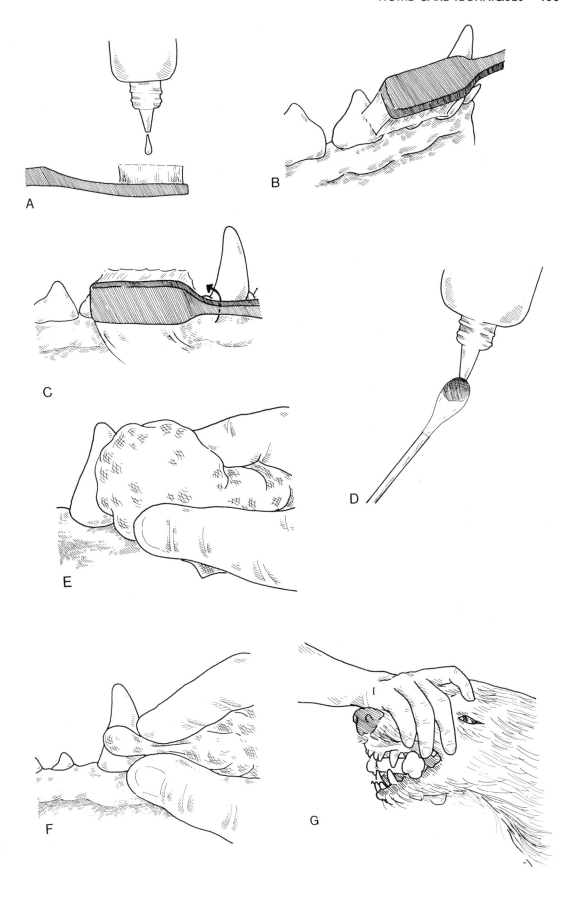

A

B

C

D

E

F

G

Home-Care Plans by Condition/Ability

Noncritical Patient

- The most important objective in the patient that is not critically ill (noncritical patient) is to start the client and patient on a brushing routine.
- Therefore, starting out with flavored water or flavored toothpaste is fine.
- Once the routine is accepted, fluoride gel is recommended.
- Treatment should be performed at least twice weekly.

Intermediate Care Category

- Patients in the intermediate category need to have plaque prevention on a higher level than the noncritical.
- They should be started out with flavored water or flavored toothpastes.
- Home care should be performed at least every other day to be effective.
- In addition, fluoride is used at least twice a week.

Intensive Care Category

- Patients in the intensive care category usually have just had some type of periodontal therapy.

- These patients are put on a routine of twice-daily rinses or brushes with a chlorhexidine solution.
- After 2 weeks, the patient is switched over to a fluoride gel or fluoride animal toothpaste, at least once a day.

References

1. Fagan DA. Diagnosis and Treatment Planning. Philadelphia: W.B. Saunders Co., 1986:785–799.
2. Page RC, Schroeder HE. Periodontitis in Man and Other Animals (1st ed.). New York: Karger, 1982:158.
3. Page RC. Keynote speech to the Academy of Veterinary Dentistry. Cincinnati: 1987.
4. Suzuki JB. Diagnosis and Classification of the Periodontal Diseases. Philadelphia: W.B. Saunders Co., 1988:195–216.
5. Mazza JE, Newman MG, Sims TN. Clinical and antimicrobial effect of stannous fluoride on periodontitis. J Clin Periodontol 1981;8:203–212.
6. Parr RW, Green E, Madsen L, Miller S. Subgingival Scaling and Root Planing (1st ed.). San Francisco: University of California, 1975:90.
7. Duke A. Dental Instrumentation and Materials. Veterinary Dentistry '89, 1989.
8. Bojrab MJ, Tholen M. Small Animal Medicine and Surgery. Philadelphia: Lea & Febiger, 1989:51.

chapter 5

PERIODONTAL THERAPY

General Comments

- Often times patients with advanced periodontal disease are presented for teeth cleaning. In these cases, more than dental prophylaxis or a "simple cleaning" is necessary to restore gingival health. The additional treatment may be broadly termed periodontal therapy.
- Antibiotics should be started preoperatively to establish a blood level prior to the initiation of periodontal therapy or surgery.[1, 2] Preferred treatment is an antibiotic by injection 1 hour prior to surgery.
- A broad-spectrum bactericidal antibiotic such as ampicillin or amoxicillin may be used in most cases. Some cases require treatment with antibiotics selective for gram-negative organisms such as cephalosporin-based agents, enterofloxin, or combinations of antibiotics.
- Antibiotics are an adjunct to treatment and prevention of secondary infections, not a cure for periodontitis.

Objectives

- Periodontal therapy has two principal objectives: (1) the eradication or arrest of the periodontal lesion with correction or cure of the deformity created by it; and (2) the alteration in the mouth of the periodontal climate that was conducive or contributory to allowing periodontal disease to become established.[3]

ROOT PLANING—CLOSED TECHNIQUE

General Comments

- Root planing is the process where residual embedded calculus and portions of the necrotic cementum are removed from the roots to produce a clean, hard, smooth surface that is free of endotoxin.[4]

Indications

- Calculus on root surface.
- Gingival recession with calculus on root surface.
- Roughening of root surface.
- Presence of periodontal pocket of less than 5 mm.

- Root planing can be performed in patients with pocket depths greater than 5 mm, but it is better to perform open techniques so that treatment may be more definitive.

Contraindications

- Nonsalvageable teeth.
- General health considerations.

Materials

- Curette; a sharp instrument is important.
- Hoes.
- Periodontal files.

Technique

- The patient should receive a preoperative antibiotic if pus is present in the pocket or if the patient has any other systemic disease.
- A routine, systematic approach should be used on each quadrant and on each tooth.
- The blade of the curette is positioned against the root surface (A).
- Root planing is performed using a curette with overlapping strokes in horizontal, vertical, and oblique directions. (See subgingival scaling technique.)
- This cross-hatch planing creates an optimally smooth surface while maintaining root anatomy.

Complications

- Deposit cannot be removed. The solution is to reposition the blade to remove less calculus per stroke, change the angle and direction of pull of the instrument, or change instruments.
- Surface is still rough after planing. The solution is to check the instrument for sharpness and replane, or if too much force has been applied causing ruffling, to use light and smooth strokes.

Aftercare—Follow-up

- Follow routine home-care instructions, pages 132 to 136.
- Antibiotics.

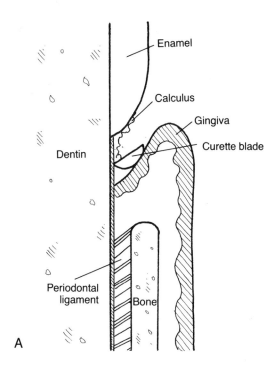

A

SUBGINGIVAL CURETTAGE

General Comments

- Subgingival curettage is the treatment of the gingival soft tissues.
- Subgingival curettage allows optimal reattachment and shrinking of the periodontal pocket.
- Subgingival curettage is usually done in conjunction with root planing.
- By performing subgingival curettage the pocket epithelium and infiltrated subepithelial connective tissues are removed without reflecting flaps, i.e., without direct vision of the surfaces to be treated.

Indication

- Removal of diseased or infiltrated soft tissues.

Contraindications

- Nonsalvageable teeth.
- General health considerations.

Objectives

- The objectives of subgingival curettage include: (1) elimination of the microorganisms that elicit inflammation; and (2) removal of diseased or infiltrated tissues.[4]

Materials

- Curette; sharp instruments are important.

Technique

- Subgingival curettage is performed with the curette held in the reverse position from normal scaling; this places the blade against the soft tissue for epithelial removal (B).
- A finger against the gingiva may be used to support the gingival tissue during the curettage.
- When the tip of the curette is used to remove the remains of the epithelial junction, a "tugging" will be felt.

Complications

- Further loosening of the teeth.
- Excessive destruction of the gingiva.
- Deepening of the periodontal pocket.

Aftercare—Follow-up

- Reexamination in 7 to 14 days; possible open surgical techniques.
- Open surgical techniques will be necessary if the gingiva does not respond to this conservative treatment.

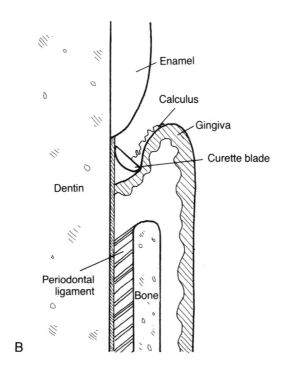

B

MANDIBULAR FRENECTOMY

Indication

- Gingival recession or pocket formation on the distal side of the canine teeth caused by the presence of the frenulum.

Contraindication

- Bleeding disorders.

Objective

- To minimize food accumulation in the anterior portion of the mouth and to improve self-cleansing of this area.

Materials

- No. 10, 15 or 15C scalpel blade and handle.
- Sharp-sharp scissors.
- 4–0 absorbable suture.
- Needle holder, thumb forceps.

Technique

Step 1—The attachment of the frenulum to the mandibular gingiva near the first premolar is cut horizontally with scissors or a blade (A).

Step 2—The cut is extended with the blade or scissors into the frenulum to release the pull of the muscular attachments. The lip will relax laterally when the attachments have been completely cut (B). A diamond shape is created by the cut surfaces.

Step 3—Suture is placed to bring the mesial and distal edges together (C). Several simple interrupted absorbable sutures are placed to prevent reattachment (D).

Step 4—The root surfaces of the canines should be planed smooth and polished.

Postsurgical Care

- Twice daily oral flushing with 0.2% chlorhexidine to keep the area clean for 2 weeks.
- Home oral hygiene to minimize progression of periodontitis.

Complications

- Reattachment of frenulum if not sutured.
- Infection.

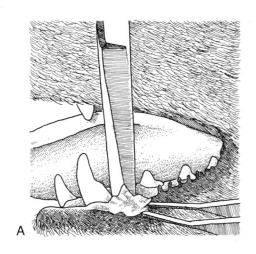

A

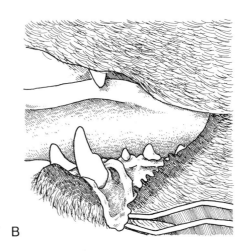

B

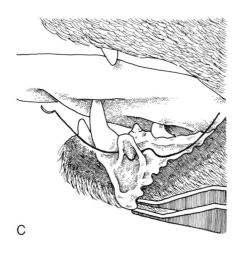

C

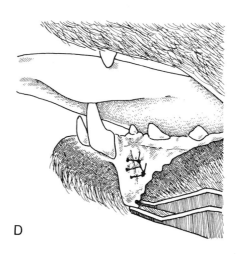

D

GINGIVECTOMY

General Comments

- Careful patient selection is necessary. Gingivectomy is only performed in patients with hyperplastic gingiva.
- This procedure is not used for treatment of deep periodontal pockets or as part of routine prophylaxis!
- Re-epithelialization takes place at the rate of 1 mm/day.

Indications

- Removal of excessive gingival tissue in cases with hyperplastic tissue (A).
- For incisional or excisional gingival biopsy.

Contraindications

- Minimal or absence of attached gingiva.
- Horizontal or vertical bone loss below the mucogingival junction.

Objective

- To remove excessive gingival tissue to achieve a clean tooth/root surface and a thin beveled gingival margin with pyramid-shaped interdental tissue.

Materials

- A No. 10, 15, or 15C scalpel blade with handle, and/or:
- Gingivectomy knives, such as Kirkland or Orban.
- Periodontal probe.
- Electrosurgery blade.
- Wet compresses to control hemorrhage.
- Hemostatic agents.

Technique

Step 1—The pocket depth and contour are determined by inserting a probe to the depth of the pocket at several areas around the tooth (B).

Step 2—The corresponding depth is measured on the outside of the gingiva using the probe (C).

Step 3—A bleeding point is made using either the tip of the probe by placing the probe perpendicular to the gingiva and applying slight pressure to make a small hole (D) or by using a small-gauge needle to create the bleeding point. These points are made around the contour of the pocket and will be used as a guide for the gingivectomy. The gingivectomy will be made at an angle apical to the bleeding point to create a beveled margin. At least 2 mm of healthy, attached gingiva must be present apical to the base of the incision.

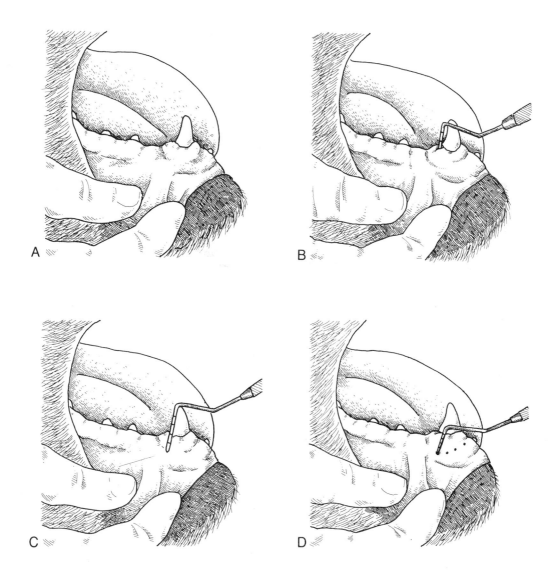

Technique *(Continued)*

Step 4—Using the cold blade or electrosurgery blade the gingiva is excised by cutting below the bleeding points with the blade held at approximately a 45° angle with the tip of the blade toward the crown *(A)*.

Step 5—The ends of the excision should be tapered into the surrounding gingiva to create the normal scalloped contour, particularly if several adjacent teeth are treated *(B)*.

Step 6—Gingival tags can be removed with the blade or a sharp curette.

Step 7—The exposed tooth/root surface can now be scaled and planed smooth *(C)*.

Step 8—Hemorrhage is controlled applying pressure with wet gauze pads or hemostatic agents.

Postsurgical Care

- Most animals eat normally following surgery. Soft food can be fed initially if necessary.
- Twice-daily oral rinses with a 0.2% chlorhexidine solution for 2 weeks by the owner at home to keep the oral cavity clean.
- Broad-spectrum antibiotic for 1 week.
- Re-examination in 14 to 21 days.
- Follow-up with home oral hygiene and dental prophylaxis as necessary for the stage of periodontal disease present.

Complications

- Inadequate beveling of the gingival margin leaving a blunted gingival margin.
- Burning the gingival tissue by using too high a setting on the electrosurgery unit. Anticipate a 1-mm sloughing of tissue even with a normal setting.
- Not leaving a 2-mm margin of attached gingiva with potential cleft formation or further retraction of less keratinized gingival tissue with bone and/or root exposure.
- Tip of electrosurgery unit touching root surface.

GINGIVOPLASTY
General Comments

- Gingivoplasty is the procedure of surgically recontouring or remodeling of the gingival surface.[4]

- Gingivoplasty and gingivectomy are often used together. Gingivoplasty is performed on hyperplastic areas without pseudopockets, and gingivectomy is performed on hyperplastic areas with pseudopockets.

Indication

- Gingival hyperplasia in interdental areas.

Contraindication

- Narrow or absent attached gingiva.

Objective

- To create a physiologic contour of the gingiva.

Materials

- Same as with gingivectomy.

Technique

- Gingivoplasty is often performed at the same time as gingivectomy.

Step 1—Using the cold blade or electrosurgery blade or loop, the gingiva is excised by cutting with the blade held at approximately a 45° angle with the tip of the blade toward the crown.

Step 2—The ends of the excision should be tapered into the surrounding gingiva to create the normal scalloped contour, particularly if several adjacent teeth are treated.

Step 3—Gingival tags can be removed with the blade or a sharp curette.

Step 4—Hemorrhage is controlled applying pressure with wet gauze pads or hemostatic agents.

Complications

- See gingivectomy.

Aftercare—Follow-up

- See gingivectomy.

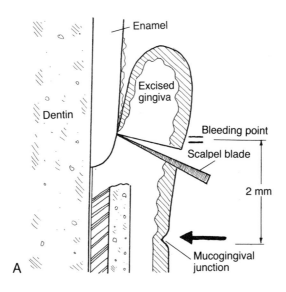

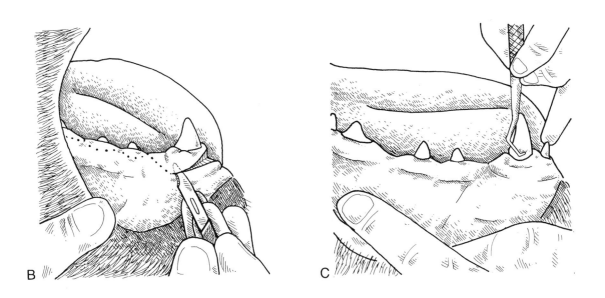

PERIODONTAL FLAP TECHNIQUES

Open Flap Curettage

General Comments

- Open curettage can provide pocket reduction and reattachment by creating access to subgingival calculus and removal of pocket epithelium.

Indications

- Local areas with suprabony pocket depths greater than 4 mm where extensive removal of pocket tissue is not required.
- To create better visualization and access for a restorative procedure.

Contraindications

- Health status of patient.
- Extensive periodontitis where additional treatment is needed.
- Deep periodontal pockets necessitating osteoplasty.

Objective

- To gain access to root surfaces to remove subgingival calculus and diseased cementum.

Materials

- No. 11, 12, 15, or 15C scalpel blade and handle.
- Mote no. 9 periosteal elevator or wax spatula.
- 4–0 or 5–0 absorbable suture.
- Needle holder, thumb forceps, and scissors.
- Sharp curettes.

Technique

Step 1—The blade is inserted into the pocket with the tip directed toward the alveolar bone *(A)* and the epithelial attachments are cut *(B)*. (The arrow points to the mucogingival junction.)

Step 2—The gingiva is elevated with the periosteal elevator lingually/palatally and labially/buccally *(C)* without exposing the marginal alveolar bone *(D)*.

Step 3—The exposed root surfaces are planed until they are smooth and hard *(E)*.

Step 4—The area is flushed with 0.2% chlorhexidine solution.

Step 5—The flap is repositioned and sutured with interrupted sutures placed interdentally *(F)*.

Postsurgical Care

- Twice daily oral flushing with 0.2% chlorhexidine solution for 2 weeks.
- Antibiotics as necessary.
- Home oral hygiene after healing to minimize future plaque accumulations.
- Follow-up examinations as necessary to monitor healing.

Complication

- Inadequate treatment in areas of more extensive periodontitis that progress.

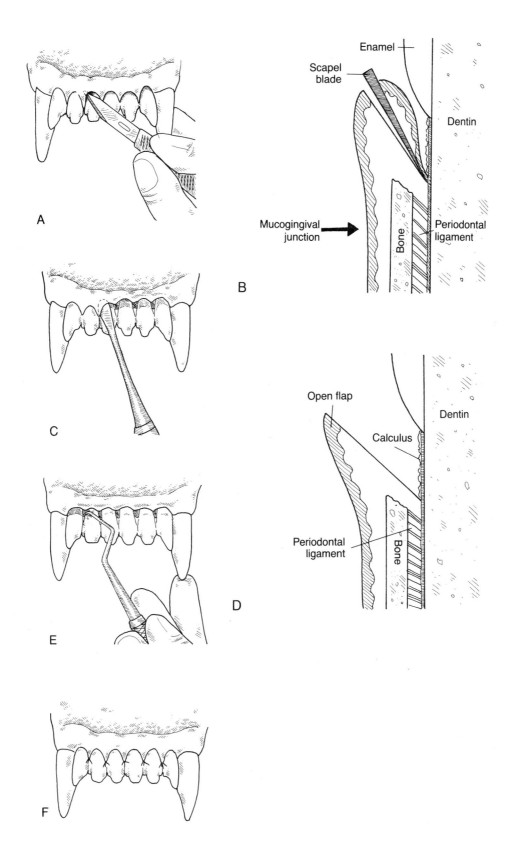

A

Scapel blade

Enamel

Dentin

Mucogingival junction

Bone

Periodontal ligament

B

C

Open flap

Dentin

Calculus

Periodontal ligament

Bone

D

E

F

Canine Teeth Palatal or Lingual Surface Flap Technique

General Comments

- Periodontal disease is often found on the palatal or lingual surface of the canine teeth.
- This area may be difficult to clean with closed techniques.

Indications

- Periodontal pockets on the palatal or lingual surface of the canine teeth deeper than 4 mm.
- To provide access for correction of osseous defects with or without grafting.

Contraindications

- Loose teeth.
- Signs of severe oronasal fistulation (nasal discharge, sneezing, penetration of probe or presences of solution in nares after irrigation of pocket).
- Secondary mandibular osteomyelitis.

Objective

- To allow access to the palatal or lingual root surface of canine teeth for planing, removal of granulation tissue, and bony correction.

Materials

- No. 10, 11, 12, 15, or 15C scalpel blade and handle.
- Mote no. 9 periosteal elevator or wax spatula.
- 4–0 absorbable suture material.
- Needle holders, thumb forceps, scissors.
- Curettes
- No. 2, 4 round burs

Technique

Step 1—The gingiva mesial and distal to the canine tooth is incised to the bone (A).

Step 2—Either an intrasulcar or reverse bevel incision is made to the level of the alveolar crest on the palatal or lingual surface (B).

Step 3—The periosteal elevator is used to elevate the full thickness gingival flap off the bone to expose the depth of the pocket (C). (The collar of tissue is removed if a reverse bevel incision was made.)

Step 4—Hemorrhage is controlled with wet compresses and direct pressure.

Step 5—Subgingival calculus, granulation tissue, and debris are removed with a curette (D).

Step 6—The exposed root surface is planed smooth.

Step 7—The area is flushed with 0.2% chlorhexidine solution.

Step 8—The desired bony corrections are made as indicated. (See sections on osteoplasty and bone grafting.)

Step 9—The gingiva is repositioned tightly against the tooth surface and sutured with interrupted sutures to the buccal gingiva (E).

Postsurgical Care

- Oral antibiotics as necessary.
- Oral flushing and swabbing initially, later gentle brushing of the palatal or lingual tooth surface to prevent plaque buildup.
- Recheck in 3 months with the patient under general anesthesia and reradiograph area.

Complications

- Puncturing into the nasal cavity during instrumentation. If only a small opening is created it may be possible to continue with the procedure and allow the defect to granulate and ossify as periodontitis heals.
- Inadequate healing of tissue with progression of periodontitis and oronasal fistula formation or mandibular bone loss and infection.

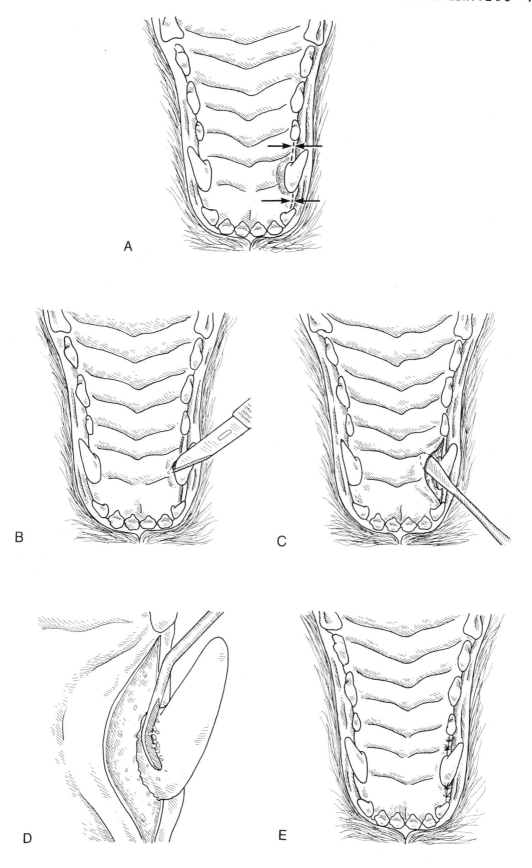

A

B

C

D

E

Reverse Bevel Flap

General Comments

- Reverse bevel flap surgery is performed to remove diseased pocket epithelium; and to gain access for root planing.
- Reverse bevel flap surgery is performed only if attached gingiva will be adequate postoperatively.
- As with all gingival surgery, the surgery is carried out from line angle to line angle. The line angle is an anatomic landmark on the tooth that represents the "corner" where two walls of the tooth meet. In *A*, "A" shows an interradicular incison and is incorrect, "B" shows a midfacial (radicular) incison and is incorrect, "C" shows an interproximal incison and is also incorrect, "D" shows a line angle incison and is correct.
- Releasing incisions are not always necessary and should not be used indiscriminately.

Indications

- Teeth that have pocket depths greater than 4 mm.
- Periodontal pockets with diseased tissue that has not responded to conservative treatment.
- Intrabony pocket formation with vertical bone loss and osseous defects in areas with sufficient attached gingiva.

Contraindications

- Deep pockets with minimal attached gingiva remaining.

- Poor owner compliance with home oral hygiene and recall dental prophylaxis.
- Health status of patient.

Objective

- To gain access to root surfaces of teeth with deep periodontal pockets (>4 mm) to remove subgingival calculus and diseased cementum, to remove diseased pocket tissue, and to correct osseous defects.

Materials

- A no. 11, 12B, 15, or 15C Bard Parker blade and handle.
- Sharp curette or scaler.
- 4–0 or 5–0 absorbable suture.
- No. 2 or 4 round bur for osteoplasty.
- Needle holder, tissue forceps, scissors.
- Molt no. 9 periosteal elevator or wax spatula

Technique

Step 1—Starting at the line angle of the healthy tooth mesial or distal to the operative area,[5] a reverse bevel incision is made extending through the gingiva *(B)* with the blade directed at the alveolar bone leaving a thin collar of marginal tissue around the teeth starting and ending at healthy gingiva *(C)*.

Step 2—Vertical releasing incisions can be made if necessary on one or both sides of the affected area to gain better access to the root surface and alveolar bone *(D)*.

Step 3—The flap is elevated with a periosteal elevator *(E)*. If minimal bony correction is needed the flap can be elevated just to expose the alveolar crest.

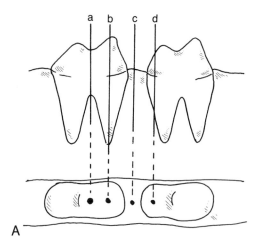

A

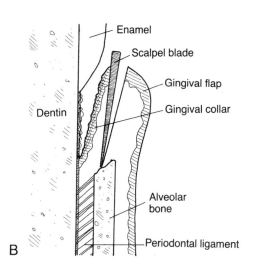

Enamel

Scalpel blade

Gingival flap

Gingival collar

Dentin

Alveolar
bone

Periodontal ligament

B

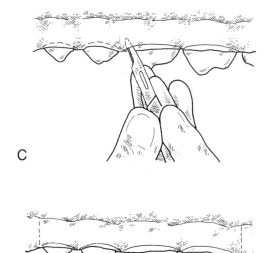

C

D

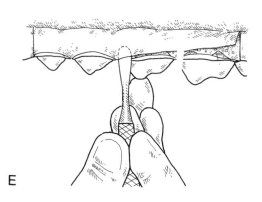

E

Technique *(Continued)*

Step 4—The collar of marginal tissue is removed by incising the attachments with the blade placed into the sulcus and horizontally at the base of the pocket and removing the tissue from the root surface with a sharp scaler or curette (*A* and *B*).

Step 5—The flap is retracted and the root surfaces are planed smooth with sharp curettes (*C*).

Step 6—Osseous defects and necrotic bone are removed with small round burs in a slow- or high-speed handpiece with saline irrigation.

Step 7—The area is flushed with a 0.2% chlorhexidine solution.

Step 8—The flap is repositioned, being sure that the bone margin is covered, and sutured interdentally with 4–0 or 5–0 absorbable suture material (*D*). The releasing incisions are sutured with interrupted sutures.

Postsurgical Care

- Soft food is recommended for 1 week.
- Oral antibiotics, continued as necessary.
- Daily oral flushing with 0.2% chlorhexidine solution for 2 weeks.
- Home oral hygiene after healing to minimize further plaque accumulation.
- Frequent follow-up examinations and prophylaxis to monitor healing progress.

Complications

- Infection.
- Dehiscence.
- Inadequate coverage of alveolar bone margin due to excessive cutting of tissue.
- Greater pocket formation.

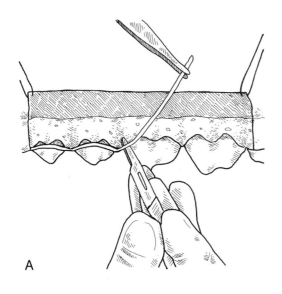

A

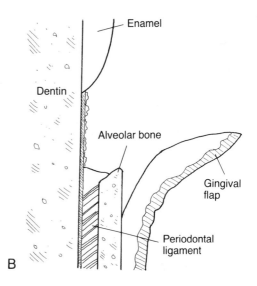

B

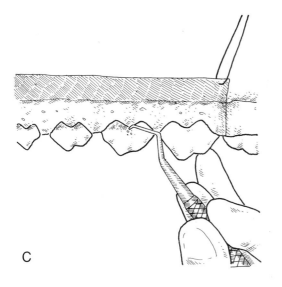

C

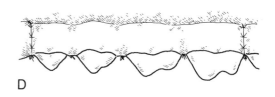

D

Apically Repositioned Flap

General Comments

- In making an apically repositioned flap, minimal gingiva is removed while making the flap.

Indication

- Areas with pocket depths greater than 5 mm where a reverse bevel flap is contraindicated (i.e., too little attached gingiva).

Contraindications

- Loose teeth.
- Lack of owner compliance with home oral hygiene or with return for recall prophylaxis.
- Health status of patient.

Objective

- To decrease pocket depth in areas with deep intrabony pockets bringing the free gingival margin just coronal to the level of the alveolar bone to allow for better self-cleansing of affected areas.

Materials

- No. 11, 12, 15, or 15C scalpel blade with handle.
- Mote no. 9 periosteal elevator or wax spatula.
- 4-O or 5-O absorbable suture.
- Needle holders, thumb forceps, scissors.
- Burs as are necessary for osteoplasty, ostectomy.
- Sharp curettes for root planing.

Technique

Step 1—The blade is inserted directly into the pocket around the involved teeth (A), and the epithelial attachments are cut buccally and palatally or lingually and interproximally (B).

Step 2—Vertical releasing incisions are made in healthy gingiva mesial and distal to the involved teeth (C).

Step 3—The gingiva is elevated apically with a periosteal elevator to expose the alveolar bone (D).

Step 4—Sharp bony edges, irregular bone margins, or necrotic alveolar bone margins

are removed with round burs and saline irrigation (E). (See osteoplasty.) Tooth supporting bone is not removed.

Step 5—Granulation tissue is removed from the gingiva by curettage and the root surfaces are planed (F).

Step 6—The surgical area is flushed to remove debris with sterile saline or 0.2% chlorhexidine.

Step 7—The gingiva is repositioned just coronal to the alveolar bone level and sutured interdentally (G).

Step 8—The vertical releasing incisions are sutured with interrupted sutures. A fold of redundant tissue may be present and will reconform during healing.

Postsurgical Care

- Daily oral flushing with 0.2% chlorhexidine solution for 2 weeks.
- Return to home oral hygiene after first week.
- Follow-up dental prophylaxis as necessary to continue oral health.
- Soft food is recommended for 1 week.
- Oral antibiotics should be continued as necessary.

Complications

- Infection.
- Dehiscence.
- Inadequate coverage of alveolar bone due to excessive cutting of tissue.
- Greater pocket formation.

CITRIC ACID

- Citric acid is applied to the root structure after any root planing procedure to enhance reattachment of gingival tissues.[6]
- Following root planing, a citric acid solution at pH 1 is applied to the dentin for 3 minutes and rinsed.

PERIODONTAL DRESSINGS

- Periodontal dressings are applied after periodontal surgery to protect gingival tissues.
- Lack of patient acceptance and of adequate adhesive areas limits their use in veterinary dentistry.

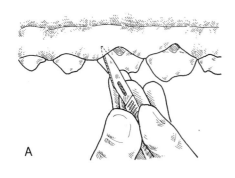

A

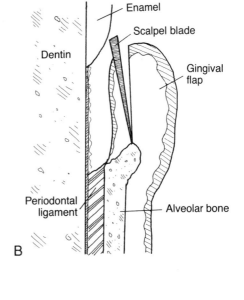

Enamel

Scalpel blade

Dentin

Gingival flap

Periodontal ligament

Alveolar bone

B

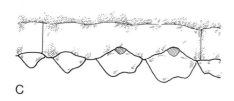

C

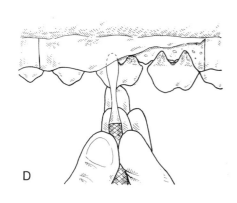

D

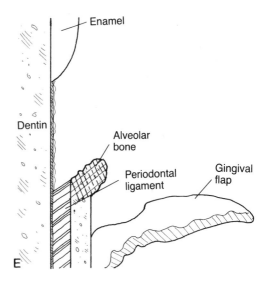

Enamel

Dentin

Alveolar bone

Periodontal ligament

Gingival flap

E

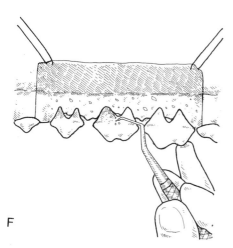

F

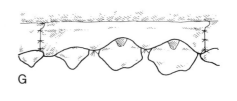

G

SOFT TISSUE GRAFTING TECHNIQUES

Pedicle Graft

General Comments

- The pedicle graft uses adjacent attached gingiva tissue to re-establish gingiva that has been lost.
- An area of exposed tissue from the graft will heal by second intention.

Indication

- For use in an area with gingival cleft formation that has an adjacent edentulous area (A).

Contraindications

- Loose tooth.
- Owner expectations.

Objective

- To establish a functional margin of attached gingiva in areas of cleft formation associated with periodontal disease or combined periodontal/endodontic lesions.

Materials

- No. 11, 15, or 15C scalpel blade and handle.
- Mote no. 9 periosteal elevator or wax spatula.
- 4-O or 5-O absorbable suture material.
- Needle holders, thumb forceps, scissors.
- Sharp curettes.

Technique

Step 1—The teeth are scaled and polished.
Step 2—A beveled incision is made along the gingival margin of the defect (B). The side adjacent to the graft is beveled externally with the side away from the graft beveled internally.
Step 3—The exposed root surface is planed smooth with a curette and the area flushed.
Step 4—A vertical incision is made at twice the cleft width from the midline of the gingival border apically to match the length of the cleft (C). A horizontal releasing incision is made along the midline of the gingiva to the depth of the periosteum.
Step 5—The portion of the graft adjacent to the cleft is elevated to the depth of the bone for the width of the cleft with a periosteal elevator while the portion of the graft away from the cleft is elevated only to the level of the periosteum.
Step 6—The graft is rotated over the cleft and sutured to the freed gingival margin with interrupted sutures (D). The sutures are placed approximately 1.5 mm apart and are tied so that the margins are just opposed (E).
Step 7—The gingival edge away from the cleft is sutured to adjacent gingiva and periosteum.
Step 8—A periodontal dressing can be applied to protect the area for a few days.

Postsurgical Care

- Antibiotics as necessary.
- Remove periodontal dressing if still present in 2 to 3 days.
- Twice daily oral rinsing with 0.2% chlorhexidine for 2 weeks.
- Continued daily home oral hygiene.
- Follow-up and frequent dental prophylaxis as necessary to maintain oral health.

Complications

- Strangulation of gingival tissue by placing sutures too closely or tightly.
- Dehiscence with failure to reform margin of attached gingiva.
- Exposure of bone with necrosis by elevating flap full thickness in area away from cleft.

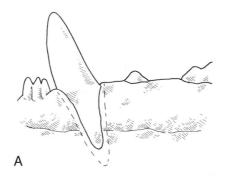

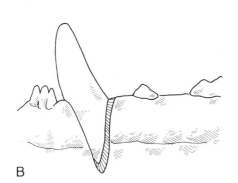

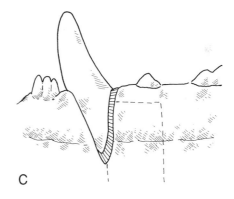

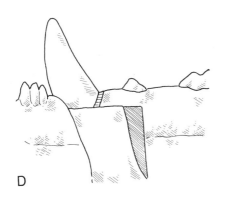

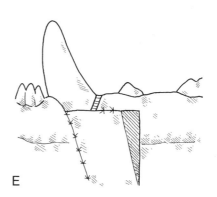

Free Gingival Graft

General Comments

- If gingival defect is related to endodontic disease, endodontic disease must be treated first.

Indications

- Individual teeth with deep cleft formation close to or beyond the mucogingival junction that are otherwise solid teeth (A).
- Where adjacent gingival tissue that could be used to cover the defect is insufficient.

Contraindications

- Owner compliance with aftercare or unrealistic expectations.
- Systemic disease.
- Untreated and uncontrolled periodontal disease.
- Other dental disease; some gingival defects are caused by endodontic disease.

Objective

- To re-establish a border of keratinized attached gingiva around a tooth with a deep gingival cleft to prolong the life of the tooth.

Materials

- No. 11 scalpel blade.
- Template made from a small piece of metal foil.
- 5–0 absorbable polyglycolic suture with swagged-on needle/reverse cutting point.
- Small periosteal elevator.
- Needle holder, thumb forceps.
- Periodontal dressing.

Technique

Step 1—The recipient site is treated by scaling and planing the exposed root surface. A reverse bevel incision is made around the gingival margin to remove pocket epithelium (B).

Step 2—A 3- to 4-mm recipient bed for the graft is created by removing all the soft tissue down to the level of the periosteum in a rectangular pattern around the defect (C). The bed should extend beyond the root surface sufficiently to allow for shrinkage during

healing. Hemorrhage is controlled with a wet gauze and pressure.

Step 3—A donor area is selected where attached gingiva is sufficient, such as the area above the maxillary canine tooth. The size of the recipient site can be measured or a template made using a small piece of aluminum foil.

Step 4—The template is placed on the donor area and the outline traced with a no. 11 blade (D).

Step 5—The donor incisions are deepened with the blade to the level of the periosteum.

Step 6—A corner of the graft is elevated with the blade (E) and tagged with a 5–0 suture with a swagged-on taper-point needle as a holder and marker.

Step 7—The remainder of the graft is elevated with the blade while tension is gently placed on the suture until the graft is free (F).

Step 8—The graft is placed over the recipient bed (gingival side up), and pressure is applied for several minutes to help create a seal and force out air and blood between the donor and recipient site.

Step 9—The edges of the graft are sutured to the surrounding gingiva with interrupted sutures, using 5–0 absorbable suture with a swagged-on taper needle, spaced 2 mm apart (G).

Step 10—A periodontal dressing is placed over the graft site to protect it for the first few days.

Postsurgical Care

- Removal of the periodontal dressing in 2 to 3 days if still in place.
- Appropriate antibiotic therapy.
- Suture removal in 10 days if using nonabsorbable suture.
- Soft food for 10 to 14 days.
- Twice daily oral flushing with 0.2% chlorhexidine for 2 weeks.
- Home oral hygiene after healing to minimize progression of periodontal disease.

Complications

- Sloughing of the graft from rough handling or poor adaptation of tissues.
- Sutures placed too tightly or closely creating loss of blood supply.
- Bone necrosis at donor site if insufficient periosteum left for healing.
- Inadequate home care.

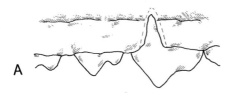

A

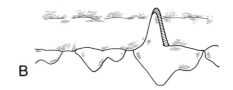

B

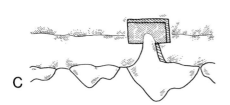

C

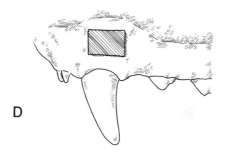

D

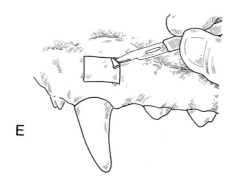

E

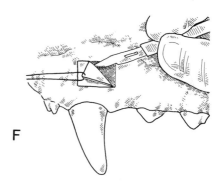

F

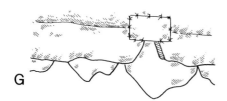

G

MANAGEMENT OF BONE DEFECTS

General Comments

- Osseous surgery techniques are used according to the degree of disease present, the experience of the practitioner, and the desire and compliance of the client.
- Management of bony defects provides an environment for better gingival healing around periodontally affected teeth with bone loss.
- These defects are further classified according to the number of remaining bony walls.
- Three-wall defect most commonly occurs in the interdental area, also called an intrabony defect (A). This condition has the best prognosis for treatment.
- Two-wall defect is the most common defect, occurring in the interdental area (B).

- One-wall defect occurs interdentally (C). This defect carries the worst prognosis for treatment.
- Osteoplasty is the technique that removes or recontours nonsupporting bone.
- Ostectomy is the technique to remove tooth-supporting bone.

Management Techniques

- Induce regrowth of bone by grafting.
- Hemisect a multiroot tooth and extract one severely affected root. Preserve the remaining root with appropriate endodontic procedure.
- Attempt to maintain pocket by frequent scaling, root planing, and plaque control.
- Extract the tooth.

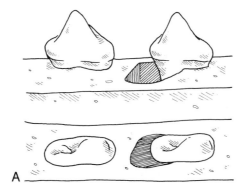

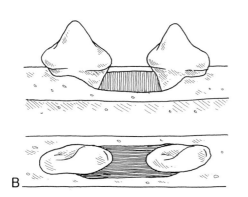

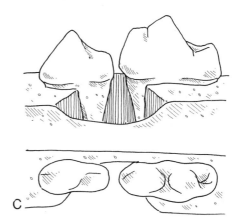

Osteoplasty

Indications

- Infrabony defect where the base of the periodontal pocket is apical to the level of the crest of the alveolar bone that results in sharp irregular bone contours.
- Thinning of bony ledges and establishing a scalloped contour to allow for periodontal flap closure.
- Irregular alveolar margins after extracting teeth.
- Leveling interdental crater formation.

Contraindications

- Health status of patient.
- Lack of owner compliance with aftercare.

Objective

- To remove necrotic, ragged alveolar bone, to improve bony contour in periodontally diseased areas allowing adaptation of the surgical flap, and to improve healing and oral hygiene.

Materials

- Materials for flap surgery.
- No. 1, 2, or 4 bur in slow-speed handpiece.
- Sterile saline.
- Small bone rongeurs (postextraction).

Technique for Osteoplasty or Ostectomy

Step 1—A full-thickness flap is prepared as previously described (*A*).

Step 2—Granulation tissue is removed, and the roots are thoroughly planed and smoothed with curettes.

Step 3—Sharp edges and ledges of alveolar bone are removed and contoured as needed with a round bur in a slow-speed handpiece with saline irrigation (*B*). Minimal bone removal is desired (*C*).

Step 4—Irregular alveolar margins are recontoured in areas of tooth extractions.

Step 5—Surgical area is lavaged with sterile saline.

Step 6—Gingiva is replaced over bone margin and sutured interdentally (*D* and *E*).

Postsurgical Care

- Periodontal dressing if desired.
- Antibiotics as indicated.
- Twice daily oral flushing with 0.2% chlorhexidine for 2 weeks.
- Home oral hygiene.
- Follow-up management/recall for dental prophylaxis.

Complications

- Excessive bone removal with loss of attachment. Supporting bone should not be removed (ostectomy).
- Excessive heat produced if inadequate irrigation or too high an RPM with bone necrosis.
- Inadequate contouring with poor gingival adaptation and poor healing or dehiscence.

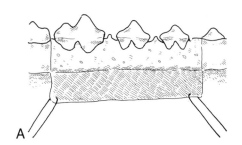

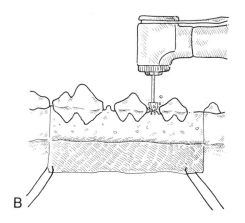

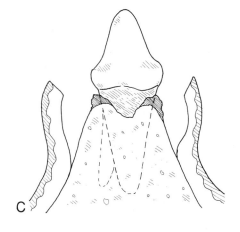

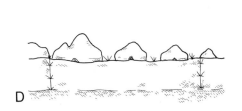

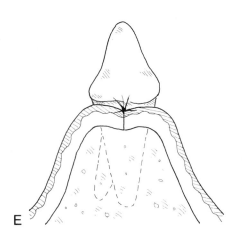

Bone Grafting
General Comments

- The benefit of bone grafting in treatment of periodontally diseased teeth is inconclusive. Bone reformation has been reported following thorough root planing and curettage after flap surgery in humans without the use of a filling material in bony defects.[4] Client compliance is extremely important to follow-up with plaque control and monitoring of the area if these procedures are to be successful.
- Can be done in conjunction with osteoplasty to improve new bone formation.

Indication

- Two- or three-wall defects where bone regeneration is desirable to maintain periodontal health of a tooth.

Contraindications

- Severely loose teeth.
- Health status of patient.
- Lack of owner compliance or patient acceptance of aftercare.

Objective

- Achieve regeneration of bone around periodontally affected teeth with bone loss using either autologous bone graft or nonvital implant material.

Materials

- Autogenous cancellous bone taken from edentulous area.
- Hydroxyapatite.*
- Polylactic granules.†

---

*Interpore 200, 18008 Skypark Circle, Irvine, CA 92714.
†Polylactic Granules, Osmed, Inc., 1669 Placenta Ave., Costa Mesa, CA. 92627.

- Materials for periodontal flap surgery.
- No. 1/2 round or No. 330 pear bur in high-speed handpiece.

Technique

Step 1—A full-thickness periodontal flap is created to expose the defect (A).

Step 2—The pocket is debrided and the root surface is planed smooth (B).

Step 3—Lateral bony projections or irregularities can be smoothed with an appropriate-size round bur in a slow-speed handpiece with saline irrigation (C).

Step 4—The bony pocket walls are fenestrated with no. 1/2 or no. 330 bur in a slow-speed handpiece to a depth of 1 to 2 mm in several places to ensure release of bone-forming elements.

Step 5—Bone grafting material is mixed with saline to form a paste and is packed into the defect to the height of the remaining bone (D).

Step 6—The gingival flap is replaced immediately and sutured interdentally (E and F).

Step 7—A periodontal dressing is placed over the graft site.

Postsurgical Care

- Appropriate antibiotics are administered.
- Periodontal dressing is removed in 7 days if still in place.
- Twice daily oral flushing with 0.2% chlorhexidine for 2 weeks.
- Follow-up plaque control; radiographs at 3 to 6 month intervals.

Complications

- Infection.
- Dehiscence.
- Progression of periodontal defect.

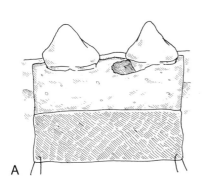

A

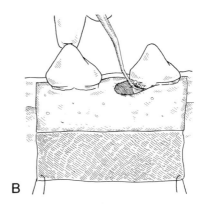

B

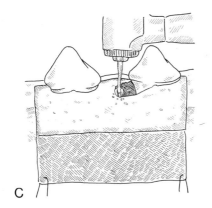

C

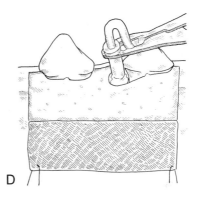

D

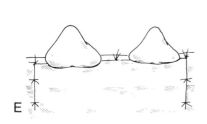

E

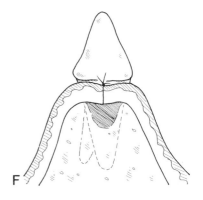

F

PERIODONTAL SPLINTING

General Comments

- Periodontal splinting is only semipermanent at best to immobilize teeth and improve gingival health, but it does not lead to any long-term stabilization.[4]
- These techniques can be used with the acrylic or composite resin alone.

Indications

- Mobile incisors with solid adjacent teeth.
- When all six incisors are slightly mobile and can be stabilized as a unit.

Contraindications

- Owner is unwilling to follow up with adequate home care or to return for office care.
- Teeth with inadequate or less than 20% bone support remaining.
- Single incisor without adjacent teeth present.
- Periodontal and endodontic involvement of a nonstrategic tooth.
- Traumatized primary teeth where the jaw is still growing.

Objective

- To stabilize loosened teeth (most commonly incisors) from bone loss to allow improved healing after periodontal treatment and/or surgery and to preserve cosmetic function.

Materials

- .010 ligature wire for figure-of-eight technique.
- Fine square orthodontic arch wire for lingual splint technique.
- Minikin pins for lingual splint technique.*
- Light-cure composite resin.
- Dental acrylic.
- Howe wire-bending pliers.
- Small wire-cutting pliers.
- Finishing burs.

Techniques

- Several techniques can be used depending upon the materials available, time needed for stabilization, and cosmetic appearance desired.

Figure-of-Eight Wiring Technique

Step 1—A no. 1/2 or 1 round bur is used in a high-speed handpiece to create a shallow groove circumferentially around each tooth at the middle of the crown (A). Do not enter the pulp chamber. (This step is optional if cosmetic appearance is not critical or splinting is temporary.)

Step 2—A .010 ligature wire is placed in a figure-of-eight pattern around the teeth in the grooves and tightened (B).

Step 3—The teeth are prepared by acid-etch technique.

Step 4—The dental acrylic or light-cure composite resin is placed over the wires and grooves and is shaped and cured (C).

Substep 1—When using dental acrylic a fine camel hair or Getz brush† is dipped into the liquid (monomer) and then into a small amount of the powder (polymer). This small amount of mixed acrylic is placed over the ligature wire. This step is repeated until the acrylic covers all the wire and the interproximal areas. It will take several minutes to harden.

Step 5—The acrylic or composite resin can be smoothed and shaped with finishing burs or sandpaper discs (D).

Step 6—The occlusion should be checked and any areas of interference adjusted.

---

*Whaledent International, 236 5th Ave., New York, NY 10001.

†Teledyne-Getz, 1550 Greenleaf Ave., Elk Grove Village, IL 60007.

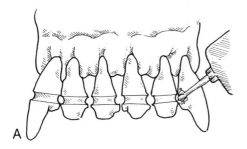

A

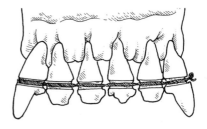

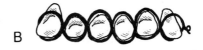

B

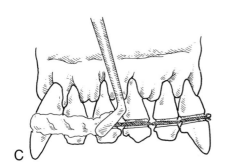

C

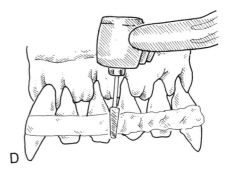

D

Lingual Wire or Pin Stabilization

• If cosmetics are important this is the preferred technique.

Step 1—A no. 33 or 34 inverted cone bur is used to make a shallow groove across the lingual aspect of the incisors coronal to the cingulum *(A)*. Do not enter the pulp chamber.

Step 2—If an arch wire is to be used it is shaped to conform to the lingual aspect of the incisors and fitted in the groove. The wire is cut and set aside.

Step 3—The teeth are prepared with acid-etch preparation. Do not etch exposed dentin.

Step 4—The wire is placed in the groove *(B)*.

Step 5—If Minikin pins are to be used, a small amount of composite resin or dental acrylic is placed in the groove first, and the pins are placed to overlap an interproximal space *(C)*.

Step 6—Composite resin material or dental acrylic is placed over the wire or pins and cured as necessary *(D)*. The material is shaped and smoothed *(E)* and occlusion checked and adjusted. The interdental spaces are left open.

Postoperative Care

• Daily home oral hygiene.
• Frequent dental prophylaxis.

• Removal of the splint when the teeth have stabilized, if the split is to be only temporary.

Complications

• Chipping of acrylic or composite with loosening of the teeth. Dental acrylic can be repaired if chipped or fractured by adding additional powder and liquid to the splint; this is less brittle than the composite resin.
• Exposure of wire leading to uncosmetic appearance for show dogs.
• Progression of periodontal disease necessitating extraction.
• Endodontic involvement caused by entering pulp chamber or thermal damage.

References

1. Grove K. Periodontal Therapy. Compend Contin Educ 1983;5(8):660–664.
2. Grove TK. Periodontal Disease. Compend Contin Educ 1982;4(7):564–570.
3. Zwemer TJ. Boucher's Clinical Dental Terminology (3rd ed.). St. Louis: C.V. Mosby, 1982:299.
4. Rateitschak KH, Rateitschak EM, Wolf HF, Hassell TM. Color Atlas of Periodontology. Stuttgart: Georg Thieme, 1986.
5. Fedi PF Jr. The Periodontic Syllabus. Philadelphia: Lea & Febiger, 1985:115.
6. Linde J. Textbook of Clinical Periodontology . Munksgaard: Munksgaard/Saunders, 1985.

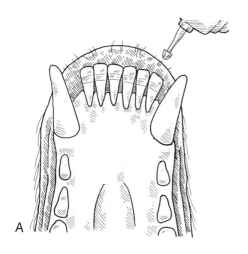

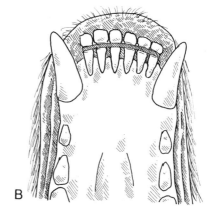

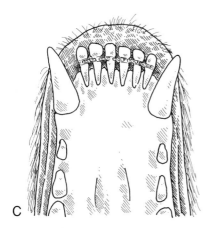

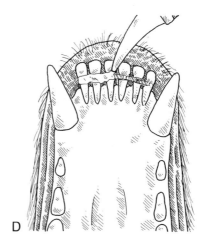

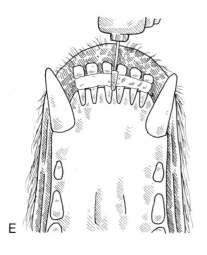

chapter 6

EXODONTICS

GENERAL COMMENTS

- Teeth should not be sacrificed unnecessarily. In years past, when veterinary dentistry was taught in veterinary curricula, exodontics was one of the primary subjects. Our predecessors learned how and where to trephine and repel equine teeth. Entire books were devoted to equine dentistry (Merillat, Louis A. Animal Dentistry and Disease of the Mouth, Chicago: Alexander Eger, 1911). As equine medicine declined, dentistry was virtually dropped from the veterinary curriculum. As we endeavor to become better able to render good dental care to our patients, let us keep in mind that exodontics is the area of dentistry we would rather practice as infrequently as possible. Most veterinarians are sensitized to the word euthanasia and do not like to perform such a procedure wantonly. It may be helpful to use the term "euthanasia" interchangeably with the word extraction. That way, every time a "tooth euthanasia = toothanasia" is performed, more sensitivity will be manifest and the practitioner will look for other more positive alternatives.
- Teeth are normally held in the alveolar bone by the periodontal ligament. In performing exodontics the periodontal ligament must be stretched and then broken or torn. If this is accomplished properly, the rest of the extraction process is easy.
- Good accessibility and exposure to the surgical site may require changing the patient's position from lateral to dorsal recumbency during the procedure and creating a gingival flap to expose the tooth and bone adequately.
- Good visibility must be maintained throughout the procedure. Lighting, suction, and position of the surgeon and patient are all factors affecting visibility.
- Gentle tissue handling is important to minimize trauma and to promote rapid healing of both hard and soft tissues.
- After the extraction, the socket is thoroughly debrided.
- Any exposed bone is covered by soft tissue and sutured if necessary.
- The practitioner should consider the need or value for preanesthetic blood sample including platelet count or estimate prior to the patient's undergoing anesthesia.

INDICATIONS

- As a general principle any tooth that is not contributing to function may need to be extracted.[1]
- Retained primary teeth (A). Two homologous teeth should never be in the mouth at the same time. If a practitioner identifies an adult tooth erupting and the primary tooth is not exfoliating naturally, it is time to extract the primary tooth.
- Interceptive orthodontics. Primary teeth are extracted when the mandible and the faciomaxillary structures are not developing appropriately and an interlock preventing normal jaw development is present.
- Supernumerary teeth (B) frequently cause crowding and interfere with occlusion and periodontal health.
- Malocclusion or malpositioned teeth, if orthodontics or other restorative methods are not desired.
- Periodontal disease. If the periodontium cannot be returned to a healthy state, extraction is better than allowing ongoing infection.
- Nonvital teeth where root canal therapy is not possible or elected.
- Teeth that have structural damage where restoration is not feasible because of the degree of destruction, the location, or economic factors.
- Retained roots or fragments.
- Resorption of root structure
- Teeth in a fracture line that interfere with bone fracture repair or healing.
- Teeth near or surrounded by oral neoplasia.
- Any dental or oral disease where owner desires less expensive or more definitive treatment.

CONTRAINDICATIONS

- Patients that are in poor health and may not tolerate the procedure.
- Malignant conditions when the patient is undergoing radiation or chemotherapy that would inhibit healing.
- Bleeding disorders that cannot be controlled.
- Patients on medications that may cause prolonged bleeding times; aspirin, anticoagulants, and anticancer drugs may be examples.

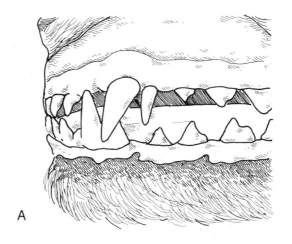

A

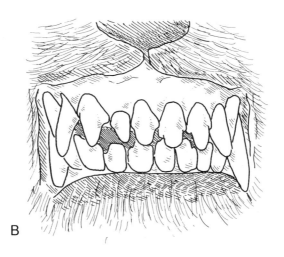

B

OBJECTIVES

- Controlled force should be used when extracting teeth.
- Adequate access to a smooth, unimpeded pathway of removal should be obtained.
- A tooth should be extracted completely with as little trauma to the oral tissues and bone as possible.
- Ideally, all the tooth's roots should be extracted.
- Elevators are used as levers to break down the periodontal ligament. Three basic types of lever are involved:[2]
  - They are used as a lever of the first class, i.e., a lever with a fulcrum between the resistance and the force (A and B).
  - A lever that is a wedge (C and D).
  - A lever that is a wheel and axle (E and F).
- Extraction forceps are used to lift the tooth out of the socket after the periodontal ligament has been torn free.

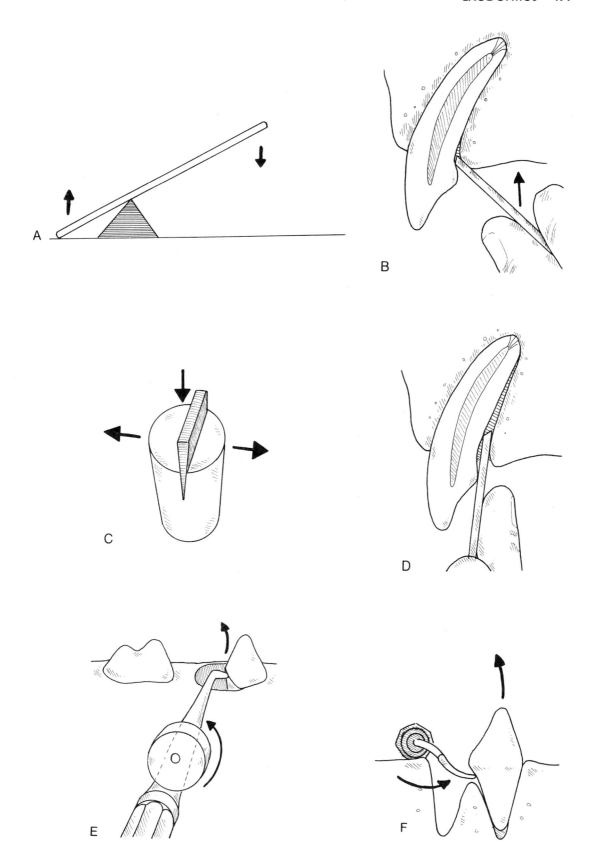

MATERIALS

- See Chapter 2 for details of specific instruments.

Simple Single-Root Extraction Pack

- Scalpel and no. 11, 15, or 15C blades.
- Molt no. 9 periosteal elevator or wax spatula elevator.
- Surgical burs and handpiece.
- Elevators.
- Extraction forceps.
- Tissue forceps.
- Needle holders.
- Scissors.
- Suture material: 3–0 or 4–0 resorbable suture, reverse cutting needle swagged on.
- Bone rongeur.

Multiroot Extraction Pack

- Items in the simple single-rooted pack.
- Cutting burs or safeside disc and handpiece.

Complicated Extraction Pack

- Items in the simple single-rooted and multiroot extraction packs.
- Root-tip picks.
- Mallet and chisel.
- Bone file or rasp.
- Bone wax.
- ADD polylactic granules.
- Surgicel or Gelfoam.

EXTRACTION OF SIMPLE SINGLE-ROOTED TEETH *(A)*

Incisors, First Premolars, and Mandibular Third Molars

Technique

Step 1—A radiograph is made and evaluated for root structure, periodontal ligament health, and surrounding bone.

Step 2—The gingiva is incised by inserting a scalpel blade into the sulcus and incising at its attachment around the tooth *(B)*.

Step 3—An elevator is used to break down the periodontal ligament by alternately stretching and compressing it. This is done by either using the elevator as a lever of the first class or as a wedge lever.

First-Class Lever

Substep 1—The blade of a concave elevator is used with the concave surface toward the tooth to be extracted and the convex surface on the adjacent tissue or tooth.

Substep 2—A rotational force is applied to the handle of the elevator *(C)*. This puts a lifting or elevating force on the tooth to be extracted. The force is held for 1 to 3 seconds, then released. If needed, a "purchase," or notch in the tooth, may be created with a bur to help give the elevator a grip on the tooth.

Substep 3—Elevating forces are repeated at several locations around the tooth *(D)*. Each time the force is applied, tooth movement should occur. At first, movement is slight. As the periodontal ligament fibers are stretched and torn, the amount of movement will increase.

Substep 4—Continue using the elevator until the tooth is mobile in its socket *(E)*.

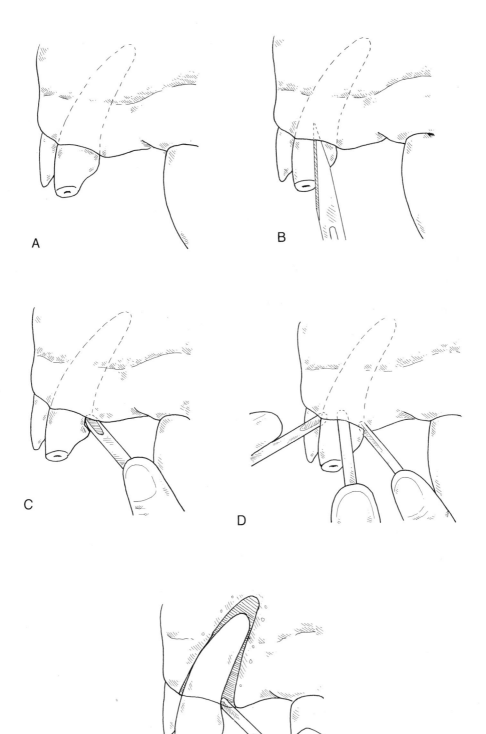

A

B

C

D

E

Wedge Lever

Substep 1—The tip of the elevator is wedged between the tooth and the alveolar bone *(A)*.

Substep 2—The periodontal ligament is stretched on the side of the tooth on which the elevator is located. Slight movement of the tooth should be noticed.

Substep 3—This is repeated at other locations around the tooth. As the periodontal ligament is stretched and broken the elevator can be inserted further into the alveolus. The process is repeated until the tooth is mobile.

- If needed, both the foregoing methods may be used in a single extraction.

Step 4—Grasp the mobile tooth firmly with extraction forceps and exert an elevating force *(B)*.

- Additional rotational or rocking force may be applied if needed in alternating directions similar to the force applied with the elevator to further break the periodontal ligament fibers.
- If elevating forces and gentle rotational or rocking forces are not facilitating the extraction, additional use of the elevator is indicated before extracting the tooth with the forceps.

Step 5—The extracted tooth should be examined to ensure that the entire root has been extracted. A radiograph may be needed to make this determination or for the medical record.

Step 6—The crest of the alveolar bone may need to be removed to facilitate suturing *(C)*. This is done by using a rongeur. This technique may increase chances of primary tissue apposition, prevent fenestrations of soft tissue by sharp bony edges, and reduce the auto-osseous remodeling period.[3]

Step 7—Gingiva is sutured using a reverse cutting needle and 3–0 or 4–0 absorbable suture material *(D)*.

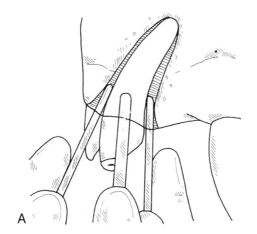

A

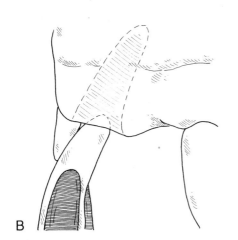

B

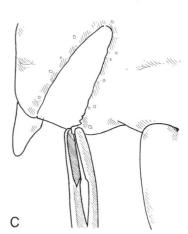

C

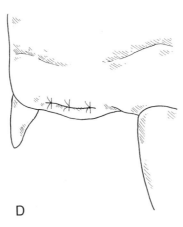

D

Complications

Complications include fractured socket, fractured or broken root tips, hemorrhage, endocarditis, secondary infections, mandibular fracture, oronasal fistula, cutting of the tooth opposing the extracted tooth into the gingiva, alveolitis, tearing of gingival tissue, inability to extract, and retained root fragment.[4]

Fractured Socket

Description

- The alveolar bone is fractured in the process of extracting the tooth[3] *(A)*.

Treatment

- Fragments that are unstable or exposed should be dissected and removed before the gingiva is closed.

Fractured or Broken Root Tips

Description

- A portion of the root is fractured and not extracted with the rest of the tooth.

Treatment

- See root-tip extraction technique.

Hemorrhage

Description

- Bleeding from the extraction site.

Treatments

Soft Tissue Hemorrhage

Pressure

- Pressure is applied with gauze sponge directly to the extraction site to allow a clot to form *(B)*.

Cold Pack

- Application of cold compresses made from ice wrapped in a gauze sponge can reduce blood flow sufficiently to allow a clot to form and at the same time retard postoperative swelling *(C)*.

Ligation

- Ligation of bleeding vessels.

Electrocautery

- Is most effective to control hemorrhage from small vessels. *Caution* must be exercised not to overcauterize or burn tissues.

Primary Closure of Site

- Suturing soft tissues over the extraction site with fine suture.

Aids for Coagulation

Gelfoam*

- These products are packed into the extraction site and act as a matrix for clot formation.

Synthetic Bone

- Packed into the extraction site to serve as a matrix for the clot to form on and then aid in the formation of new bone.
- The cube form is preshaped and is placed into the socket *(D)*.
- The granular form is inserted into the socket *(E)*.
- Is either polylactic† or hydroxyapatite.‡

Hemorrhage of Bone

Crushing Bone

- Rongeurs may be used to crush the bone.

Packing with Gauze

- The socket may be packed with gauze or a coagulation-enhancing material such as Gelfoam or Surgicel.

Sterile Bone Wax§

- Sterile bone wax may be placed into the alveolus on bleeding bone.

Endocarditis

Description

- If the tooth being extracted is abscessed or severely affected by periodontal disease, a transient bacteremia should be expected.

Treatment

- If anticipated, pretreatment with an appropriate antibiotic is warranted.

---

*Upjohn Company, 4000 Portage Road, Kalamazoo, MI 49001.

†Osmed, Inc., 1669 Placenta Ave., Costa Mesa, CA 92627.

‡Interpore 200, Interpore, 18008 Skypark Circle, Irvine, CA 92714.

Secondary Infections

Description

- Secondary infections creating osteomyelitis or suppurative arthritis.
- Although infrequently diagnosed as direct sequelae of extractions the practitioner should be aware that these occur.
- Signs include fever, reluctance or inability to eat, resistance to examination, depression, and lack of healing.

Treatment

- Antibiotics, radiographs, and surgical intervention may be in order in cases of osteomyelitis to debride diseased bone and to cover exposed bone with soft tissue.

Mandibular Fracture

Description

- The severity of bone damage can be evaluated with a preoperative radiograph (*F*). If severely infected or radiographically thin bone is found, advise the client of an increased possibility of fracture. The amount of force used in extractions must be limited.
- A diseased mandible, once fractured, is often difficult to repair. It may never heal.

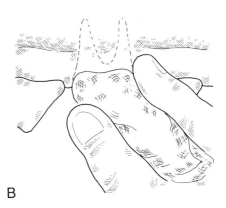

B

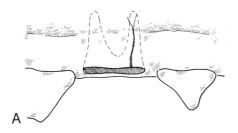

A

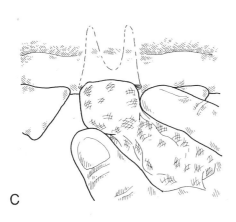

C

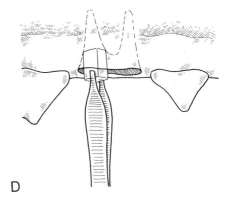

D

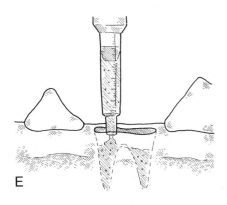

E

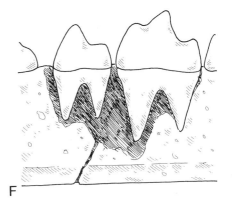

F

Treatment

- Best to prevent.
- See Chapter 10.

Oronasal Fistula

Description

- A hole between the oral and nasal cavity may be present and not detected, or it may be created in the process of extraction.

Treatment

- Important to explain possibility to owner before extracting tooth.
- See page 198 for oronasal fistula repair.

Alveolitis—Painful Socket

Description

- Inflammation or infection of the empty socket after extraction.

Treatment

- Best to prevent at time of extraction by debriding necrotic or infected tissues.
- Antibiotic therapy after extraction.
- Irrigation.

Opposite Tooth Cutting into Extraction Site or Lip

Description

- Most often seen when a canine tooth is extracted. The lip or cheek is not held away from the gingiva and the opposing tooth strikes it. It may only pinch the lip or it may puncture or lacerate the lip.

Treatment

- The occlusion of the opposing tooth must be changed. This can be treated by:
- Amputating the opposing tooth to a level that does not trap the lip. This will also require pulp capping if the pulp chamber is exposed.
- Orthodontically moving the opposing tooth to a position that will not impinge upon the soft tissue.
- Extracting the opposing tooth.

Tearing of Gingival Tissue

Description

- Happens as the tooth is extracted if its gingival attachment is not incised completely.

Treatment

- Suturing gingiva.
- Prevention by completely severing the gingival attachment.

Ankylosis

Description

- Periodontal ligament space is not visible on radiograph.
- No tooth movement with the elevator because of ankylosis.

Treatment

- See buccal flap procedure.
- Using bur and high-speed handpiece to pulverize root.

Large Tooth Surface

Description

- Tooth root surface so large that the practitioner is unable to exert enough force with the elevator to stretch/break down the periodontal ligament.

Treatment

- See buccal flap procedure.

Aftercare—Follow-up

- The client should be instructed to cleanse the area of extraction daily with a water-based mouthwash such as Maxiguard, CET Spray, or Listerine, chlorhexidine, or iodine solution.
- Appropriate antibiotics are administered.
- The patient should be examined at 10 to 14 days by the doctor to determine whether healing has been normal and is complete or whether further treatment is indicated.

General Comments

Caution

- Heavy rotational or rocking force should never be applied, to prevent fracturing the root tips in the socket.

Dental Radiology

- Any time we are not sure that we have removed all the root, a radiograph should be taken. It is much better to find a piece of root at the time of extraction than to have to go back later.
- The practitioner should always weigh the risk of leaving a portion of the root against the damage that may occur to tissue in extracting it.
- If the bone around the fractured root appears healthy on a radiograph and considerable tissue damage would be created by extracting it, then a decision may be made to leave the fractured root.
- This should be annotated in the dental record/chart and complications and follow-up discussed with the client.

Canine Tooth Extraction

General Comments

- Extraction will take one of two forms depending upon how well the tooth is attached. If the attachment has been weakened sufficiently to allow some mobility, the tooth can be extracted in a manner similar to that of any single-rooted tooth. If the attachment is solid, as with normal periodontium, it will be best to lay a gingival flap and remove the buccal plate of bone.

Indications

- Same general indications as previously mentioned.
- Disarming a vicious or biting dog or cat if amputation and pulp capping are not desired.

Contraindications

- With a fractured mandible or faciomaxillary complex, extraction of a canine tooth may need to be postponed.

Technique

- See simple-single root extraction technique, pages 178–182.
- See gingival flap buccal plate technique, pages 192–194.

Complications

Tongue Hanging Out of Mouth

Description

- When lower canines are extracted, the tongue may not be held in the mouth all the time.

Treatment

- Discuss possibility with client prior to extraction; this may give added reasons to perform alternative treatments to extraction.
- Osseous integrated implant is the only treatment.
- Cheiloplasty may be attempted, but difficult to obtain success and healing.

Trapping Lip between Gum and Mandibular Canine Tooth

Description

- After the extraction of the maxillary canine tooth, the maxillary lip may be caught and pinched between the mandibular canine and gingiva of the maxilla.
- This may be very uncomfortable for the patient.

Treatment

- Amputation and pulp capping of mandibular canine tooth.
- Extraction of the mandibular canine tooth.

EXTRACTION OF TEETH WITH MULTIPLE ROOTS

Maxillary Second and Third and Mandibular Second, Third, and Fourth Premolars, as well as Mandibular First and Second Molars (A)

General Comments

- The indications, contraindications, and objectives are the same as for single-root extractions.
- If the multirooted tooth is first divided, its extraction is no more difficult than a simple single-rooted tooth.

Materials

- The same as single-root extraction.
- High- or slow-speed handpiece.
- Bur or safeside disc for sectioning teeth.

Technique

Step 1—The gingival attachment is incised with an elevator or blade (B).

Step 2—Evaluate and determine whether the tooth can be elevated easily. The elevator can be used in the furcation to gain good purchase. If it can, it is extracted using the same techniques and principles as used in the simple single-root extraction. If elevation is not easily performed, the tooth should be divided, separating each root.

Step 3—A crosscut fissure bur is used in either a high-speed handpiece or slow-speed handpiece to cut through the tooth (C). This leaves each root separate.

Step 4—Elevate each root as if a simple single-root extraction (D), except neither root is extracted all the way until the other root has been elevated (E).

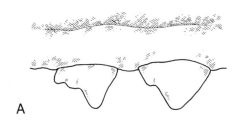

A

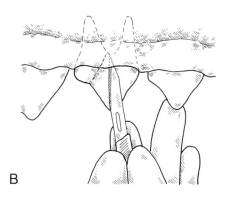

B

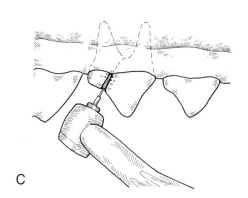

C

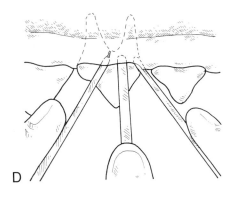

D

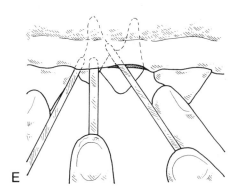

E

Technique (Continued)

Step 5—Once both roots are luxated in the sockets, each is extracted using extraction forceps as in a simple, single-root extraction *(A* and *B)*.

Step 6—The alveolus is curetted and debrided of necrotic and/or infected tissues.

Step 7—The alveolar crest is reduced using a rongeur or a bur in a handpiece *(C)*.

Step 8—The gingiva is approximated over the extraction site with 3–0 or 4–0 resorbable suture *(D)*.

Complications

- Root-tip fracture is more likely if the periodontal ligament is strongly attached and the roots are not extracted separately.
- Fracture of one root if the division is not made completely.

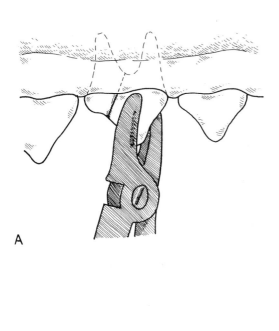

A

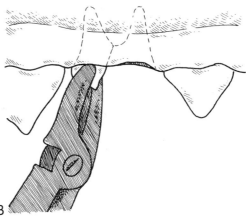

B

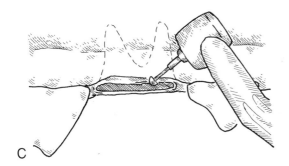

C

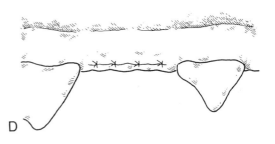

D

Maxillary Fourth Premolar

Additional Considerations

- Each root is separated using a crosscut fissure bur in a handpiece (A).
- The palatine root is separated by cutting in the fissure created by the base of the large mesial cusp and the palatine cusp.
- The mesial and distal roots are separated by cutting from the fissure between the two large cusps in an apicomesial direction.
- Each of the divided roots is elevated using elevators and working around the roots in the same manner as in a single-root extraction. Personal preference dictates the order of elevation.
- After all three roots are mobile, extraction forceps are used on the individual roots.

Maxillary First and Second Molar

Additional Comments

- Each root is separated using a crosscut fissure bur in a handpiece (B).
- The palatine root is separated from the rest of the tooth by cutting with a crosscut fissure bur in the distomesial fissure created by the mesial-distal cusps and the palatine cusp.
- The mesial and distal roots are separated by cutting apically through the fissure formed by the large cusps in an apical direction.

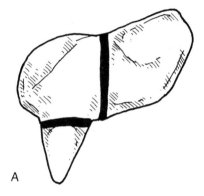

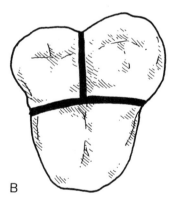

GINGIVAL FLAP/BUCCAL PLATE TECHNIQUE

General Comments

- This technique is used in difficult extractions.
- This process is more involved; therefore, simpler techniques should be attempted first.

Indication

- On all types of teeth where movement is not created with the elevator because the root is too large, the root is hooked, or the root is ankylosed.

Contraindication

- Any extraction that may be accomplished with conventional extraction techniques.

Objective

- Removal of a buccal plate of bone to facilitate the extraction of the root with minimal trauma.

Materials

- Multiroot extraction pack.

Technique

Step 1—A radiograph is taken and evaluated prior to extraction.

Step 2—Incise around the gingival margin with a scalpel blade (A).

Step 3—Make releasing incisions at the distal edge of the canine tooth (B).

Step 4—Elevate the gingiva from the buccal bone beyond the end of the jugum (bony prominence covering the root) (C).

Step 5—The outline of the juga is cut through the bone with a bur and high-speed handpiece (D). Alternatively, a chisel and

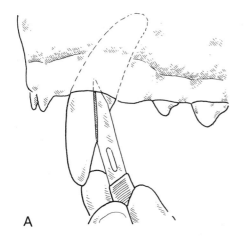

A

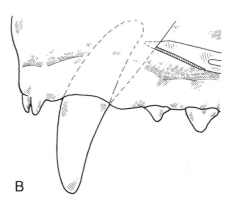

B

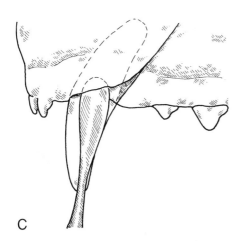

C

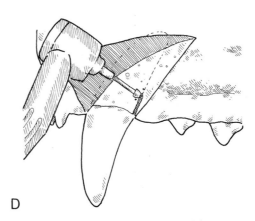

D

Technique *(Continued)*

mallet may be used. This frees the buccal bony plate from the rest of the facial bone. An elevator can be used to remove the freed bony plate *(A)*.

Step 6—An elevator can now be used as a wedge around the mesial, lingual, and distal surfaces to break the periodontal ligament or ankylosis from the lingual surface of the root structure *(B)*.

Step 7—As the tooth is loosened, the elevator is changed from a wedge to a lever of the first class.

Caution: Care is taken not to twist the crown of the tooth too far buccally in order to maintain the thin alveolar bone at the apical end of the palatal wall of the root. If this bone is damaged, an oronasal fistula may be created.

Step 8—Extraction forceps are used to grasp the tooth *(C)*, and the tooth is rocked in a twisting motion on its long axis until it is extracted. If rocking/twisting does not readily extract the tooth, further use of the elevator is required as in steps 6 and 7.

Step 9—Any sharp bony projections are smoothed using a bur or rongeur *(D)*. The alveolar crest may also be decreased if needed to facilitate suturing.

Step 10—Gingival tissues are approximated and sutured in place using 3–0 or 4–0 resorbable suture material *(E)*.

Complications

- Fracturing the root with too much force.
- Fracturing more of the buccal bone than is necessary if the overlying bone was not adequately cut.
- Creation of an oronasal fistula as the maxillary canine tooth is extracted by fracturing the bone between the alveolus and the nasal cavity as the crown is rotated buccally during the extraction process or by uncovering existing pathology.
- Fracturing the mandible.

Aftercare—Follow-up

- Pain should be considered and controlled with softer diets and drugs if warranted. Remember that frequently we are unable to recognize or diagnose chronic pain in our patients. It may be better to err on the cautious side and administer pain-relieving drugs if not contraindicated.

- The client should be instructed to cleanse the extraction site at least once a day.
- Antibiotics should be administered.
- The patient should be examined by the doctor in 10 to 14 days to determine whether healing has progressed normally and is complete.
- Periodontal dressings may be applied.

DENTAL PULVERIZATION

General Comments

- Occasionally, stubborn roots, root tips, or feline teeth that have been resorbed to a point of fragility cannot be extracted with elevators and extraction forceps.
- In these cases, a high-speed handpiece and pear-shaped, round, or crosscut fissure bur in standard length or operative length can be used to pulverize the remaining root.
- This is a particularly effective technique in the cat.
- The root tip is much harder than bone, and the bur tends to bounce off and has a different feel and drilling sound than bone when pulverizing.
- The root tip does not bleed; adjacent bone does.
- The root tip is white; adjacent bone has a slightly different color.

Indication

- Pulverization is used when having difficulty extracting with elevators.

Contraindication

- This technique will not be as fast as an elevated extraction and thus is not preferred.

Objective

- Remove all the retained or ankylosed root fragment.

Materials

- Same as complicated extraction.
- Magnification, additional light, forced air, or suction may improve visualization.

Technique

Step 1—A radiograph is made to evaluate the size and length of the root(s).

Step 2—The crown of the tooth is cut off at the gingival line.

Step 3—The bur is used to carefully remove root structure.

Step 4—A radiograph is taken to demonstrate that the entire root has been removed.

Complications

- Penetration into adjacent structures such as nasal passages, sinus, mandibular canal.
- Forcing a root fragment into nasal passages, sinus, or mandibular canal.
- Overheating tissue. Use plenty of water spray to keep the tissues cool. The smell of burning bone can indicate future problems with necrotic bone and slow healing of extraction sites.

Aftercare—Follow-up

- Reexamine in 7 to 10 days to evaluate healing.
- Antibiotics may be prescribed.

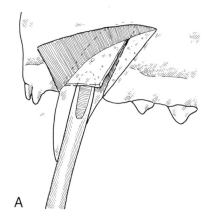

A

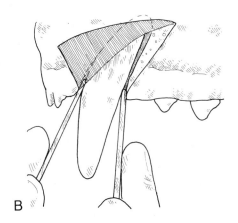

B

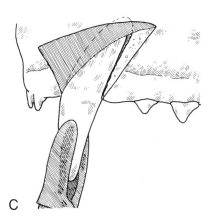

C

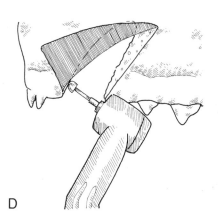

D

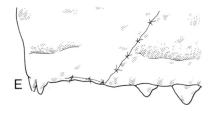

E

EXTRACTION OF RETAINED ROOT-TIP FRAGMENTS

General Comments

- Root-tip fragments may occur due to trauma, cavities, and resorption of the crown or as complications of extractions *(A)*.

Indication

- If the root-tip fragment can be visualized, it should be extracted.

Contraindication

- If the risk of tissue damage is greater than the advantage gained by extraction, then the root fragment may be left and closely monitored.

Objective

- Removing the entire root tip without excessive damage to adjacent tissues.

Materials

- Same as single-root and multiroot extractions.
- The fine root-tip picks are particularly effective.
- Magnification, additional light, forced air, and suction improve visualization.

Techniques

- Of the several techniques for removing root tips, pulverization *(B)* (page 194) and buccal plate removal (page 192) have been described.
- Root-tip picks can be used as a wedge to expand bone and tease the root fragment out of the socket *(C)*.
- In a multirooted tooth, the interradicular septum can be pulverized with a bur on a high-speed handpiece to break down one wall of the alveolus. The root fragment may then be avulsed into the created space.

- An oversized endodontic file can be used to retrieve the root fragment by inserting the file into the root canal and twisting to lock the file in place.

Complications

- Repelling the tooth fragment into the nasal cavity, sinus, or mandibular canal.
- Creating tissue damage (nerve, bone, or vascular).
- Additional hemorrhage.

Aftercare—Follow-up

- Monitor the healing process.
- Same as with other extractions.

EXTRACTION OF PRIMARY TEETH

General Comments

- The roots of primary teeth are both longer and thinner than those of permanent teeth; thus, they are more easily fractured.

Indications

- When the adult tooth is erupting and the primary tooth has not been lost.
- Proper time is as soon as the adult tooth is noticeable, whether it has erupted through the gingiva or not.
- If the mandible and the facial maxillary complex are not developing properly, the primary teeth may be extracted to allow independent growth of the two jaws. See interceptive orthodontics, page 366.

Objective

- Remove the primary tooth and root without damaging the adult tooth or other oral structures.

Materials

- Single-rooted extraction pack (page 178).

Technique

Step 1—Radiograph the tooth (teeth) to be extracted for identification of the shape and length of the root(s).

Step 2—Using an elevator as a wedge lever, elevate around the tooth. With primary teeth it is important to elevate to the point that the periodontal ligament is broken and the tooth is free in the alveolus.

Step 3—Extraction forceps are used to lift the tooth out of the socket. Rotational forces should not be used. They will usually cause root fracture.

Step 4—A radiograph is made if any doubt exists that the entire root was extracted.

Complications

- Fracture of the root.

Aftercare—Follow-up

- Monitor healing.
- Monitor eruption of the adult tooth.

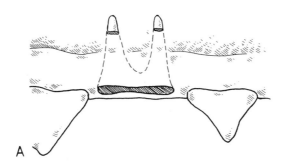

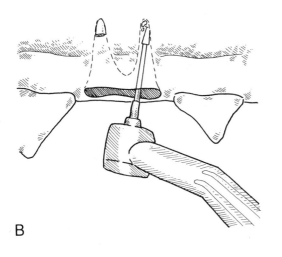

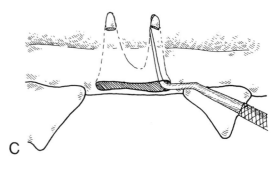

ORONASAL FISTULA REPAIR

General Comments

- Severe periodontal disease creating a palatal pocket and loss of the bone on the palatal side of the root may be noted radiographically or by irrigation of the sulcus resulting in irrigant dripping out the nose. Many clients will report chronic sneezing in patients.
- If an oronasal fistula is created by an extraction, it should be repaired.
- Traumatic avulsion of a canine tooth can create an oronasal fistula.
- Ideally the repair should place an epithelial layer in both the oral and nasal cavities.
- The flap must not have any tension on it after it is sutured in place.

Indication

- A communication between the oral and nasal cavities.

Contraindication

- Severely infected tissue; best to wait to do reparative surgery.

Materials

- Complicated extraction pack.

Techniques

Single-Flap Technique—Buccal Sliding Flap

- Usually used for smaller fistulas. If the fistula is large or chronic, then the double-flap method is recommended.

Step 1—The margins of the fistula are debrided of necrotic and epithelialized tissue (A).

Step 2—Releasing incisions are made (B). The mesial incision is started at the gingival ridge mesial to the fistula and continued apically into the buccal mucosa. The distal incision is started at the gingival ridge in the area of the mesial line angle of the first premolar and continued apically into the bucal mucosa. The incisions should be diverging apically.

Step 3—A reverse bevel incision is made at the buccal edge of the fistula connecting the releasing incisions. The palatal margin can be elevated slightly with a blade to facilitate suturing (C).

Step 4—The gingival flap with its periosteum is elevated apically (D). Enough tissue should be elevated for the flap to be placed over the fistula without retracting. This will ensure that there will not be tension when the sutures are placed.

Step 5—The alveolar bone may need to be recontoured for better positioning of the flap. This can be done with a small rongeur, chisel, or curette.

Step 6 (optional)—Synthetic bone, polylactic acid crystals, or tetracycline may be packed into the oronasal fistula prior to suturing.[5]

Step 7—Place the flap over the defect and suture with 3–0 or 4–0 suture (E).

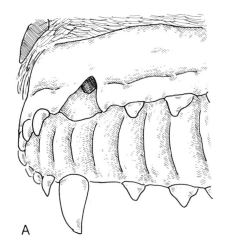

A

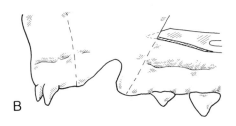

B

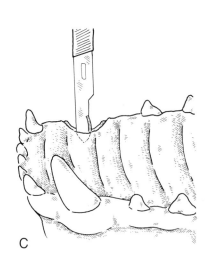

C

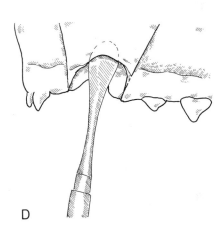

D

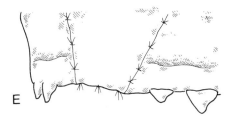

E

Double-Flap Techniques

- These methods are more complicated and are usually used for large defects or when the simple technique has failed.

Double-Flap—Palatal and Buccal Sliding Flap

Step 1—A full-thickness palatine flap is created by making parallel incisions from mesial and distal borders of the fistula to the midline on the palate where they connect (A). This should create a flap large enough to fit over the fistula, and after suturing, not have tension on the suture lines.

Step 2—The palatine flap is elevated and inverted over the fistula (B). This inversion places the epithelium of the flap on the nasal side of the fistula (C).

Step 3—The palatine flap is sutured to the mucosa at the edges of the fistula using 3–0 or 4–0 absorbable suture (D).

Step 4—A sliding flap is created, placed over the palatal flap, and sutured (E), as described in the buccal sliding flap technique (page 198), or if more tissue is needed, a labial buccal pedicle flap may be created.

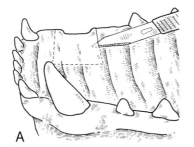

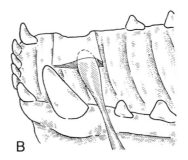

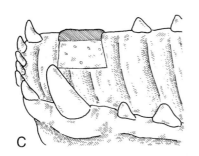

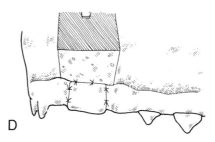

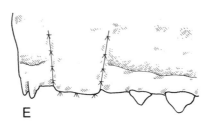

Double Flap—Palatal and Labial Buccal Pedicle Flap

Step 1—A palatal flap is created using steps 1 to 3 of the previously described double-flap, palatal and buccal sliding flap technique.

Step 2—An incision is made along the mucogingival junction from the area of the distal edge of the jugum, extending mesially to create a flap long enough to completely cover the defect from where the palatal flap is taken (A). This usually is near the midline. A second incision is made, one and one-half times the diameter of the fistula, this incision is made parallel to the initial releasing incision on the mucogingival junction. A third incision is made perpendicularly, connecting the two releasing incisions.

Step 3—Starting at the midline (B), the flap is elevated (C).

Step 4—The pedicle flap is sutured over the palatal flap using simple interrupted sutures (D).

Step 5—The edges from the two releasing incisions are sutured together (E).

Complications

- It is important to tell the client before extracting teeth that an oronasal fistula may be a possibility.
- With any flap technique, a suture dehiscence or infection is a possibility.

Aftercare—Follow-up

- Maintain on an antibiotic.
- Area may need cleansing, but this can disturb the healing process. Using a water irrigation device or water spray bottle may be beneficial.
- Doctor recheck at 2- to 3-day intervals if in doubt. It is better to recognize trouble early than to find it when the surgery has completely fallen apart.
- The client should be warned not to put tension on the graft site by pulling on the patient's lip while cleansing the area or looking at the surgical site.

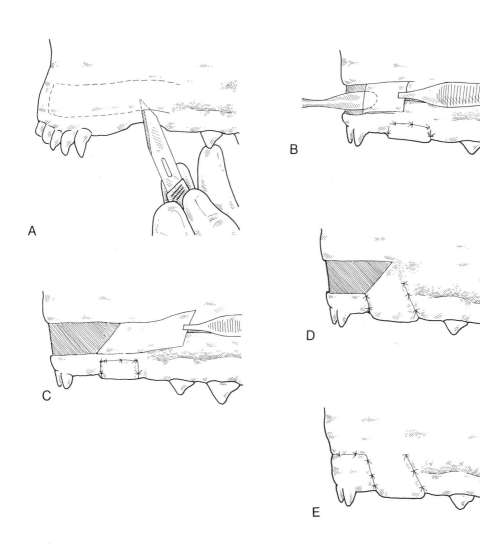

IMPACTED, UNERUPTED, OR EMBEDDED TEETH

General Comments

- An impacted tooth is one whose path of eruption is blocked or impaired.
- If the opposing tooth is erupted, then impaction should be suspected, and if the homologous tooth (on the other side) is erupted, then impaction is almost certain.
- If a tooth is expected to erupt, it is called an unerupted tooth. Frequently this is determined by noting progress in the eruption process clinically. If the eruption process has ended and the tooth is located beneath the mucosa, it is called an embedded tooth. This term is usually applied to teeth associated with some abnormality, i.e., supernumerary, mesiodens, or pathologic states.

Indications

- In general, most impacted teeth should be removed.
- To prevent infection (perioconitis) and follicular pathologic processes—odontogenic cysts and neoplasms.
- The presence of infection or disease due to the impaction.
- To assist in maintaining occlusion.

Contraindications

- Before the root has developed sufficiently for adequate extraction.
- If there is an increased risk of injuring an adjacent significant structure (nerve tissue, vascular tissue, other teeth).
- When the patient's general health is not sufficient to tolerate the procedure.

Objective

- Extractions with minimal damage to other oral structures.

Materials

- Complicated extraction pack.

Technique

Step 1—A radiograph is made to identify the location of the impacted tooth (A).

Step 2—Releasing incisions are created to adequately expose the area, and the buccal gingiva is elevated (B).

Step 3—The bone covering the tooth is removed with a bur and high-speed handpiece (C) or chisel and mallet. This will create access to the crown and root surfaces.

Step 4—The tooth may be sectioned for a stepwise removal of the tooth and to create space for elevation and instrumentation (D).[6]

Step 5—Once this space is created then the remaining tooth structures can be displaced, elevated, and extracted (E).

Step 6—The flap is sutured using simple interrupted suture.

Complications

- Delayed healing due to improper closure or poor flap design.
- Fracture of the mandible when too much bone is removed.
- Infection of soft tissue or bone.

Aftercare—Follow-up

- Standard postsurgical follow-up.

References

1. Waite DE. Principles of exodontia. In: Waite DE ed. Textbook of Practical Oral and Maxillofacial Surgery. Philadelphia: Lea & Febiger, 1987:81–91.
2. Peterson LJ, Ellis E III, Hupp JR, Tucker MR. Contemporary Oral and Maxillofacial Surgery. St Louis: C.V. Mosby Co., 1988.
3. Maretta SM, Tholen M. Extraction techniques and management of associated complications. In: Bojrab MJ, Tholen M eds. Small Animal Oral Medicine and Surgery. Philadelphia: Lea & Febiger, 1989:75–95.
4. Dorn AS. Complications of Dental Extractions. Chicago: Surgical Forum, 1989.
5. Mulligan TW. Oral/Nasal Fistula Repair. New Orleans: Nabisco, 1988.
6. Pedersen GW. Oral Surgery. Philadelphia: W.B. Saunders Co., 1988:69–71.

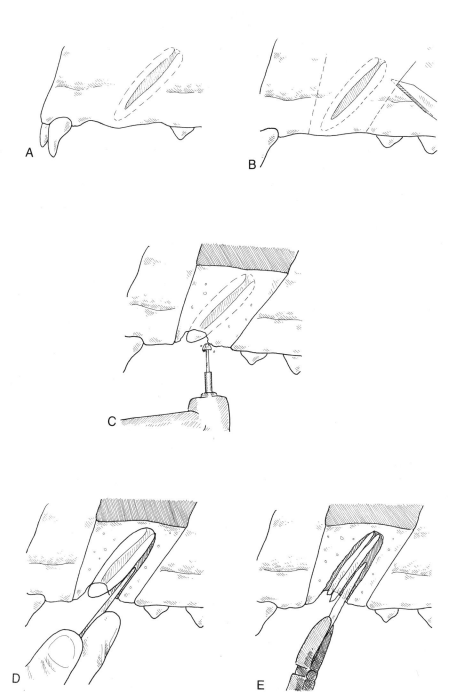

chapter 7

ENDODONTICS

General Comments

- The objective of endodontic therapy is to maintain a vital tooth or, failing that, to alleviate discomfort and infection from the tooth and periapical tissues by obliteration of the root canals.[1]

INDIRECT PULP CAPPING

General Comments

- Indirect pulp capping is indicated when a cavity or restorative preparation comes within 1 to 2 mm of the pulp.
- During deep-decay-type cavity preparation, a layer of carious dentin can be left over the pulp. This layer will be sterilized with the application of calcium hydroxide.[2]

Indications

- Deep cavity preparations where a pink color is seen over the pulp.
- Extensive crown restorations on vital teeth.

Contraindications

- Direct pulp exposure.
- Nonvital tooth restorations.
- Radiographic evidence of apical pathology.

Objective

- A protective layer of calcium hydroxide or glass ionomer is placed over areas of a restorative or cavity preparation close to the pulp tissue to protect the pulp from thermal or chemical injury and to prevent sensitivity.

Materials

- Fast-setting calcium hydroxide Life,* Dycal,† Pulpdent paste‡) or glass ionomer cavity liner.

*Kerr/Sybron Manufacturing Co., P.O. Box 455, Romulus, MI 48174.
†Caulk/Dentsply, Lakeview and Clark Avenues, Milford, DE 19963.
‡Pulpdent, Watertown, MA 02272–0780

- Injection syringe or plastic working instrument.
- Materials, instruments, and equipment needed to prepare and complete a cavity preparation or restoration (see Chapter 8, pages 275 to 286).

Technique

Step 1—The cavity preparation or restoration site is flushed with sterile saline to remove dentinal debris and is air dried (A).

Substep 1—A dentin tooth conditioner is applied to the dentinal surface with a Getz brush for the manufacturer's recommended time, rinsed with water, and air dried (B).

Substep 2—For deep cavity preparations, it is desirable to use both a calcium hydroxide and glass ionomer cavity liner. The calcium hydroxide should be placed first. The tooth conditioner can be used over the calcium hydroxide product to prepare the dentinal walls for the glass ionomer.

Step 2—The cavity liner is applied over the base of the cavity or restorative preparation in a thin layer and is allowed to dry using a Getz brush or plastic working instrument (C). Bonding of the final restoration will be inhibited if the liner coats the walls of the cavity preparation (D). If the walls are inadvertently coated, they should be prepared again.

Substep 1—When using a light-cured glass ionomer liner, the material is cured with a visible light gun for the prescribed length of time (E).

Step 3—In deep restorations, another layer of a glass ionomer can be placed to reduce the thickness of the final restoration (F). This reduces the polymerization shrinkage that occurs as the restoration material cures.

Step 4—The restorative procedure is continued (G), as described in Chapter 8, pages 275 to 286.

Postoperative Care

- Follow-up radiographs at 6 and 12 months to evaluate pulp chamber size and evidence of apical abscess formation by comparison with other teeth.

Complications

- Entering pulp chamber during cavity preparation.
- Not allowing enough room for the final restorative material.
- Covering the walls of the preparation with the liner.
- Loss of restorative material due to poor retention.

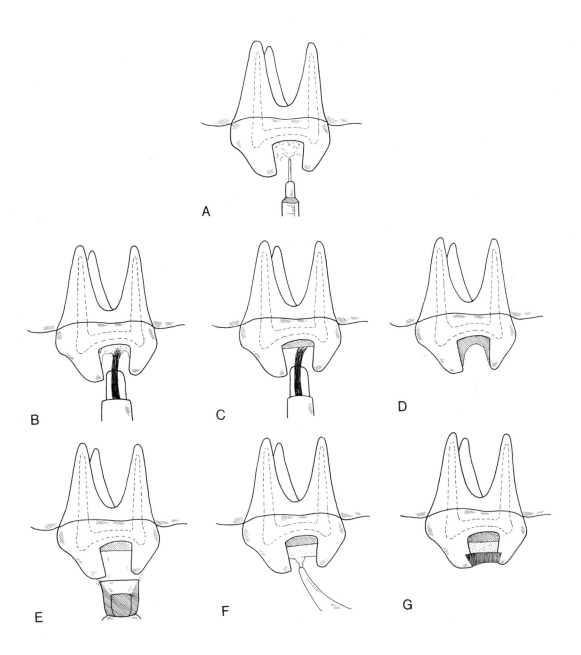

VITAL PULPOTOMY WITH DIRECT PULP CAPPING

General Comments

- In patients younger than 18 months of age it is frequently desirable to achieve additional dentinal formation to increase the strength of a tooth that has been fractured.
- In recent fractures, vital pulpotomy with direct pulp capping is the treatment of choice.
- Patients that have received this treatment should be followed closely with radiographs to monitor changes in pulp health.
- Root canal therapy is indicated if pulp death is evident on follow-up.

Indications

- Fractured tooth crowns with pulp exposure of less than 2 weeks' duration in patients younger than 18 months of age.
- Fractured tooth crowns with pulp exposure of less than 48 hours' duration in patients over 18 months of age.
- Disarming animals by shortening the crowns of teeth used for biting.
- In patients with malocclusion to shorten the tooth crown to eliminate interference with other teeth or soft tissues.
- Accidental exposure of pulp during deep cavity or restorative preparation.
- Hemisection of vital multirooted teeth with extraction of one diseased or injured root when the remaining roots and crown are salvageable.

Contraindications

- Pulpal death.
- Pulp exposure for longer than 2 weeks in an animal of any age.
- Fractures of the primary teeth.
- Severely traumatized or grossly contaminated pulp where the pulp is unlikely to survive.

Objective

- Protect the pulp and stimulate repair with secondary dentin by using a calcium hydroxide preparation directly on the pulp tissue and by placing a restoration over the pulp access site.

Materials

- Diamond disc or no. 701 crosscut, tapered fissure bur for shortening the crown.
- Round, pear, or tapered fissure burs of various sizes in high-speed handpiece.
- Sterile saline.
- Sterile paper points.
- Calcium hydroxide paste (HypoCal,* Pulpdent paste).
- Intermediate filling material (Life, Dycal, IRM†).
- Injection syringe.
- Restorative material of choice is discussed in Chapter 8, pages 275 to 286.

Technique

Step 1—The oral cavity is disinfected by flushing with an antiseptic solution (0.2% chlorhexidine). Aseptic technique is used throughout the procedure.

Step 2—The tooth crown is shortened (A and B) using a diamond disc in a slow-speed handpiece with water irrigation to keep the tooth cool. (When disarming animals, the biting teeth are shortened to the level of the adjacent teeth (C).)

Step 2 (alternate)—A no. 701 crosscut, tapered fissure bur in a high-speed or slow-speed handpiece with water cooling can also be used to amputate a tooth crown (D) or to hemisect a multirooted tooth (E).

---

*Ellman, 1135 Railroad Avenue, Hewlett, NY 11557
†Caulk/Dentsply, Lakeview and Clark Avenues, Milford, DE 19963-0359

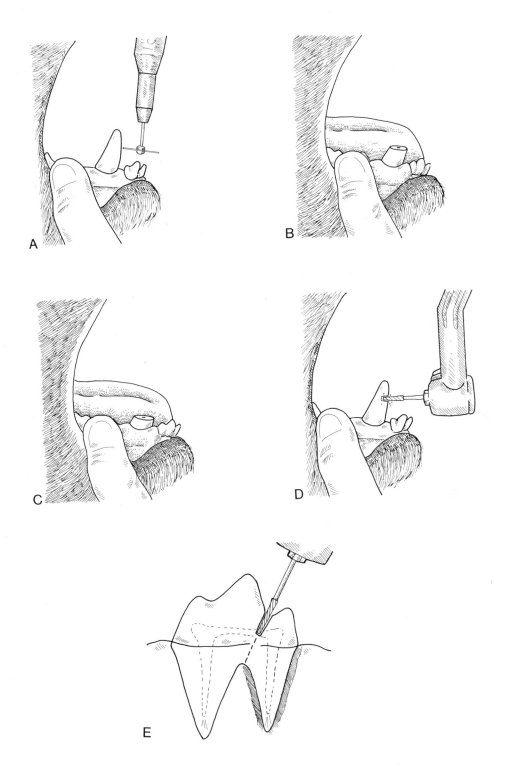

Technique (Continued)

Step 3—A bur of approximately the size of the diameter of the pulp chamber (round, pear, or tapered fissure) is used in a high speed handpiece to remove approximately 5 mm from the coronal portion of the pulp of the amputated tooth (A).

Step 4—Hemostasis is achieved with sterile saline lavage and using the blunt end of multiple sterile, dry paper points (B). Leaving a paper point in place for 2 to 3 minutes is often sufficient to control hemorrhage. In cases with persistent hemorrhage, lavage with a local anesthetic solution containing epinephrine can be used.[3] Caution should be used if using a halothane (Fluothane) anesthetic agent.

Step 5—When bleeding is controlled, calcium hydroxide paste is applied over the exposed pulp for a depth of 1 to 2 mm using the applicator syringe provided (C). The paste is tamped against the pulp stump with the blunt end of a paper point.

Step 6—An intermediate filling material (glass ionomer or resinated calcium hydroxide) is placed over the calcium hydroxide paste with an injection syringe or jiffy tube and is allowed to cure (D).

Step 7—The pulp access (cavity) opening is prepared for the desired filling material (E), and the restoration is completed (F).

Postsurgical Care

- Postoperative antibiotics for 7 days.
- Radiographic follow-up at 6 month and 12 months or at appropriate intervals is necessary to detect pulp death and subsequent apical changes indicating the need for a root canal. (Compare with contralateral tooth.)

Complications

- Loss of restorative material with possible contamination of pulp.
- Tooth discoloration due to hemorrhage from pulp seeping into dentinal tubules coronal to pulp amputation. (Bleeding through intermediate filling material necessitates redoing the procedure.)
- Pulp death, which may lead to apical abscessation.
- Pulpitis, which causes pain and may be difficult to detect because our patients cannot talk!
- Internal resorption of the pulp chamber or root canal.

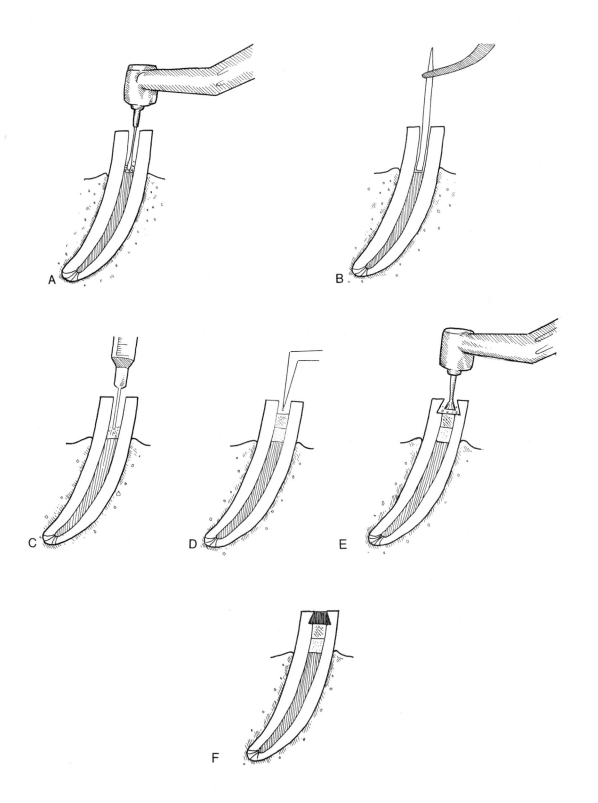

APEXIFICATION/ APEXOGENESIS/HARD TISSUE FORMATION

General Comments

- Apexification is the process of stimulating the formation of a closed apex when a necrotic pulp is present in a young permanent tooth.
- Apexogenesis is the stimulation of root end closure in traumatized young permanent teeth with vital pulp.
- The calcium hydroxide paste can be removed and replaced during the healing period if there is no radiographic evidence of hard tissue formation.
- Hard tissue formation is usually seen in 3 to 6 months.
- Length of time to apexification has not been documented in dogs but can take up to 18 months in humans.[2]
- The prognosis is guarded in immature animals because of the fragility of the thin tooth wall that is subject to fracture with minimal trauma.

Indications

- Fractured tooth crowns with severely traumatized or necrotic pulp in animals with a weak apical seal (younger than 18 months).
- Root perforations caused by overinstrumentation during endodontic therapy.

Contraindications

- Mature teeth with solid apex will not need apexification; conventional endodontic therapy will usually be successful.
- Noncompliance of client to return for follow-up radiographs and completion of root canal.

Objective

- To induce closure of the apical third of the root canal or formation of a calcified barrier at the apex to allow for future obturation of the canal.

Materials

- Calcium hydroxide paste (Pulpdent Paste, Hypo-Cal).
- Lentulo spiral filler.
- Endodontic files and stops.
- Sterile water or saline.
- Sterile paper points.
- Needle and endodontic syringe.
- Sterile cotton pellets.
- Fast-setting cement base (Dycal, Life, IRM).
- Restorative material of choice.

Technique

Step 1—A radiograph is taken to examine root length and apical closure or lucency.

Step 2—Access to the pulp chamber is made as per standard endodontic treatment (see page 218).

Step 3—A small file is placed into the canal to the approximate apical limit (A), and the tooth is radiographed again to determine a working length of the files 2 mm short of the apex to prevent injury to the apical tissues.

Step 4—The root canal is filed and shaped in a standard manner (B), described (see nonsurgical root canal, page 220), using only sterile water or saline for irrigation.

Step 5—The canal is dried using the blunt end of sterile paper points (C) to avoid perforation into the apex.

Step 6—The canal is filled with calcium hydroxide paste by using a spiral filler with a stop at the working length (D) or a sterile needle with an endodontic syringe.

Step 7—The calcium hydroxide paste is forced into the apex by placing a cotton pellet over the paste and using a blunt plugger to condense it apically (E). The cotton pellet is removed with an endodontic file or broach.

Step 8—The calcium hydroxide paste is removed 3 mm from the access area (F), and a fast-setting cement base is placed over the paste.

Step 9—A restoration is placed according to standard techniques.

Postoperative Care

- Follow-up radiographs are taken every 3 months to evaluate apical closure or root healing.

- When the desired hard tissue formation or apical closure is seen, the calcium hydroxide paste is removed and the canal is flushed with sodium hypochlorite and dried. Obturation can be completed using a technique to fill a larger canal adequately (chloropercha, inverted cone, or thermoplasticized gutta percha techniques).

Complications

- Because the restoration may need to be replaced, be careful to use restorative material that can be removed with the least damage to the tooth.
- Chronic abscess formation or drainage due to the thin wall of the tooth.
- Penetration of the seal obtained when refilling the canal.

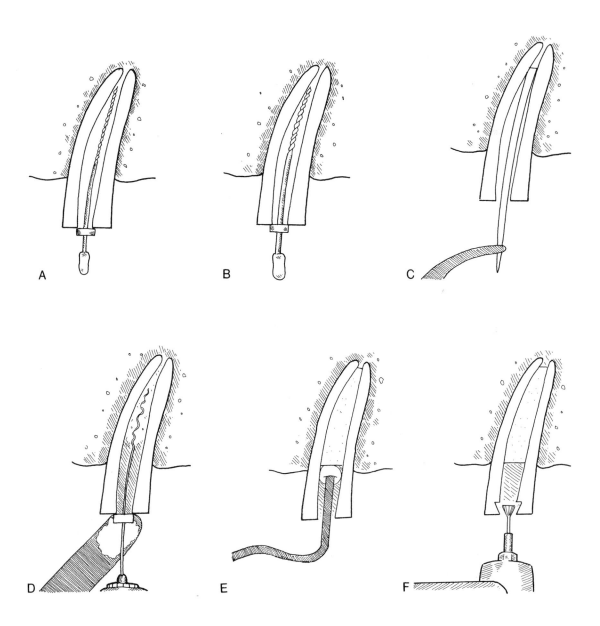

NONSURGICAL ROOT CANAL

General Comments

- When the tooth pulp has been traumatized, the pathogenesis culminates in apical root end resorption and abscess formation in the surrounding osseous tissue.[4, 5]
- Patients requiring root canal therapy may present with a variety of signs.
- They may be asymptomatic.[6]
- They may show signs such as fever, localized facial edema, a draining tract out of the skin or orally, reduced biting pressure (some trainers report that attack dogs bite and release as they bite—"typewriting"), and reluctance to eat (or pick up the food; they start to chew and then drop the food).

Indications

- Fractured crown with pulp exposure (A and B).
- Worn tooth with pulp exposure (C).
- Deep carious lesion with pulp exposure (D).
- Discolored tooth with pulp death (E).
- Reimplantation of avulsed/luxated tooth.

Contraindications

- Fractured primary teeth.
- Teeth with an incomplete apex.
- In adult teeth of young animals when the pulp chamber is large and the dentinal layer is thin.
- Fractured crown with vertical root fracture.
- Tooth with internal resorption creating a thin wall.
- Old animals with inaccessible or sclerosed root canals.
- Severe apical changes involving more than one third of the root.
- Systemic disease such as heart disease, diseases that slow healing such as diabetes, and terminal cancer.

Objective

- To remove diseased or necrotic pulp tissue and achieve a hermetic seal at the apex to preserve a tooth.
- Root canal therapy consists of three basic parts: (1) accessing the pulp canal; (2) cleaning and shaping the canal; and (3) obturation (filling) of the canal. Each of these parts will be covered as a general procedure. Following will be guidelines to adapt these general principles to individual tooth types.

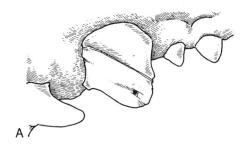

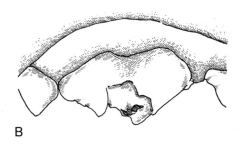

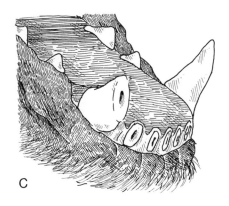

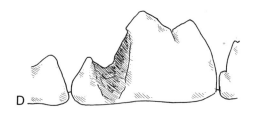

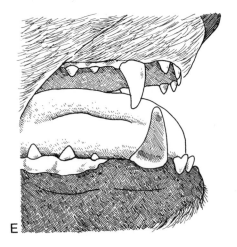

Coronal Access to the Pulp Chamber

General Comment

- The coronal access is the first step to root canal therapy. The access may already be present in the case of a fractured tooth, or it may need to be made.

Objective

- To obtain straight-line access to the apical (toward the apex) third of the root canal in order to allow for free instrumentation of the canal, preservation of tooth structure, and at the same time shaping the access to the width of the pulp chamber so the coronal walls do not deflect the instruments during preparation.

Materials

- No. 2 or 4 round bur, no. 330 pear bur, or no. 701 or 701L crosscut tapered and fissure bur for high- or slow-speed handpiece.
- Intraoral x-ray film.

Technique

Step 1—A preoperative radiograph is taken to identify landmarks and to evaluate canal size and position.

Step 2—Evaluate the tooth clinically to determine root angulation, cusp position, and surface anatomy to guide position and angulation of the access preparation. (Access to specific teeth is outlined later in this chapter under specific tooth type.)

Step 3—The oral cavity is disinfected with 0.2% chlorhexidine solution.

Step 4—Using the desired bur, a hole is drilled through the enamel layer with the drill positioned perpendicular to the tooth surface (A). (This step is eliminated if the fracture site allows straight-line access to the pulp.)

Step 5—The drill is repositioned to align vertically with the canal, and the access cavity is continued to be cut (B).

Step 6—The access cavity is deepened until the pulp canal is entered (C). (When using a high-speed handpiece, a change in resistance and a higher-pitch drilling noise is noted when the pulp canal is reached.)

Step 7—The access can be enlarged using a no. 701L bur and shaped to expose the entire width of the pulp chamber to accommodate the endodontic files by using a no. 701L bur without ledging (D).

Complications

- Removal of too much dentin at the cervical margin will weaken tooth structure and may lead to fracture of the tooth (E).
- Incorrect alignment of the drill with the root canal will cause perforation of the root or cervical area (F).
- Inability to achieve pulp exposure (palatal root of upper carnassial tooth).
- Ledge formation leading to excessive stress or bending of files during filing (G).

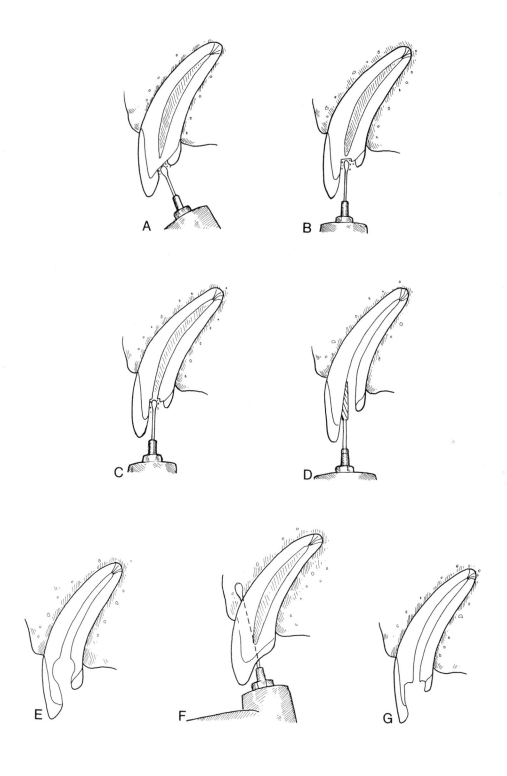

Cleaning and Shaping the Canal

Objective

- To debride the root canal by removing all pulp tissue and to shape it for obturation by the use of endodontic files, and to disinfect the canal by the use of disinfectant flushing solutions.

Materials

- Endodontic files/reamers with rubber endodontic stops (45-mm K-files* are minimum size for canine teeth).
- Broaches.
- Intraoral x-ray film.
- Syringes with blunt-end 27-gauge irrigation needles.
- Hydrogen peroxide.
- Sodium hypochlorite solution (dilutions range from practitioner to practitioner by individual preference, from 1 part sodium hypochlorite to 1 part water to a ratio of 1:3).
- EDTA preparation (R-C Prep†).
- Paper points.
- Ruler/measuring device/endodontic ring.
- Dressing forceps.
- Gates Glidden reamers.

Technique

Step 1—Removal of pulp tissue. Vital pulp tissue is removed from the canal by inserting the largest broach that will fit loosely in the apical third of the canal, twisting past 360°, and pulling it out with attached pulp tissue (A).

- This step can be repeated several times with a clean broach.
- In large canals, two or three broaches can be placed and rotated simultaneously to ensnare the pulp tissue.
- While treating the same patient, pulp material may be removed from the broach by

*Brasseler, Savannah, Georgia 31419
†Premier, Norristown, PA 19404

passing it through a rubber glove or rubber dam. Broaches are intended to be disposable and appropriately discarded as a "sharp" after use.

Step 2—Length determination. A small-diameter endodontic file (usually size 10, but 06 and 08 sizes are available) with a preplaced endodontic stop is inserted into the root canal 2 mm short of the estimated canal length, as determined from a preoperative radiograph (B).

Step 3—A radiograph is taken to verify the file depth (how far the file has penetrated) and the working length (how far the file should penetrate). The ideal working length is 1 mm short of the apex. The file may be inserted further and additional radiographs may be taken until the working length is achieved. Once the working length is achieved, the endodontic stop is moved until it contacts the crown with the file at the appropriate position, and the length is noted and recorded. To avoid confusion as to the measurement, the stop should be perpendicular to the file, not at an angle.

- Subsequent files are fitted with endodontic stops at the predetermined file length (C). If the file is not close to the desired position, it is adjusted and a repeat radiograph is taken until the correct position is achieved.

Step 4—Filing. The canal is cleaned and shaped using the files in an appropriate manner (push-pull only for Hedström files (D) and either push-pull or push-rotate clockwise 90° and pull for reamers and K-files (E)). The files are used in sequential order, with each file inserted to the predetermined length and drawn against the sides of the canal in all directions until it moves freely.

Substep 4—An EDTA preparation can be used to help soften the dentin and lubricate the files by placing a small amount in the canal with a curved-tip syringe or by placing a small amount on an endodontic ring and running the tips of the files through it before entering the canal. When using these preparations, make sure all the chemical is removed from the canal in the filing/irrigating process.[7]

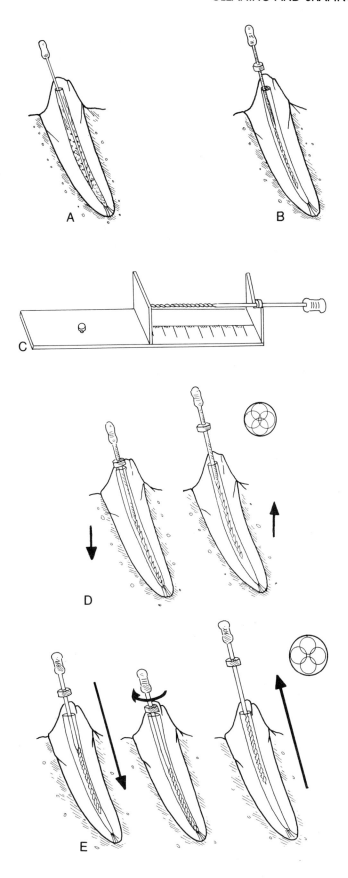

Technique *(Continued)*

Step 5—Irrigation. The canal is irrigated between file sizes using a syringe with a blunt tipped needle *(A)*. The needle is inserted into the canal so it does not bind. Irrigating solutions used are sodium hypochlorite and hydrogen peroxide.

Step 6—Recapitulation. Periodically a smaller file should be used to remove any dentinal filings packed into the apical portion of the canal by larger files *(B)*.

Step 7—Shaping. The canal is shaped by using either standard (rigid-core technique) or step-back (tapered, flared, serial, telescoping, or funneling) technique.

Substep 1—Standard technique *(C)*. (Ideal for straight, narrow canals.) To prepare a canal that has the same size, shape, and taper as a standardized instrument. Each size file is placed to the working limit as the canal is cleaned and shaped *(D, E, and F)*. Cleaning and shaping continue until clean white dentinal filings are seen on two to three successive file sizes *(G)*, and the next-size file binds before reaching the working length *(H)*.

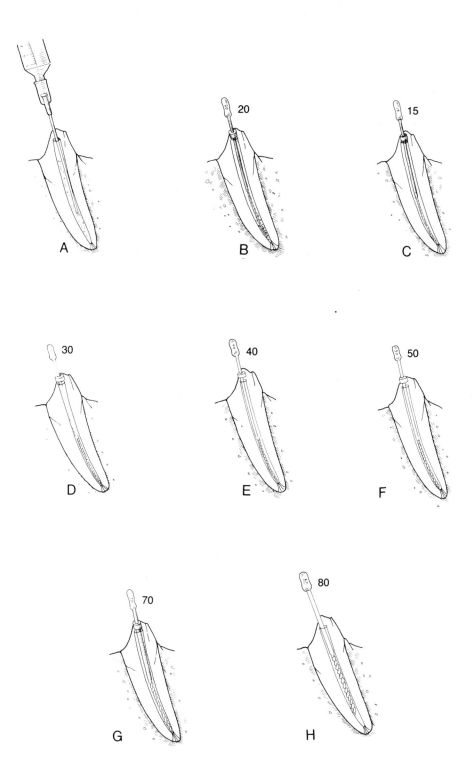

Technique *(Continued)*

Substep 1 (alternate)—Step-back technique *(A to D)*. Filing is started in the standard manner until the first file that binds at the apical limit is reached. Filing is continued in the standard manner for one or two more increases in file size. Next, the taper or funnel shape is created by placing the subsequent file sizes 1 to 1.5 mm short of the previous file length. For curved canals or large-diameter canals, a sweeping motion is made with the file along one side of the canal at a time to create a smooth, tapered canal.

Substep 2 (alternate)—Between each step-back file and the last full-length file, a smaller file is used to clean accumulated debris from the terminal portion of the canal. This is called recapitulating.

Substep 3 (alternate)—Between each file size, the root canal is irrigated with sodium hypochlorite. A Gates Glidden reamer can be used to complete the coronal taper *(E)*.

Step 8—Disinfection. The canal is irrigated with sodium hypochlorite.

Step 9—Drying. The canal is dried by successively inserting paper points into the canal with dressing forceps *(F)*. The canal is dry when a paper point remains dry after insertion into the canal. When wet, the paper point has a grayish appearance, as compared to the white of a dry paper point.

Postoperative Care

- The canal is obturated with a root canal sealer and filling material of choice.

Complications

- Perforation of the root apex with a file. This should be followed radiographically and may need retrograde filling (see page 254).
- Breaking a file in the canal. If the canal is clean, one option is obturation with paste, leaving the broken file in place. If this is not possible, a retrograde filling is indicated.
- No general rule says how long an endodontic file may be used. To prevent breaking files in the pulp chamber, the safest practice would be to dispose of the file after every use. However, this is seldom economically feasible. Without doubt, files should be discarded when acute bends, deformation, or reverse twists are noted. Endodontic files should be treated as "sharps" and disposed of according to local regulations.
- Incomplete filing leaving remnants of pulp tissue or contaminated dentin leads to failure with apical abscess formation and will require a repeat root canal procedure or a retrograde filling (see page 254).
- Inadequate shaping leads to difficult or incomplete obturation. The canal is reshaped with a Gates Glidden reamer or larger files.

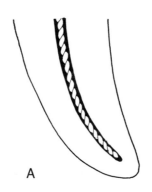

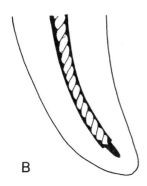

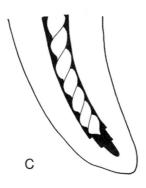

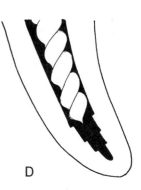

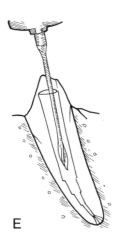

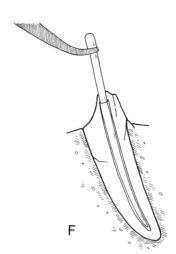

Treatment of Persistent Pulp Hemorrhage

General Comments

- The root canal must be completely dry before obturation for the procedure to be successful.
- Persistent hemorrhage may occur during a root canal on teeth with fresh fractures.
- If hemorrhage does not stop with flushing, try blotting or use of epinephrine on a paper point inserted into the canal.
- An alternative method is to mummify the bleeding vessels with a formaldehye preparation; the final filling is completed at a second visit.

Indication

- Persistent hemorrhage after complete filing of a canal in a freshly fractured tooth.

Contraindications

- Open apex.
- Fractured root (class B fracture).

Objective

- To treat persistent apical hemorrhage during root canal therapy by fixing residual apical vessels with the use of formocresol.

Materials

- Formocresol.
- Cotton pellet or paper point.
- Temporary cavity material (Cavit*).
- Sterile saline.
- Sterile paper points.

Technique

Step 1—The canal is irrigated with sterile saline (A) and is dried with sterile paper points (B).

Step 2—A paper point or small cotton pellet is dipped in the formocresol solution, blotted dry, and placed into the canal with a dressing forceps (C). (The paper point can be cut short to fit entirely into the canal.)

Step 3—The access opening is sealed with a temporary cavity filler (D).

Postoperative Care

- The animal is reanesthetized in 2 to 3 weeks. The temporary filling material is removed with a bur and the paper point or cotton pellet is removed with a broach or small file. The canal can now be obturated as desired.

Complication

- Failure of the client to return when requested, with subsequent irritation of apical tissues by formocresol.

---

*Premier, Norristown, PA 19404

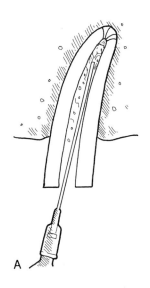

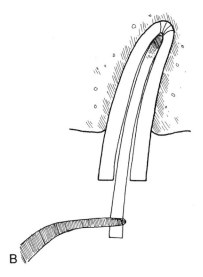

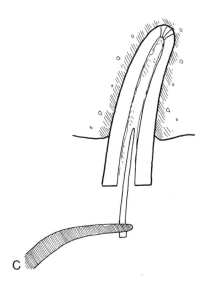

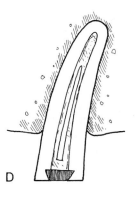

A

B

C

D

Obturation

General Comment

- Obturation is filling of the prepared root canal to obtain an apical seal.

Contraindications

- Persistent hemorrhage (see p. 226).
- Open apex (see surgical root canal).

Objective

- To fill the entire root canal system and any accessory canals completely and densely with nonirritating inert material resulting in a fluid-tight seal.

Materials

- All materials may not be needed, depending upon the method used.
- Root canal sealer (zinc oxide-eugenol product).
- Gutta percha points.
- Root canal pluggers or condenser.
- Root canal spreaders.
- Dressing forceps.
- Source of flame.
- Glass slab
- Mixing spatula.
- Spiral fillers.
- Files.
- Chloroform.
- Eucalyptus.
- Alcohol in dappen dish.
- Heated gutta percha applicator.
- Electrically heated plugger.
- Zinc oxide-eugenol applicator.

Obturating Techniques
Application of Sealer

- The root canal sealer is a zinc oxide-eugenol-based preparation that is placed into the canal first in any filling technique. It is mixed to a thick consistency and is placed into the canal using one of the following methods:

  1. A spiral filler with a reduction gear on a slow-speed handpiece is loaded with the paste and inserted into the canal to depth; it is activated and moved in and out to distribute the paste along the canal walls.

  2. Using a file two to three sizes smaller than the last file to reach the apical limit, the file is placed into the sealer paste, is inserted into the canal to the apical limit, is rotated counterclockwise to coat the walls, and is withdrawn (A). Loading the file and inserting are continued until the walls and the apex are coated.

  3. The sealer paste can be injected into the canal using pressure with a syringe and blunt-end needle (B).

  4. The sealer paste can be placed on the master gutta percha cone after sizing and inserted into the canal with the cone.

Advantages

- Improved apical seal.
- Bacteriostatic.
- Radiopaque.

Disadvantages

- Some toxicity to tissues if forced periapically.
- Soluble when exposed to oral or tissue fluids; therefore, if used as the only obturant, may "wash out" and fail.

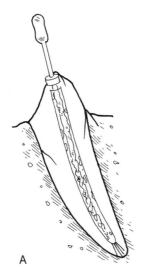

A

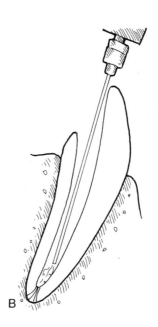

B

Injection or Spiral Filling

- A mixture of zinc oxide powder and eugenol liquid (zinc oxide eugenol [ZOE]) is spatulated on a glass slab until smooth and the consistency is such that a thread of material is formed when the spatula is elevated off the slab 1 to 2 cm *(A)*.

Spiral Filling Technique

Substep 1—A spiral filler is placed in a reduction gear contra-angle on the slow-speed handpiece. Spiral fillers come in several sizes, and one is chosen that can be inserted to the apical limit of the canal without binding.

Substep 2—The tip of the spiral filler is loaded with the ZOE mixture *(B)*, and the spiral filler is placed into the canal to the apex.

Substep 3—The rotary movement is then activated, and the spiral filler is carefully moved back and forth in the canal without completely withdrawing it to fill the canal with paste filler *(C)*. A spatula with additional paste on the tip is held near the access opening to place paste filler continuously into larger canals.

Substep 4—When the canal is full, paste will be extruded out around the access opening(s) as the filler is moved towards the apex *(D)*. The slow-speed handpiece with reduction gear must be set to rotate in a forward direction (clockwise) for proper filling.

Complication

- Binding and breaking the spiral filler in the canal if the spiral filler is too large in relation to the canal diameter.

Injection Technique

Substep 1—A 3-ml syringe is loaded with the zinc oxide-eugenol paste, and a blunt-end or notched-end needle is placed into the canal to the apical limit *(E)*. The needle is slowly withdrawn as the paste filler is injected into the canal.

Substep 2—Premade injection guns have cannules of premixed root canal filler (Pulp canal sealer,* Endoseal System,† Endoseal†) that can be used to inject the paste into the canal under pressure.

Advantages

- Faster fill technique.
- Fewer materials needed.

Disadvantages

- Potential for inadequate fill and air bubbles; accessory canals not filled.
- Without a denser filling material such as gutta percha, ZOE may be resorbed at the apex losing the fluid-tight seal.
- Shrinkage of zinc oxide-eugenol paste after setting, leading to microleakage if the paste is used as the only obturator.

---

*Kerr, Romulus, MI 48174
†Centrix, Milford, CT 06460

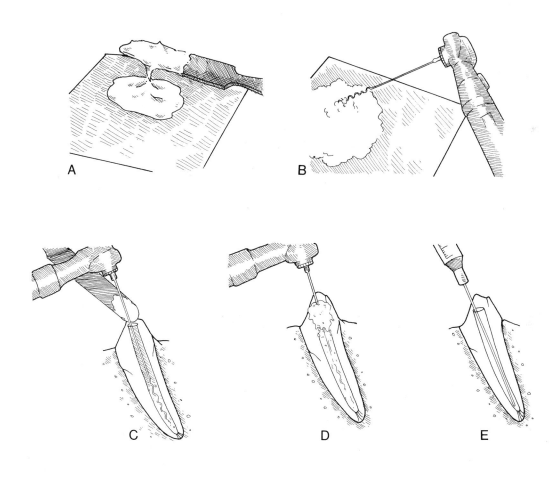

Application of Solid Filling Material

General Comments

- Many types of techniques have been developed to fill the root canal with solid filling material.
- Because of the variety of situations, each practitioner should have a variety of techniques available.
- A three-dimensional fill is desired.[8]

Single-Cone Technique

- A dry gutta percha or silver cone equal to the size of the last file used during instrumentation is placed into the canal to the apex. There should be a little resistance or "tugback" felt when removing it.
- A radiograph is taken with the point in place to check for position and fill (A and B). The entire canal should be filled. When the appropriate position is achieved, the gutta percha point can be marked at the coronal access by pinching with dressing forceps. If a stiffer gutta percha point is desired, the point may be soaked in alcohol prior to insertion.

- A root canal sealer is placed in the canal as a liner using a method described previously.
- The point is placed into the canal and pushed in with a plugger or condenser until the pinch mark is at the desired level (C).

Advantages

- Provides a dense filling material at the apex to provide a longer-term success rate.
- Can provide sufficient fill in smaller, shorter canals prepared with standard technique.

Disadvantages

- Inadequate procedure in larger, longer canals because only the apical 2 to 3 mm of canal is solidly filled.
- The single-cone technique has a greater amount of leakage than techniques condensing gutta percha.
- Difficult to force smaller gutta percha point (less than 30) to the apical limit. Alcohol use helps to stiffen the gutta percha.

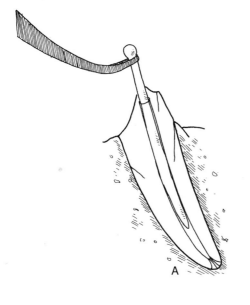

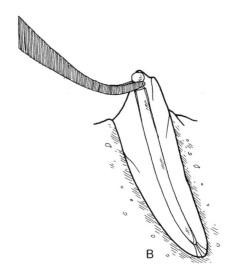

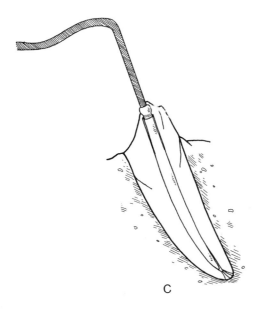

Cold Lateral Condensation

- The canal is shaped in a step-back technique creating a flare of the coronal limit of the canal.
- A root canal spreader is chosen that can be inserted to within 1 to 2 mm of the working length of the canal alongside the master cone *(A)*. Larger files or reamers can be used as spreaders in longer canals. The spreader must not be wider than the canal because it may cause excessive lateral force and breakage of the root.
- A standardized gutta percha point (master cone) is placed in the canal and checked for a snug fit 1 mm short of the apical limit of the canal *(B)*. Use a point the same size as or one size smaller than the last file used. The length of the point is marked by pinching the cone with dressing forceps at the level of the access hole.
- A root canal sealer is placed into the canal as previously described.
- The master cone is placed slowly into the canal to the predetermined length.
- A root canal spreader is inserted along the master cone to within 1 to 2 mm of the working length with apical pressure only *(C)*.
- The spreader is rotated on its axis clockwise and counterclockwise several times and is removed.

- An accessory gutta percha point slightly smaller than the spreader is immediately placed into the space created by the spreader.
- These two steps are repeated until it is impossible to insert an accessory cone further than 2 to 3 mm into the canal *(D)*.
- The excess gutta percha is removed with a heated instrument below the access opening *(E)*.
- A radiograph is taken to confirm a complete fill.

Advantages

- Provides more complete obturation of canal with inert filling material.
- Gutta percha is moved into apical stop during condensation to prevent overfill.

Disadvantages

- Takes more time.
- Need variety of gutta percha sizes and spreaders. Most spreaders used in human dentistry do not reach desired limit in longer canals.
- Vertical root fracture may occur if excessive lateral force is applied.

Complications

- Splitting of root by overinstrumentation.
- Inadequate fill of canal.

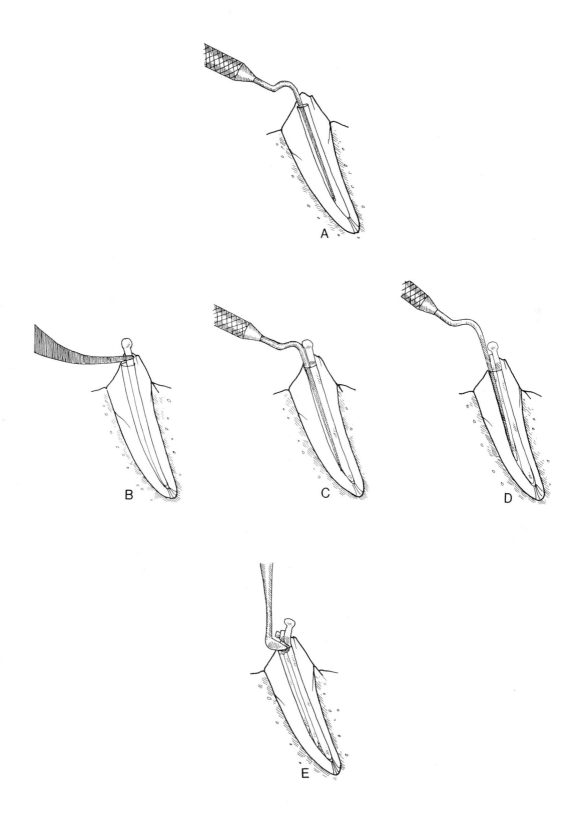

Warm Lateral Condensation

- The warm lateral condensation technique uses the same instruments as cold lateral condensation. In addition, a heated carrier is used to soften the gutta percha to allow further condensing of gutta percha against the canal walls.
- The canal is prepared and shaped in a step-back technique with coronal flare.
- A master cone is fitted, sealer is applied to the canal, and the master cone (A) and several accessory points are placed as in the cold lateral condensation technique.
- A carrier (spreader) is warmed in a flame (B) and is inserted into the gutta percha in the canal (C). It is rotated and moved up and down continuously to keep it from sticking to the gutta percha and dislodging it as the spreader is removed. (An electrically heated spreader, Touch and Heat,* simplifies this technique.)

---

*Analytic Technologies, Redman, WA 98052

- A cold lateral spreader is inserted into the space created and is removed (D).
- An accessory point is inserted and the process is repeated until the canal is full (E).
- The excess gutta percha is removed with a heated instrument below the coronal access opening (F).
- A radiograph is taken to confirm the fill.

Advantages

- A denser fill and elimination of irregularities (caused by accessory canals, lateral canals, or filing procedure) are achieved.
- The microleakage potential is reduced.

Disadvantages

- Time consuming.
- Accidental removal of gutta percha from canal with heated carrier. (This can be overcome by proper technique and experience.)

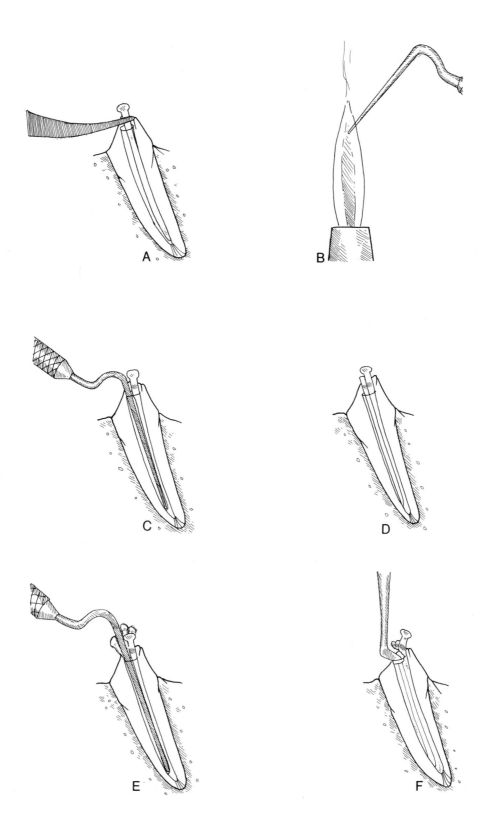

Vertical Condensation

- After placement of a single cone in the canal, a root canal plugger or condensor is used against the end of the point to push it apically.
- As a complete filling technique, a set of spreaders with depth markings is required and the canal is prepared in step-back technique *(A to C)*. (The spreaders should reach the desired length and be wide enough to cover as large an area of gutta percha as possible at the desired depth.)

Substep 1—A master cone is fitted, the canal is lined with sealer, and the master cone is seated *(D)* as described under the single-cone technique.

Substep 2—The coronal portion of the cone is removed with a hot instrument *(E)*.

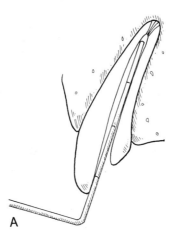

A

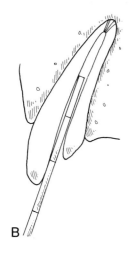

B

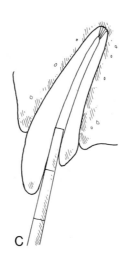

C

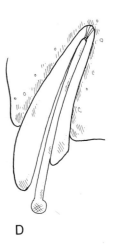

D

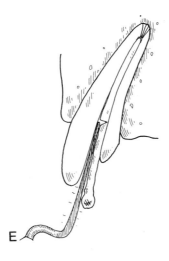

E

Vertical Condensation *(Continued)*

Substep 3—A heat carrier (spreader or plugger) is warmed in a flame, inserted into the coronal third of the gutta percha, and removed *(A)*. (Some gutta percha will be removed with the instrument).

Substep 4—A vertical plugger of the appropriate length and width is inserted, and the gutta percha is condensed apically *(B)*.

Substep 5—An additional piece of gutta percha 3 to 4 mm in length and matching the width of the canal is inserted into the canal *(C)*, and the process is repeated until the canal is full *(D)*.

- 4- to 5-mm increments of plasticized gutta percha can be inserted into the canal with a special device (see thermoplasticized gutta percha technique) and condensed apically with an appropriate-size plugger for the entire fill or in addition to a master cone.

Advantage

- Complete obturation of canal apex and accessory and lateral canals.

Disadvantages

- Time consuming.
- Requires variety of pluggers and spreaders and is more technically complicated.
- Greater chance of overfill.
- Available commercial spreaders are not sized for large canine teeth.

Lateral and Vertical Condensation

- The two previous techniques are used together to achieve complete fill of the canal.

Advantage

- Complete obturation of canal with gutta percha.

Disadvantage

- Time consuming.

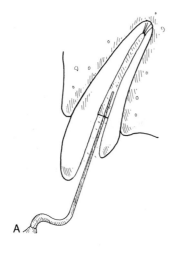

A

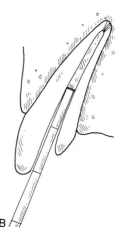

B

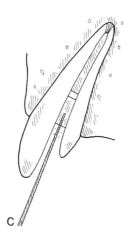

C

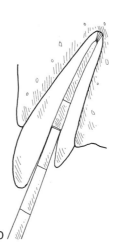

D

Chloropercha/Eucapercha Technique

- This technique uses chloroform or warm oil of eucalyptus as a solvent to soften gutta percha and allow its condensation into canal irregularities.
- Several large standardized gutta percha points are placed in the solvent to produce a thick paste similar in consistency to zinc oxide-eugenol. This paste is used as a sealer with a master cone and lateral condensation technique.

Advantage

- The softened gutta percha can be forced into fine, tortuous canals.

Disadvantages

- Chloroform is a reported carcinogen; however, this does not appear to be a problem in the amounts used.
- Gutta percha is less solvent in oil of eucalyptus.

Softened Gutta Percha Condensation (Chloroform Dip Technique)

- This technique is useful when the apex is open or the apical portion of the canal is irregular (A).
- A master cone is fitted that stops 2 to 4 mm short of the apex (B). A pinch mark is made with dressing forceps at the desired working length determined by previous radiographs.

- The apical 2 to 3 mm of the master cone is dipped in chloroform for 1 to 2 seconds (C).
- Wet the canal with irrigant (sodium hypochlorite or saline) to prevent sticking to the walls. The cone is inserted into the canal and is tamped apically with a plugger until it goes to the working length (D). (The cone can be removed, dipped in chloroform, and retamped until the working length is achieved; make sure it is reinserted in the same direction each time.) Confirm the fill with a radiograph. The cone can be 1 mm short of working length.
- The shaped cone is removed and is allowed to dry for several minutes.
- The apical third of the cone is coated with sealer and the cone is inserted into the canal to the set length (E).
- The canal is filled using lateral condensation; coat each accessory point with sealer prior to insertion (F).
- A radiograph is taken to confirm the fill.

Advantage

- Adequate apical seal obtainable in irregularly shaped canals.

Disadvantages

- Chloroform is reported to be a carcinogen.
- Shrinkage of the gutta percha as the chloroform evaporates may lead to microleakage.

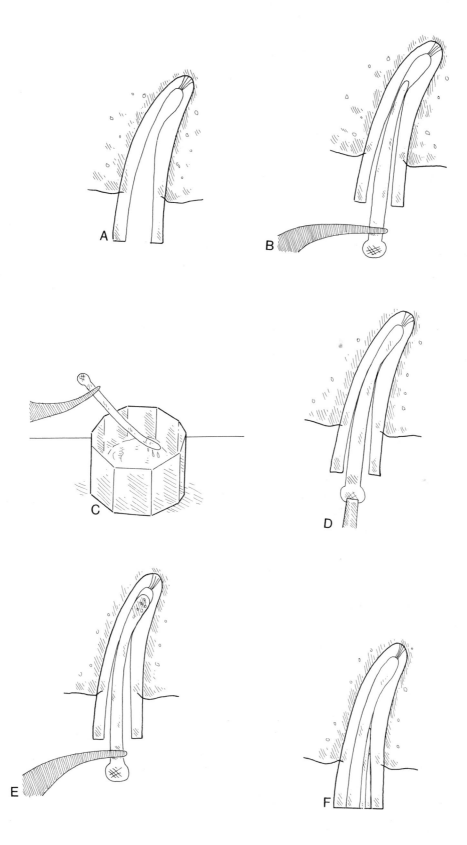

Custom Point Fill

- A custom point fill is used in canals that are larger than the largest standardized gutta percha available.
- Several large cones are softened in a flame *(A)*.
- The softened points are rolled to a cone shape between two glass slabs *(B)*.
- When the point is the approximate size of the canal, it is cooled in water and trial fitted *(C* and *D)*. The process is repeated until the cone fits 1 to 2 mm from the apex.
- The custom cone is used as the master cone, and warm or cold lateral condensation techniques are used to fill the canal completely.

Advantage

- Allows obturation of large canals.

Disadvantages

- Time consuming rolling gutta percha to proper size.
- Gutta percha must be softened sufficiently to minimize seams or apical voids. It is difficult to remove them all with this technique.

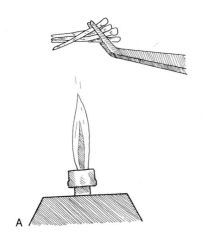

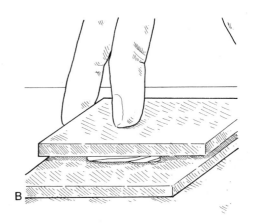

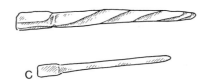

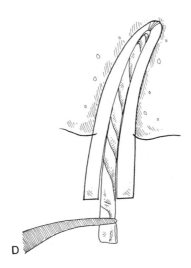

Thermomechanical Condensation (McSpadden Method)

- A McSpadden compactor, which looks like a Hedström file but with reverse flutes, is used in a slow-speed handpiece and is inserted alongside a master gutta percha cone placed 1 to 2 mm short of the apex. The compactor chops up the gutta percha, thus plasticizing it and forcing it apically and laterally.
- A master cone is fitted in the canal, which has been prepared in a step-back technique, 1.5 mm short of the apex (A).
- The McSpadden compactor selected is the same size as the last file that came 1 to 1.5 mm from the apex. The working length is marked on the compactor.
- The master cone is coated with sealer and is inserted into the canal.
- The compactor is inserted alongside the cone until resistance is felt and is rotated at maximum speed (B).
- After 1 second the compactor is advanced apically to the predetermined length and is slowly withdrawn while rotating.
- Accessory points can be dipped in sealer and placed alongside the master cone and a larger compactor used until the canal is full (C).
- A radiograph is taken to confirm the fill.

Advantage

- Rapid condensation technique forcing softened gutta percha into canal irregularities.

Disadvantages

- Breakage of compactor tip in canal.
- Heat generation.
- Compactor is not long enough for use in canine teeth.

Broken-Instrument Technique

- If an instrument tip is broken off inside the canal and cannot be retrieved, and an apical seal is believed to be achieved, it can be left in place and a filling technique used to fill around it if the canal has been completely cleaned (D).
- The "instrument misadventure" must be noted in the chart.
- The client must be informed and follow-up radiographs taken at 6 months or earlier if the condition is not resolving normally.

Advantage

- Do not have to remove a broken file tip.

Disadvantages

- If the canal is not adequately prepared, the procedure can lead to failure.
- If a larger file tip is broken, it may not allow fill around it, necessitating apicoectomy with retrograde filling.

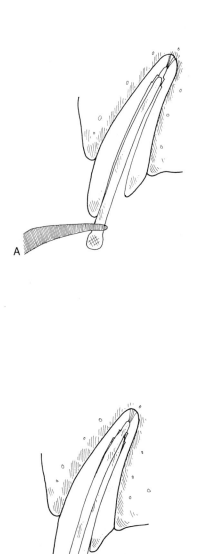

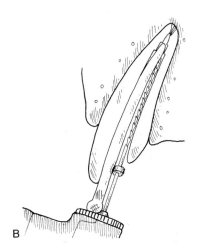

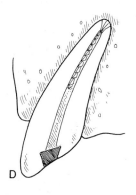

Inverted Cone

- Some canals may have a wider apical portion that makes it difficult to fill with standard-size cones (feline canine teeth).
- Root canal sealer is placed as previously described.
- Place a gutta percha cone with the rounded end toward the apex *(A)*.
- Using lateral and/or vertical condensation techniques, the remaining canal is filled with accessory gutta percha points *(B)*.

Advantage

- Allows fill of atypical root canals using standard gutta percha and root canal sealer.

Disadvantage

- Time consuming.

Orthograde Amalgam

- A technique that can be used when trying to fill a large open canal, as in an immature canine tooth, to provide greater strength for future restorations.[9]
- Amalgam is mixed and placed into the canal with an amalgam carrier *(C)*.
- The amalgam is condensed vertically with custom-made amalgam condensors *(D)*. (Condensors must be sized to reach the length and width of the canal.)
- These two steps are repeated until the canal is full.

Advantage

- Makes a stronger tooth when dentinal development is minimal.

Disadvantages

- Amalgam can be extended beyond apex if apical development is incomplete.
- Will discolor tooth.
- Amalgam may expand and fracture tooth.
- Need adequate-length condensing instruments for complete fill.

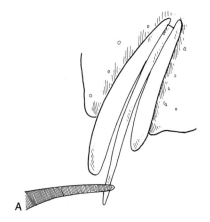

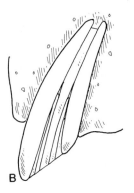

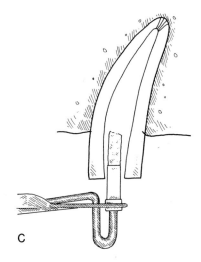

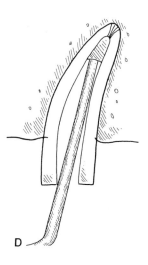

Thermoplasticized Gutta Percha

- A special device (Ultra Fil,* Obtura II†) is used to heat gutta percha that is injected into the canal with a pressurized syringe. The canal must be filed to a size 60 or 70 to allow the needle to be inserted near the apex.
- Root canal sealer is placed in the canal with a file or spiral filler.
- A cannule of gutta percha is heated and loaded into the syringe.
- The needle (22-gauge) of the cannule is placed into the canal to within 1 mm of the apex.
- Melted gutta percha is slowly injected into the canal as the needle is withdrawn *(A)*.
- In longer canals a few millimeters of gutta percha are placed in the canal *(B)*. After cooling for 20 to 30 seconds, a root canal plugger is used to push the gutta percha apically *(C)*.
- This step is repeated until the canal is full *(D)*.
- Final condensation is done with a root canal plugger to ensure an apical seal *(E)*.
- Excess gutta percha is removed from the access opening with a heated instrument *(F)*.

Advantages

- Rapid filling method in larger canals.
- Can fill accessory or lateral canals.

Disadvantages

- Not applicable in small canals because the cannule needle is equivalent to a size-60 file.
- Needle of cannule is not long enough for most canine teeth, so must be combined with the vertical condensation technique to fill long teeth completely.

---

*Analytic Technologies, Redman, WA 98052
†Texceed Corp, Costa Mesa, CA 92626-4532

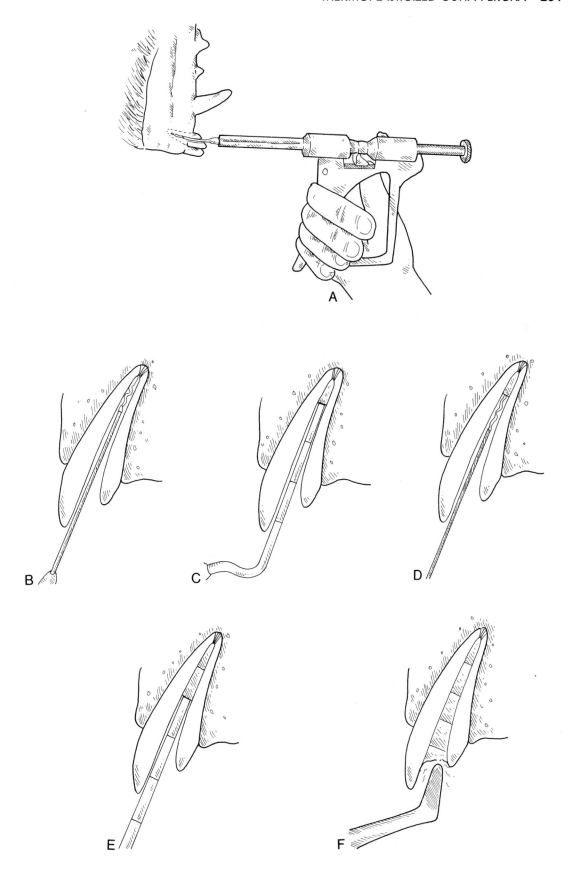

A

B

C

D

E

F

Obturation with Thermafil*

General Comments

- The Thermafil system uses a stainles steel carrier to which a rubber stopper and thermally plasticized gutta percha have been applied.
- After standard endodontic preparation, the gutta percha on the carrier is warmed and the carrier is inserted into the treated canal.
- The carrier is either broken off in the canal or is slowly withdrawn while the access to the canal is sealed with the rubber stopper, keeping the gutta percha from being withdrawn.
- Thermafil is available either in specific carrier sizes or in an assortment of sizes.
- The carrier sizes are from standard file size 20 to 140.

Advantages

- Thermafil allows filling of narrow, medium-length canals where using standard gutta percha techniques may be difficult.
- Thermafil provides a good apical seal.
- Although relatively rare in the dog and cat, if lateral canal or apical canals are present, Thermafil provides introduction of gutta percha into these secondary canals.

Disadvantages

- The carriers are manufactured only in 25-mm lengths; therefore, canals longer than 25 mm cannot be treated.
- The carriers are expensive, and using the system is moderately technique sensitive.

Technique

- Although several variations exist, two basic techniques are used with Thermafil.

Method 1—Break-off Technique

Step 1—A standard parallel endodontic filing technique is used.

---

*Tulsa Dental Products, Tulsa, OK 74136

- The canal length is measured and the length and file size are recorded.

Step 2—A light coating of zinc oxide and eugenol is placed in the canal.

Step 3—A carrier, the same size as the last file used, is selected.

- With a tapered fissure bur (for example, a no. 701) a notch is placed through the gutta percha and into the metal carrier.
- Difficulty arises in notching the carrier enough to break when the carrier is inserted into the canal, but not to weaken to the point that the carrier breaks prior to insertion into the full length of the canal.

Step 4–After the notch is cut, the carrier is warmed with a flame.

- The gutta percha should be softened, but not burned.

Step 5—Once the gutta percha is soft, the carrier is gently but firmly inserted into the root canal length.

- The carrier is inserted to the previously measured depth of the canal.
- A radiograph is taken to verify that the carrier is at the apex.

Step 6—Once you are satisfied with the location, the carrier is twisted counterclockwise.

- The carrier fractures, and the handle and shaft portion of the Thermafil carrier are removed.
- A final radiograph is taken.

Complications

- If the apex is not reached, the fractured end of the carrier may be pushed further in with an endodontic plugger or by using the previously discarded carrier handle. An alternative to forcing the carrier further into the canal would be to retrieve the carrier. Without (and even with) carrier-recovering instruments, this may be difficult.

- Carrier removal at a future date may be difficult. Initial caution in measuring the root canal length and accurate notching of the carrier will prevent the metal portion of the canal from extending into the pulp chamber.
- Should the cut portion of the carrier protrude from the pulp chamber, the excess portion should be cut off with a bur in a high-speed handpiece.

Method 2—Carrier Removal

Step 1—The canal is conventionally filed; the length and size of the last file used is recorded.

Step 2—A light coating of zinc oxide and eugenol is placed in the canal.

Step 3—A carrier the same size as the last file used is selected.

- The Thermafil carrier is not notched with this technique.

Step 4—The Thermafil gutta percha is warmed with a flame.

Step 5—The carrier is inserted into the canal; the rubber stopper on the Thermafil carrier is pushed down the carrier with cotton pliers to cover the access site.

Step 6—The carrier is withdrawn from the canal while the cotton pliers hold the rubber stopper over the access hole to prevent gutta percha from escaping from the canal.

- This forces the gutta percha to fill the void caused by the removal of the carrier.

Step 7—The gutta percha is further condensed with a plugger.

- A spreader and accessory points may be used to fill the canal if necessary.
- A radiograph is taken to ensure that an apical seal has been formed.

Complications

- Withdrawal of gutta percha when carrier is removed.
- Voids in gutta percha.

Restoration of Coronal Access

- The access site is restored using a technique discussed in Chapter 8.

Postoperative Care

- Soft food for 48 hours.
- Follow-up radiographs are recommended at 6 months, 1 year, 2 years, and 5 years.
- Antibiotics should be prescribed for 1 week.
- Minimize aggressive chewing activity.

Complications of Nonsurgical Endodontics

- The primary complication of a nonsurgical endodontic procedure is failure of the procedure related to operator failure to perform the procedure properly.
- The tooth may be asymptomatic and therefore radiology is important in diagnosis of a failed treatment. The radiograph may demonstrate that the lesion has remained the same, has enlarged, or has only diminished in size slightly, and total healing has not occurred.
- Common causes of procedure failure are incomplete obturation and inadequate apical seal, pathologic or iatrogenic root perforation, and broken instruments in the canal.
- Other nonoperator causes of failure are external root resorption, coexistent periodontal-periapical lesions, or endodontic disease in adjacent teeth.

SURGICAL ENDODONTICS (Apicoectomy with Retrograde Filling)

General Comments

- The teeth most commonly requiring apicoectomy are the upper and lower carnassial teeth and upper and lower canines.
- A surgical root canal can only be successful if the basic tenets of canal cleaning and shaping have been accomplished.
- All roots should be treated either nonsurgically or surgically in multirooted teeth.
- The palatal root of the upper fourth premolar cannot be accessed. It can be resected and extracted if necessary to save the tooth. If adequately filled it can be left.
- Having a skull for reference of anatomic features and comparison with preoperative radiographs can help to locate the root apices.

Indications

- Teeth with an open apex and periapical infection that do not respond to conventional treatment.
- Perforation of apex with file during standard preparation that leads to clinical or radiographic failure.
- Broken file tip wedged in canal allowing inadequate preparation and filling that leads to clinical or radiographic failure.
- Failure of standard root canal procedure resulting in clinical or radiographic failure (inadequate obturation, overfill, root perforation, etc.). May need to redo standard root canal first if canal is markedly underfilled.
- Coronal approach impossible (narrow canals, aberrant canal formation, pulp stones, or calcified canal).
- Horizontal fracture of root tip.

Contraindications

- Health status of patient.
- Difficult access (palatal root of maxillary fourth premolar).

Objective

- To ensure a seal of the root canal system at the apex by exposing the apical area and sealing the canal with a retrograde filling.

Materials

- Instruments and materials for standard endodontic preparation.
- No. 10 or 15 scalpel blade with handle.
- Periosteal elevator.
- Flap retractors.
- No. 701, 2, 4, 33½, or 34 bur.
- Small bone rongeurs.
- Dental excavator.
- Bone curette.
- Dressing forceps.
- Cotton pellets, sterile gauze squares, hemostatic agent.
- Sterile saline.
- Retrograde amalgam carrier if amalgam technique is used.
- Amalgam plugger and carver if amalgam technique is used.
- Nonzinc amalgam if amalgam technique is used.
- Amalgamator if amalgam technique is used.
- Amalgam well if amalgam technique is used.
- IRM or EBA Cement.*
- 4-0 absorbable suture material with swagged-on taper needle.
- Needle holders, scissors, thumb forceps.

---

*Getz, Elk Grove Village, IL 60007

Technique

Step 1—Conventional root canal therapy is performed first. (Retreatment and refilling of the canal may be first treatment option if failure is due to inadequate obturation, etc.)

Step 2—The mouth is disinfected with 0.2% chlorhexidine, and aseptic technique is followed.

Step 3—The tooth apex is located by feeling the bulge of the root (jugum) under the alveolar mucosa and is exposed by incising the soft tissue over the apex with a semilunar incision. The incision is made through the periosteum. (The area can be infiltrated with lidocaine with epinephrine to enhance hemostasis.)

Substep 1—A preoperative radiograph is taken to locate the apex with anatomic references.

Access Sites

- Access to the maxillary canine tooth (*a*) is made with an incision starting mesial to the root in the alveolar mucosa and extended distally to the level of the distal root of the second premolar with the depth of the curve at the distal third of the root (*A*).
- Access to the maxillary fourth premolar (*b*) is made with a semilunar incision through the alveolar mucosa starting at the level of the third premolar and extending distal to the first molar with the depth of the curve at the distal third of the root. (Do not disturb the infraorbital nerve exiting above the mesial buccal root.)
- Access is made to the first mandibular molar either intraorally, with a semilunar incision starting at the level of the fourth premolar and continuing distal to the second molar with the depth of the curve at the distal third of the root (*B*), or through a ventral approach to the ramus of the mandible.

- Access to the mandibular canine teeth is made through a ventral approach to the mandible (*C*).

The maxillary canine tooth is used as an example for a surgical root canal.

Substep 2—An incision is made through the alveolar mucosa and periosteum over the tooth to be treated (*D*).

Step 4—The gingiva and periosteum are reflected off the bone (*E*). The bulge over the root is palpated, and the apical area is determined by comparing with file length used in preparation of canal to locate the apex. Retractors are placed to keep the soft tissue out of the way.

Step 5—The bone is drilled away in a small circle encompassing the apex to expose the distal 4 mm of the root with a high-speed no. 2, no. 4 round, or no. 330 pear bur with sterile saline irrigation (*F*). If a draining fistula is present, the bone will be soft and can be removed wih a rongeur or bone curette.

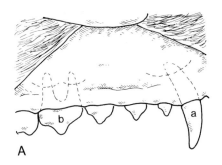

A

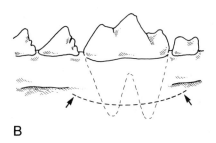

B

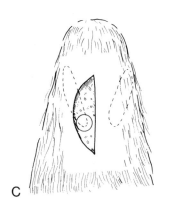

C

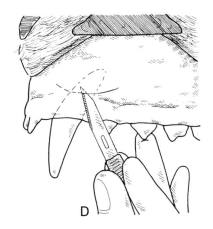

D

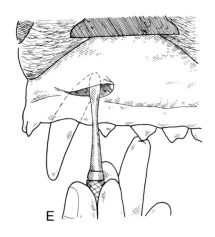

E

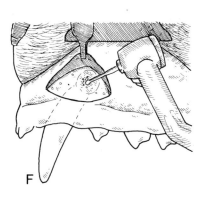

F

Access Sites (Continued)

Step 6—The soft tissue in the apical area is curetted away from the bone with a surgical excavator or sharp curette (A).

Step 7—The apex is resected at a 45° angle to the long axis of the tooth with a no. 701 tapered fissure or no. 330 bur in a high-speed handpiece with sterile saline irrigation (B). This creates an oval opening of the pulp canal and exposes the canal filling material.

Step 8—The surgical site is flushed liberally with sterile saline to remove debris.

Step 9—Hemorrhage is controlled by packing the area around the apex with sterile cotton pellets soaked in a hemostatic agent or using bone wax.

Step 10—The opening into the canal is undercut with a no. 33½ or no. 34 inverted cone bur in a slow-speed handpiece to make adequate retention for the filling (C). This preparation should extend 2 to 3 mm into the canal.

Step 11—The area is flushed, dried, and repacked with cotton pellets or bone wax to keep the area dry and to allow entrapment of amalgam particles (D). The cotton pellets or bone wax are removed prior to closure.

- Many filling materials have been proposed to seal the apex. Amalgam has been used for years,[10-12] and zinc-free amalgam has been recommended because of the moist enviroment in which the restorative material is placed. Most recently, IRM or EBA cement has been recommended.[13]

Step 12—If amalgam is used, the amalgam is mixed in an amalgamator, is placed in the opening with the retrograde amalgam carrier, and is condensed with a small plugger (E). If IRM or EBA is used, it is mixed and placed into the opening with a Centrix syringe.

Step 13—The filling material is carved smooth with a carver and allowed to set.

Step 14—The hemostatic packing is removed and the area is flushed with sterile saline or 0.2% chlorhexidine.

Step 15—the flap is closed with interrupted sutures using 3-0 to 4-0 absorbable suture material (F).

Step 16—A postoperative radiograph is taken to verify the seal.

Postoperative Care

- Antibiotics for 1 week.
- Follow-up radiographs at 6 months.
- Soft food for 3 to 5 days.

Complications

- Drilling into nasal cavity around maxillary canine. (This will generally heal with the closure of the flap.)
- Injury to infraorbital nerve during access to mesial root of upper carnassial tooth.
- Disruption of retrograde filling due to inadequate preparation, placement, condensation, or finishing.
- Infection.

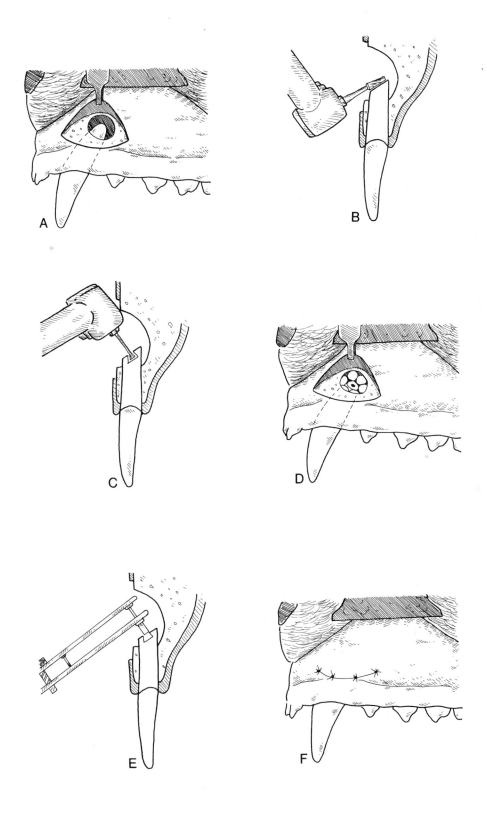

Variations with Individual Tooth Types

Incisors

Access Opening

- If the crown is fractured or worn (*A*), the opening to the pulp canal can be enlarged with a no. 2 round or no. 330 pear bur in a high- or slow-speed handpiece.
- If the crown is intact, the access hole can be made on the lingual surface between the crown tip and the cingulum (*B*). The bur is directed toward the center of the tooth along the long axis to avoid penetration of the root.

Filing and Irrigation of the Canal

- Smaller and shorter files are used to clean and prepare incisor canals. The root of the third maxillary incisor curves dramatically, and it may be necessary to prebend the files to reach the apex (*C*).

General Comment

- Incisor teeth can be done relatively quickly. In small dogs it may be difficult to enter the canals of the central incisors and 06 and 08 files may be necessary to start filing. Generally, the canal is filed to size 35 to 40 for the average-size dog.

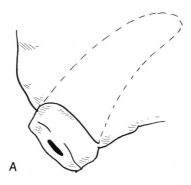

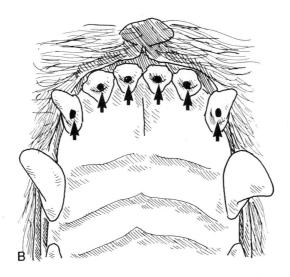

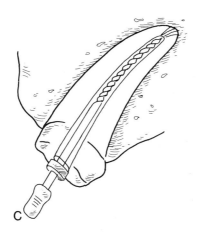

Canine Teeth
Access Opening

- An access hole can be made at the fracture site by enlarging the pulp canal opening with a no. 2, no. 4 round, or no. 330 pear bur in a high-speed or slow-speed handpiece (*A*). This access may be sufficient in fractured teeth with little remaining crown. A separate access hole is made on the mesial surface of the tooth 2 to 3 mm above the gingival margin in a line with the root canal visualized on a preoperative radiograph in intact teeth or teeth with distal crown fractures to allow complete instrumentation of the entire canal length without undue bending of files (*B* and *C*). The access hole begins with an initial cut made perpendicular through the enamel; the bur is then turned apically to intersect the pulp chamber in a straight line.
- Access holes must be large enough to allow instrumentation without removing excessive tooth structure.

Filing and Irrigation

- Filing and irrigation are completed as previously decribed; 40- to 60-mm files or reamers are necessary to reach the apex in large dogs. In older dogs it may be necessary to enlarge the coronal portion of the canal with a Gates Glidden reamer on a slow-speed handpiece to eliminate binding of the larger files.
- Alternating between file types can be beneficial in completing the instrumentation and ensuring a clean canal.
- Wide pulp canals in younger dogs necessitate circumferential filing to remove all pulp remnants and softened dentin.
- The average canal size ranges from no. 25 × 23 mm in small dogs to no. 50 × 36 mm in large dogs.[14]

Filling Techniques

- Those most beneficial are spiral filling, lateral condensation with multiple gutta percha points, combinations of lateral and vertical condensation with standard gutta percha, and thermoplasticized gutta percha techniques.
- Large canals in young dogs can be filled with amalgam or Core Paste.*

----

*Denmat, Santa Maria, CA 93456-9967

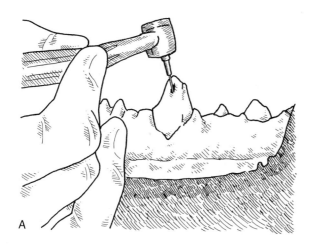

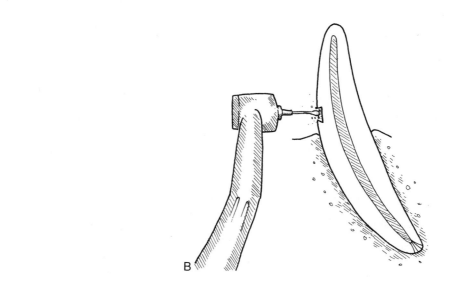

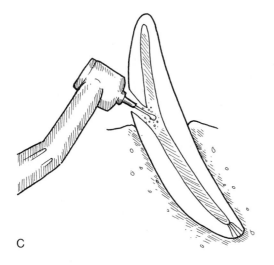

Teeth with Two Roots

Access Openings

- Openings need to be made into each root (*A*). Premolars can be accessed from fracture site, or a separate hole is drilled into the crown over each root. The least amount of tooth surface as possible should be removed in making the access. Some authors advise opening up the common pulp chamber to allow removal of pulp tissue.
- In a molar, access is made into the mesial root by drilling a hole just lingual to the small fissure on the buccal surface of the tooth (*B*). The distal root is accessed by a hole drilled in the center of the occlusal surface. Comparing the anatomic features to a radiograph helps direct proper site and angle of access hole.
- The roots may be filed one root at a time or simultaneously (*C*).

Restoration

- Amalgam is the material of preference for restoration of the mandibular molar to withstand the occlusal and shearing pressure placed on tooth.

Teeth with Three Roots

Maxillary Fourth Premolars

Access to Mesial-Buccal Root

- The mesial-buccal root can be accessed by drilling a hole at the point of intersection of a line about two thirds the distance between the fissure and the waist of the tooth and one quarter the distance from the gingival margin to the full length of the normal cusp tip.

Palatal Root

Transcoronal Approach (Eisner)

- The palatal root can be accesssed through this same hole by directing the file towards the palatine root (*D*).[15]

Three Access-Hole Approaches

- The palatal root can also be accessed by drilling directly over the palatal cusp close to the notch created by the large cusp surface. This is more difficult, particularly in older dogs.
- A third approach to the palatal root is to create a groove between the mesial root access hole and the palatal cusp across the surface of the tooth. This will allow visualization of the common pulp chamber, and the files can then be directed into the palatal root.

Palatal Root Amputation

- If the palatal root cannot be accessed or if root perforation occurs in attempts to locate the canal, it can be sectioned and removed and the common pulp chamber filled with a restorative.

Access to Distal Root

- The distal root access hole is drilled halfway between the distal surface of the tooth and the fissure and halfway from the gingival margin to the crown tip. These holes are made large enough to allow free instrumentation of the canals.

Molar Teeth

- Access holes to the three-rooted molar teeth are difficult and are best made on the occlusal surface after careful study of preoperative radiographs and study teeth or skulls.

Filing and Irrigation

- Filing and irrigation of all three roots are completed using 21- to 30-mm files as previously described. The distal root is generally larger and may often be filed to size 80. The mesial-buccal root averages size 30 to 35 and the palatal root 25 to 30.[14]

References

1. Wiggs RB. Standard Endodontics. Las Vegas: Veterinary Dentistry '90, 1990:51.
2. Messing J, Stock C. Color Atlas of Endodontics. St. Louis: C.V. Mosby Co., 1988:170, 176.
3. Grossman LI, Oliet S, Del Río CE. Endodontic Practice (11 ed.). Philadelphia: Lea & Febiger, 1988:106.
4. Rubin LD, Maplesden DC, Singer RR. Root canal therapy in dogs. VM/SAC 1978;73(5):593–589.
5. Ridgeway RL, Zielke DR. Nonsurgical endodontic technique for dogs. J Am Vet Med Assoc 1979;174(1):82–85.
6. Goldstein GS, Anthony J. Basic Veterinary Endodontics. Compend Contin Educ 1990;12(2):207–217.
7. Products PD. Premier R-C Prep Instructions for Use. Norristown, PA: Premier.
8. Anthony JMG. Endodontic Filling Techniques. New Orleans: Veterinary Dentistry '89, 1989:29.

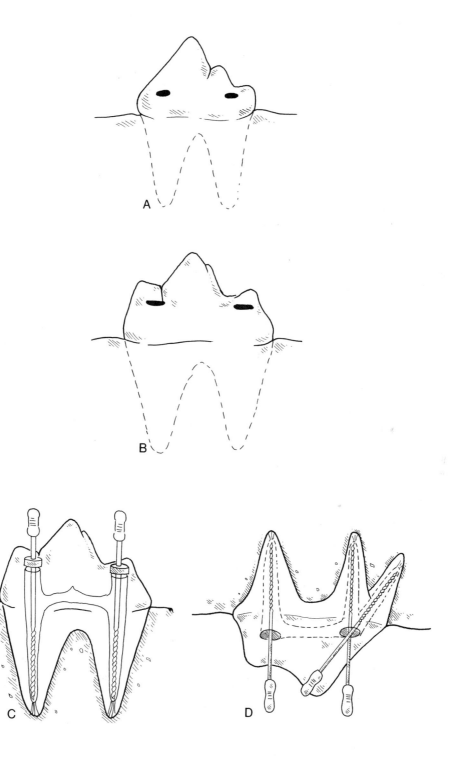

9. Fahrenkrug P. Crowns: Indication, Preparation, Proceedings. New Orleans: Nabisco, 1988.
10. Ross DL, Myers JW. Endodontic therapy for canine teeth in the dog. J Am Vet Med Assoc 1970; 157(11):1713–1718.
11. Taylor RA, Raymond P. Endodontia in the dog. VM/SAC 1972;67:1197–1200.
12. Lawer DR. Root canal with retrograde amalgam filling. Ca Vet 1979; Mar:11–15.
13. Emily P. Surgical Endodontics. Las Vegas: unpublished, 1990.
14. Eisner E. 353 Sequential Endodontic Cases: A Retrospective Study of Dogs and Cats in Veterinary Practice. New Orleans: Nabisco, 1989:33–37.
15. Eisner E. Transcoronal approach to the palatal root of the maxillary fourth premolar in the dog. J Vet Dent 1990;7(2).

chapter 8

RESTORATIVE DENTISTRY

GENERAL COMMENTS

- Teeth are restored both in an attempt to return the tooth to normal function and appearance and after endodontic therapy has been performed.

CLASSIFICATION OF LESIONS

- Various classification systems have been designed to communicate the extent of a dental lesion. One of the early classification systems was developed by G.V. Black. Black's system classifies cavities based on the location of the lesion.
- Cavities are defects in the tooth surface from any cause (such as a carious lesion, fracture, or abrasion).

Classification by Location of Lesion

Class 1—Cavities beginning in structural defects in a tooth's pits and fissures (occlusal surface) (A).

Class 2—Cavities in the proximal surfaces of premolars and molars (B).

Class 3—Cavities in the proximal surfaces of the incisors and canines that do not involve the removal and restoration of the incisal angle (C).

Class 4—Cavities in the proximal surfaces of the incisors and canines that involve the removal and restoration of the incisal angle (D).

Class 5—Cavities that are not pit cavities in the gingival third of the crown of the labial, buccal, or lingual surfaces of the teeth (E).

Class 6—Defects on the incisal edges of anterior teeth or the cusp tips of posterior teeth (F).

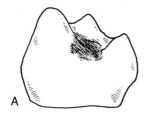

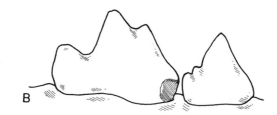

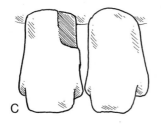

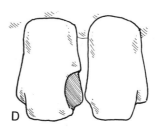

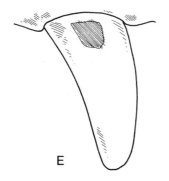

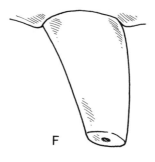

Classification by Extent of Fracture

- Although Black's system classifies the cavities by location, the system does not classify the extent of the lesion. Basrani has developed a classification system that accomplishes this goal.[1] This system is amenable to discussing treatment plans as well.

Class A1 Crown Fractures— Enamel

Description

- Fractures that involve only chips of enamel *(A)*.

Treatment

- In the dog, follow radiographically every 6 months to 1 year; root canal therapy is indicated if there is any sign of pulp death.
- In the cat, root canal therapy is recommended because most chip fractures will lead to pulp death and apical abscess formation.
- If on the cusp, crown therapy may prevent further damage.

Class A2a Crown Fractures— Enamel and Dentin

Description

- Fractures that have entered the enamel and dentin but have not entered the pulp *(B)*.

Treatment

Dog

- If enough dentin remains, indirect pulp capping and restoration with a glass ionomer, composite resin, or crown therapy.
- If very close to the pulp, pulp capping or root canal therapy followed by glass ionomer, acrylic, or crown therapy.

Cat

- Root canal therapy followed by glass ionomer, acrylic, or crown therapy.

Class A2b Crown Fractures— Enamel and Dentin

Description

- Fractures that involve enamel and dentin and have invaded the pulp.

Treatment

Young Animal (Younger than $1\frac{1}{2}$ Years) *(C)*

- Pulp capping followed by glass ionomer, acrylic, or crown restoration if the fracture is less than 2 weeks old.
- Extraction or root canal therapy and reinforced crown techniques if the fracture is open over 2 weeks (prognosis guarded; see Chapter 7, page 210).

Older Animal (Older than $1\frac{1}{2}$ Years) *(D)*

- Pulp capping if less than 48 hours.
- Root canal therapy followed by glass ionomer, acrylic, or crown restoration if pulp exposed longer than 48 hours.

Class B Crown Fractures—Root Fractures

Description

- Fractures involving the roots of teeth *(E)*.

Treatment

- If the fracture is in the coronal third of the root, endodontic therapy followed by a post in the endodontic system of both pieces of the tooth may be attempted (prognosis guarded).
- If the fracture is in the middle third of the root, extraction is necessary.
- If the fracture is in the apical third of the root, a surgical root canal and extraction of the apical fragment can be done.

Class C Crown-Root Fractures

Description

- Fractures involving both the crown and root *(F)*.

Treatment

- Most of the time, extraction is the best alternative.
- Root canal therapy followed by bonding of the split root may be attempted.

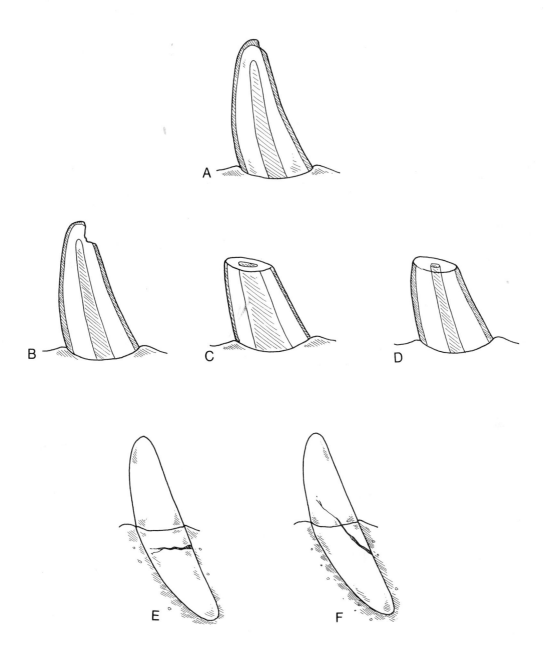

RESTORATIVE TECHNIQUES— GENERAL

Cutting Techniques

- Cut "away from" the enamel; i.e., when doing a crown preparation, cut in a counterclockwise rotation (the bur is rotating clockwise).
- When drilling into teeth, an intermittent pressure is applied. The time period is two counts on to one count off in order to limit heat generation and keep up bur speed.
- The operator should be aware of the change in pitch in the handpiece as an indication of pressure placed on the tooth. A higher pitch indicates a higher speed, which is desirable.

Cavity Preparation Techniques

- The outline of the preparation is made using a round bur or a tapered fissure bur to a depth of at least 1.5 mm.
- The retention is created using an inverted cone or pear-shaped bur.
- Additional retention can be made by making retention grooves in the base of cavity walls (intersection of wall and floors) with an appropriate-size round bur.
- The walls and floors may be smoothed with chisels or hatchets.
- Any carious dentin or poorly supported tooth structure should be removed.

RESTORATIVE MATERIALS

General Comments

- Through the years, many types of dental materials have evolved for the dental profession.

- The ideal material for restorative work would form a chemical bond to the enamel and dentin, would not distort after placement, would not break or fatigue, would have a high impact strength, would have the same coefficient of expansion as dental structures, and would wear at the same rate as the teeth.
- Unfortunately, this material does not exist at this time.[2]
- Given the different functions of different teeth and the areas to be restored, obtaining the best results from the materials available requires paying attention to the properties of each material.
- Restorative materials to be used should be picked by the conditions to be restored in order to maximize the desirable properties and minimize the undesirable properties of the material.
- The restorative materials and techniques discussed in this chapter can be classified as plastics (or restorative resins), glass ionomers, amalgams, and crown restoratives.
- It is important to store restorative materials correctly. An improper storage environment can rapidly destroy the material. The first thing one should do when receiving a material is to note the expiration date and read the package insert, paying particular attention to use and storage.
- Simplified, restorative dentistry can be broken down into five steps:

  1. Preparation of the surface.
  2. Placement and curing of the bonding agent.
  3. Placement and curing of the restorative agent.
  4. Shaping of the restoration.
  5. Smoothing of the restoration.

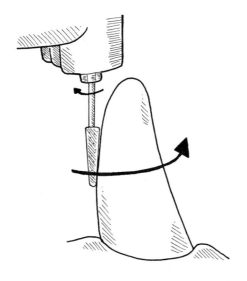

Plastics

General Comments

- As in the rest of our world, dentistry has been dramatically changed by the development of synthetic plastics.
- Dental plastics are polymers created by a series of chemical reactions combining large numbers of similar smaller molecules (monomers) into a compound of high molecular weight.[3]
- Throughout the "life" of the material, the polymerization process continues.
- Polymerization is a continuous reaction that is never entirely complete.
- The polymerization reaction is started either chemically or by light.
- Chemical-cure plastics usually come in two parts that, after mixing, cause molecules to join and the material to harden.
- Acrylic resins can be generally classified as filled or unfilled.
- Unfilled resins do not have fillers; they flow readily, are translucent, and are used to coat "cavity" preparations prior to the application of the filled resins.
- The unfilled resins are applied to prevent microleakage and promote the attachment of the restorative material to the tooth.
- Applying an unfilled resin to an acid-etched surface creates microprojections of resin into the tooth's crystalline structure.
- The filled resins contain fillers and are less viscous, opaque, harder, and have better wearability.
- The filled resin is bonded onto the unfilled resin.
- Fillers added to the filled resins give them hardness, strength, color, resistance to temperature change, wearability, and control of polymerization shrinkage.[4]
- Composite resins contain at least 60% (usually 70 to 80%) inorganic filler (quartz, lithium, or silica) by weight.
- The filler particles are described according to size: conventional (20 to 35 μm), intermediate or macrofilled (1 to 5 μm), microfilled (equal to or less than 0.04 μm), and hybrid (containing either a conventional or intermediate particle in addition to a microfilled).[4]
- The conventional and macrofilled compounds are more resistant to fracture and can be exposed to more "wear and tear."
- The disadvantage of the macrofilled compounds is a decreased ability to be polished because of larger particle size, and they become pitted with wear.
- Microfilled compounds polish to a very smooth surface; however, their disadvantage is that they tend to fracture more easily and are used in areas with less exposure to wear.
- In an attempt to reach a compromise between the microfilled and macrofilled qualities, hybrid compounds were developed to combine smoothness with durability.
- Both filled and unfilled resins cure by either chemical reaction or light exposure.
- Some products require the use of a "bonding agent" prior to the application of the unfilled resin to improve bonding to the tooth structure. Many types of systems are used for bonding agents, and the practitioner should refer to the instuctions on the restorative kit for specific instructions.
- Care should be used with unfilled resins or bonding agents to apply only a thin film to the tooth.

Indications

- Restoration of a damaged tooth crown.
- Restoration of access holes after endodontic therapy.
- Bonding wires for fracture repair and splinting teeth.

Contraindication

- Patients who will be chewing rocks, bones, etc.

Materials

- Flour pumice.
- Prophy cup.
- Slow speed-handpiece.
- Mixing pad.
- Mixing spatula.
- Centrix syringe.
- Brushes/sponges.
- Acid-etch materials.
- Plastic working instrument.
- Light-curing gun (light cure).
- High-speed handpiece.
- Smoothing/polishing materials.

Technique

- Although many different applications and variations of chemical and light cure restorations exist, the following is a step-by-step method for placement using a two-rooted tooth that has undergone endodontic therapy as an example.

Step 1—Preparation of the Surface

- Step 1, preparation of the surface, is common to both chemical-cure and light-cure restorations.

Substep 1—Prepare the filling site with the following considerations:

- All unsupported enamel should be removed using a chisel or sharp curette (*A* and *B*).
- Margins should be made at sites least susceptible to caries.
- The preparation may include deep grooves on the side or base for retention.
- The border of the preparation should not terminate on cusps.[5]

Substep 2—Clean the surface with flour pumice (not prophy paste, which may contain fluoride and glycerin) (*C*).

Substep 3—Wash with water and air dry (*D*).

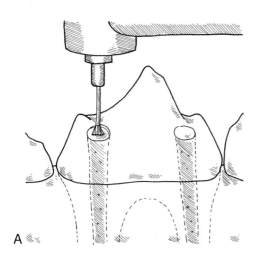

A

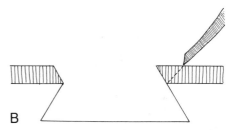

B

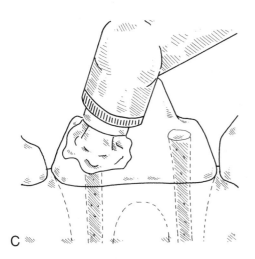

C

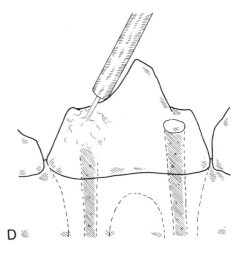

D

Step 1—Preparation of the Surface *(Continued)*

Substep 4—Acid etch the enamel with 38 to 50% phosphoric acid gel for 30 to 60 seconds. Either a sponge *(A)* or a brush *(B)* may be used.

Substep 5—Wash with water for at least 20 seconds *(C)*.

Substep 6—Dry the surface with oil and moisture-free air for at least 20 seconds *(D)*.

- The area to be restored should have a chalky white appearance; if it does not, the surface should be re-etched.
- It is important to keep the surface free from chemicals, saliva, blood, and other contaminates that interfere with bonding.
- Contamination is the most common reason for restorative failure.
- If contamination occurs, the surface should be reprepared, although a shorter etching time may be used.

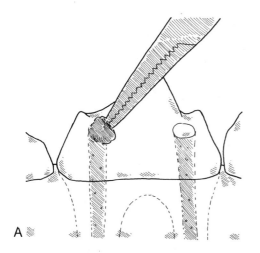

A

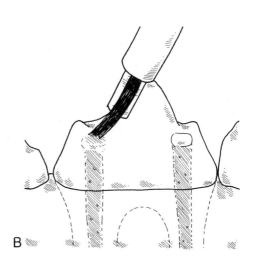

B

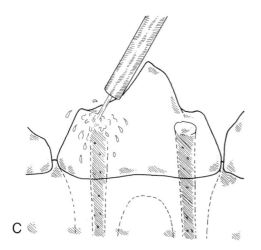

C

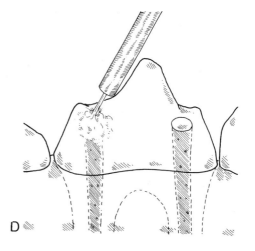

D

Step 2—Application of the Bonding Agent

- These steps vary with the manufacturer (Table 8–1). Some first apply a chemical to enhance bonding of the unfilled resin; others mix chemicals and the unfilled resin.
- The following procedure is for first mixing and applying a bonding agent followed by mixing and applying a restorative resin.

Substep 1—Bonding agent solution A is dropped into a dappen dish (A).

Substep 2—Bonding agent solution B is dropped into the same dappen dish (B). (Exact proportions of the two solutions are used according to the manufacturer's recommendations.) The solutions are mixed with a brush (C).

Substep 3—A thin coat of bonding agent is applied to the prepared surface (D).

Substep 4—A gentle stream of air is blown over the surface to minimize the thickness and eliminate pooling of the bonding agent (E).

Table 8–1. BONDING AGENTS

Chemical-Cured Bonding Agents	
Name	*Manufacturer*
Bonding Agent	Johnson & Johnson
Bonding Agent Self Cure	L. D. Caulk
Etch-Prep	Schein
Dentin Bonding Agents	
Name	*Manufacturer*
Bondlite	Kerr
Clearfil New Bond	J. Morita
Gluma	Columbus
Mirage-Bond	Chameleon
Scotchbond II	3M
Tenure	Den-Mat
XR Bonding System	Kerr

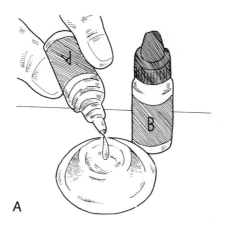

A

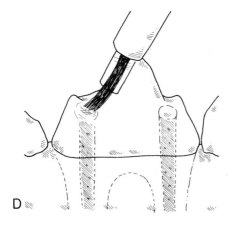

B

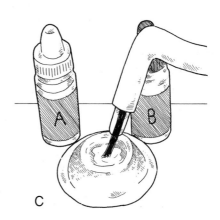

C

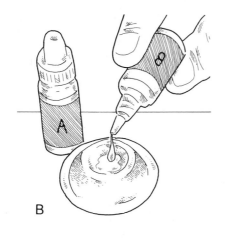

D

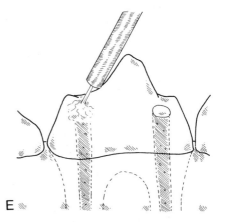

E

Step 2—Application of the Bonding Agent *(Continued)*

Substep 5—The unfilled resin is placed onto a brush *(A)* and is brushed onto the tooth *(B)*.

Substep 6—A gentle stream of air is directed onto the unfilled resin covered tooth surface to thin the layer of resin and to eliminate pooling *(C)*.

Step 3—Application of the Restorative Agent

Chemical Cure

- The chemical-cured, filled resin (Table 8–2) is mixed as directed by the manufacturer.

Substep 1—Equal portions of the filled resin are placed on a slab *(D)*.

Substep 2—The restorative material is spatulated in a figure-of-eight spatulation method.

- The mixing should be thorough and take 15 to 20 seconds.

Substep 3—Transfer the mixed resin to the site with a plastic filling instrument *(E)*.

Table 8–2. CHEMICAL-CURED COMPOSITE RESINS

Conventional Fillers	
Name	*Manufacturer*
Concise	3M
Adaptic	Johnson & Johnson
Profile	S.S. White
Simulate	Kerr
Intermediate or Macrofilled Fillers	
Name	*Manufacturer*
P10	3M
Cervident	S.S. White
Powder Lite	S.S. White
Extra Smooth	Den-Mat
Ultra Bond	Den-Mat
Marathon	Den-Mat
Class II	Den-Mat
Microfilled Fillers	
Name	*Manufacturer*
Finesse	L. D. Caulk
Silar	3M
Isocap	Vivadent
Isopast	Vivadent
Hybrid Filler	
Name	*Manufacturer*
Miradapt	Johnson & Johnson

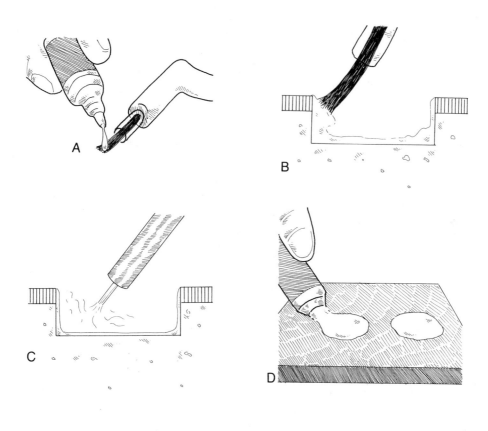

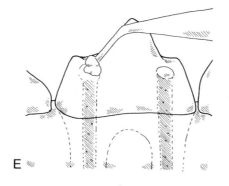

Step 3—Application of the Restorative Agent *(Continued)*

- The material may also be transferred to the site using an injection syringe.*
- The injection syringe is loaded by scooping the material into the plastic tip off either the spatula or the glass slab *(A)*.
- The rubber plunger is placed into the plastic tip on top of the restorative material *(B)*.
- The material is injected into the restoration site *(C)*.

Substep 4 (optional)—A Mylar strip is placed over the site to conform the material to the tooth shape *(D)*.

Light Cure

- Some light-cure products require mixing (substeps 1 and 2); others may be used directly without mixing (Table 8– 3).
- The unfilled resin may also need light curing prior to the application of the filled resin.

Substep 1—Equal portions of the filled resin are placed on a slab.
Substep 2—The restorative material is spatulated.
Substep 3—Transfer the mixed resin to the site with a plastic filling instrument or injection syringe.
Substep 4—Shape the restorative material with a plastic working instrument.
Substep 5 (optional)—Place a Mylar strip over the site to conform the material to the tooth shape.
Substep 6—Cure the restorative material for 30 to 60 seconds according to the depth of the restoration and the product used *(E)*. The thickness of restorative material should be no more than 3 to 4 mm at a time without curing. The deeper the fill, the longer the cure time required.

- Additional layers of restorative material can be placed on top of the cured material for deep restorations.

---

*Centrix II Syringe, Milford, CT 06460

Complications/Cautions

- It is important when using light-curing units to use appropriate protective glasses or shields.
- Light emission requires that the light be close to the restoration (less than 1 mm).
- To ensure a full cure, cure everything at least 60 seconds.

Table 8–3. LIGHT-CURED RESTORATIVES

Conventional Fillers	
Name	*Manufacturer*
Command	Kerr
Nuva Fil PA	L. D. Caulk

Intermediate or Macrofilled Fillers	
Name	*Manufacturer*
Aurafil	Johnson & Johnson
Command	Kerr
Estilux	Kulzer
Extra Smooth	Den-Mat
Ful-fil	L. D. Caulk
Healthco VLC	Healthco
Ultra Bond	Den-Mat
Prisma Fil	L. D. Caulk
P30	3M
Visio Fil	ESPE/Premier

Microfilled Fillers	
Name	*Manufacturer*
Adaptic LCM	3M
Durafil VS	Kulzer
Heliosit	Vivadent
Heliomolar	Vivadent
Helioprogress	Vivadent
Opalux	Coe
Pekalux	Columbus
Prisma Microfine	L. D. Caulk
Silux	3M

Hybrid Fillers	
Name	*Manufacturer*
Adaptic II	Johnson & Johnson
APH (All Purpose Hybrid)	L. D. Caulk
Bis Fil P	Biscol
Bis Fil M	Biscol
Command Ultrafine	Kerr
Herculite XR	Kerr
Lumifor	Columbus
Mirage	Chameleon
P50	3M
Perfection	Den-Mat
Prisma APH	L. D. Caulk
Profile TLC	S.S. White
Occlusin	Coe
Silux Plus	3M
Ultra Bond	Den-Mat
Visarfil	Den-Mat

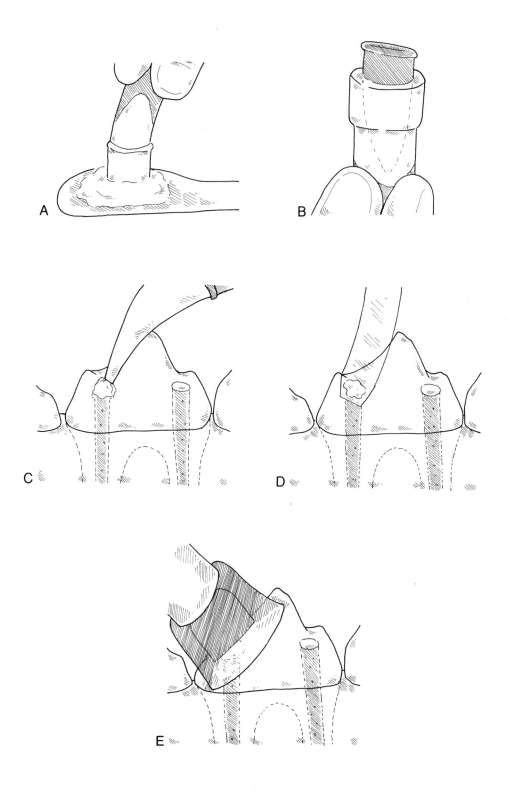

Step 4—Shaping the Restoration

- The material is shaped with finishing diamond burs, 12-blade carbide finishing burs, or fine particle stones (see pp. 38, 39, 46, and 47).

Step 5—Smoothing the Restoration

- Once the material has hardened, the restoration is smoothed with sandpaper discs or strips or with fine particle stones.

Sanding Discs

Description

- Plastic or sandpaper circular discs are held by a mandrel and driven by a contra angle and slow-speed handpiece.
- Paste lubricants/polishing agents are available to aid in smoothing.

Advantage

- Quick reduction of tooth surface.

Disadvantage

- Being circular, they may not fit into all areas of the restorative surface.

Finishing Strips

Description

- Thin plastic sanding strips.

Advantage

- Useful in conic shaped teeth such as canine teeth to smooth rapidly.

Disadvantage

- Will not fit into all spaces.

Nonadhesive Strips

Description

- Do not contain adhesive to hold particles. This decreases the number of particles that break free and readhere to the strip, to become captured particles.
- Captured particles have the potential to damage the surface being finished by leaving deep grooves.
- Thin, flexible strips to smooth down the tooth surface.

Advantages

- Easy interproximal access.
- Readily contours to the shape of the tooth.

Complications

- Microleakage is recognized by a black line between the restorative material and the tooth occurring some time after restoration.
- In the case of vital teeth, sensitivity can result from microleakage.
- The three main factors that cause microleakage are: (1) poor technique; (2) shrinkage of the restorative material occurring with polymerization; and (3) the inability of the resin to chemically bond to the tooth structure.
- Acid etching may cause dentinal sensitivity in vital teeth. Etching, if performed, should be carried out with the milder acids called "dentin conditioners."

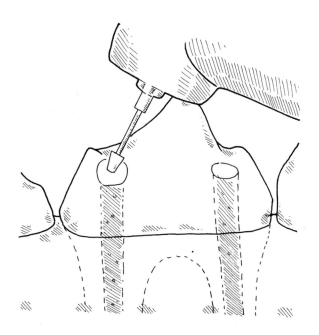

Product Options

Repair of Defective Composite Resin Restorations [6]

General Comments

- The trauma of use may cause defects in the acrylic restoration.
- The overall strength of the repair may not be as strong as the original restoration.

Indication

- Fractured acrylic restoration.

Contraindication

- Fracture of tooth that may require more than conservative restoration.

Materials

- Same as with composite restoration.

Technique

Step 1—The restoration is probed to discover any defects that may not be visualized.

Step 2—A water-cooled, inverted-cone carbide bur is used to remove defective resin. A slight undercut may aid retention.

Step 3—A coarse diamond is used to roughen the entire surface of the remainder of the restoration to eliminate superficial resin that has been exposed to the oral environment.

Step 4—A phosphoric acid gel is spread over the entire preparation for 30 seconds and rinsed with water for 30 seconds.

Step 5—An unfilled resin is applied over the surface and blown with compressed air to a thin layer.

Step 6—The filled resin is mixed, placed into an injection syringe, and injected into the restorative site.

Step 7—The resin is allowed to cure. If using a light-cure restorative material, the curing light is held from the side in an attempt to cure from the restorative margins first.

Step 8—The surface is recontoured and smoothed as described under finishing techniques.

Glass Ionomers

General Comments

- Glass ionomers are sold in kits that may contain powder (in various shades), liquid, measuring scoops, varnish, etching agent, and mixing pads.
- The powder is an aluminosilicate glass.
- The anhydrous form contains acid in the powder.
- The hydrous form contains acid in the liquid.
- When the powder and liquid are mixed together, chemical reactions bond the restoration to tooth structure and harden the compound.
- Light-cure and dual-cure glass ionomer restorative materials are available.
- Glass ionomers can be classified as type I (luting) or type II (lining, restorative, or core) (Table 8–4).
- Type I glass ionomers are finely grained and are used for cementing (luting) crowns, bridges, and other castings.
- Type II glass ionomers are used as restorative materials.
- Type II glass ionomers are coarser than type I and therefore are not suitable for cementation purposes.
- Restorative glass ionomers can be used as a base or as the sole restorative.
- Glass ionomers are biocompatible and do not require placement of obtunding base material to protect the pulp, except in case of direct pulp exposure.
- Nonencapsulated forms are mixed with a spatula and pad.
- The encapsulated type requires a special tool to break the internal separation between the liquid and powder, an amalgamator to mix the compound, and a special syringe to apply the mixture.
- A problem with glass ionomer compounds is their lack of wearability. In an attempt to increase wearability, some manufacturers have added metals to the mixture. Most commonly, silver is added; gold, copper, and zinc have been suggested as possible alternatives.

- Upon mixing nonencapsulated forms, the material is either transferred to an injection syringe and squeezed into the prepared cavity or placed with a plastic working instrument.
- Once hardened, the surface can be smoothed with a diamond finishing bur, irrigated with copious amounts of water.
- The restoration should not be smoothed with a carbide bur.
- If water is not used, cocoa butter can be used as a lubricant.
- Without a lubricant, the material will overheat, desiccate, and weaken.
- Glass ionomer restorative materials have the advantage of forming a chemical as well as a mechanical bond to teeth.
- Glass ionomers slowly release fluoride.
- The expansion coefficent is the same as that of the tooth.

Indications

- Cementing (luting) crowns and onlays, orthodontic appliances.
- Lining glass ionomers are used as a foundation upon which other materials, such as plastic resins, are applied.
- Core glass ionomers are used as a base or to build up material around a post to support a laboratory-manufactured crown.
- They can also be used in combination with light-cure restoratives to reduce the amount of light-cure restorative required and to decrease the potential for polymerization shrinkage.
- Type II glass ionomers are ideal for repair of cervical erosive lesions,[7, 8] as well as for filling of root canal access points on nonocclusal areas.

Contraindication

- Because these materials are less durable than other restoratives, glass ionomers are not recommended on high-wear surfaces.

Materials

- Power equipment (air preferred).
- Glass or paper slab.
- Spatula.
- Centrix syringe or Jiffy tube.
- Glass ionomer.

Table 8–4. GLASS IONOMER RESTORATIVE MATERIALS

Type I: Luting or Cementing	
Name	Manufacturer
Chemical Cure	
Ceramchem	Healthco
Glassic	Stratford Cookson
Glasslute	Pulpdent
Fuji I	G.C. International
Ketac Cem	ESPE/Premier
Shofu Type I	Shofu
Light Cure	
Vitrabond	3M
Zionomer	Den-Mat
Type II: Glass Ionomers—Core	
Name	Manufacturer
Ceracore	Healthco
Glasscore	Pulpdent
Ketac Silver	ESPE/Premier
Miracle Mix	G.C. International
Shofu Base Cement	Shofu
Zionomer Core	Den-Mat
Type II: Glass Ionomers—Lining Ionomers	
Name	Manufacturer
Ceramlin B	Healthco
G.C. Lining Cement	G.C. International
Gingiva Seal	Parkell
Glassline	Pulpdent
Ketac Bond	ESPE/Premier
Shofu Lining	Shofu
Shofu Base	Shofu
3M Ionomer	3M
Zionomer Lining	Den-Mat
Type II: Glass Ionomers—Restorative	
Name	Manufacturer
Ceramfil	Healthco
Chemfil II	DeTrey/Dentsply
Fuji Cap	G.C. International
Fuji Type II	G.C. International
Ketac Fil	ESPE/Premier
Shofu Type II	Shofu

Technique for Restoration After Root Canal Therapy

Step 1—Preparation of the Surface

Substep 1—In most situations, cavity preparation will be the same as a standard preparation for composite resins *(A)*.

- In the treatment of nonocclusal, class V lesions, the creation of an undercut may not be necessary.

Substep 2—The surface is cleaned with flour pumice (without fluoride or glycerin) with a prophy cup.

- Etching/conditioning of nonvital dentin to remove the smear layer that forms during preparation is controversial.

Substep 3—The cavity is dried with an air source or blotted dry with paper points.

Substep 4—The cavity preparation agent (usually a mild acid) is applied *(B)*.

Substep 5—After 15 seconds the cavity preparation agent is washed off with water *(C)*.

Substep 6—The area is dried.

- Unlike with all other restoratives, it is important that the cavity not be "bone dry." Although there should be no pools of water in the preparation, the area should not have the chalky white appearance of a completely dried tooth. If overdried, the preparation should be rehydrated with water.
- Once the area has been prepared, it is important to prevent contamination. If contaminated, the area must be reprepared.

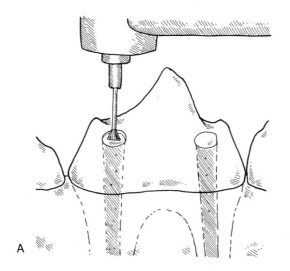

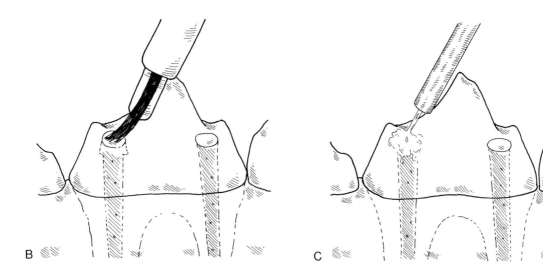

Step 2—Application of the Bonding Agent

- In this case, it is the glass ionomer applied in step 3.

Step 3—Application of the Glass Ionomer

- Glass ionomer restorative material is quickly mixed according to the manufacturer's instructions. Although the ratios may vary by manufacturer and the amounts by case, the following substeps apply.

Substep 1—The powder is "fluffed" (shaken) with the lid closed and level scoops of the powder are measured and placed preferably on a heavy glass slab (A).

Substep 2—The appropriate number of drops of liquid are dripped out; be careful to avoid air bubbles that may distort the measurement (B).

Substep 3—First the powder is divided in half, and then one of the halves is split into quarters (C).

Substep 4—Half the powder is pulled into the liquid and is rapidly mixed (D).

Substep 5—Half the remaining powder is pulled into the liquid (E), and in turn the final quarter is mixed in (F). A figure-of-eight motion is used to mix the glass ionomer (G).

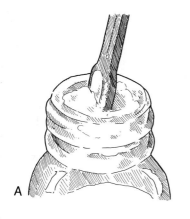

A

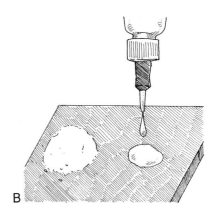

B

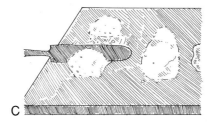

C

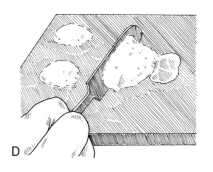

D

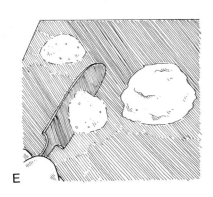

E

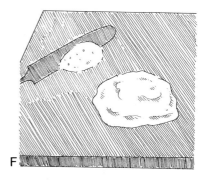

F

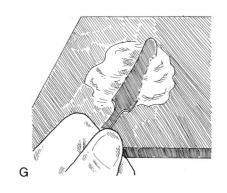

G

Step 3—Application of the Glass Ionomer *(Continued)*

- Once the material is applied to the cavity. manipulation is limited.

Substep 6—The mix is loaded into the curved tip of the injection syringe *(A)*.

Substep 7—The tube is pushed down over the plug *(B)*. The tube and plug are loaded into the syringe.

Substep 8—The restorative material is injected into the cavity to be filled *(C)*.

Step 4—Shaping the Restoration

Substep 1 (optional)—The glass ionomer is covered with a Mylar strip as it is setting up to prevent moisture contamination *(D)*. A condenser may be placed over the Mylar strip to conform the restorative material to the tooth structure *(E)*.

Substep 2—The edges of the material (flashing) are painted with a varnish *(F)*. If a Mylar strip is not used, the restorative material must be coated with a layer of varnish after it begins to harden.

- Alternatively, the liquid component of a light-cure resin can be painted on to protect the glass ionomer as it sets.

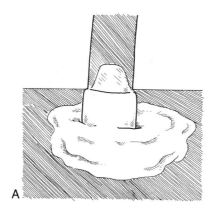

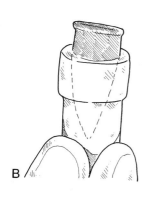

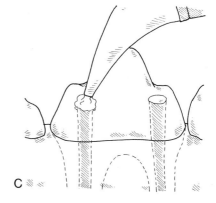

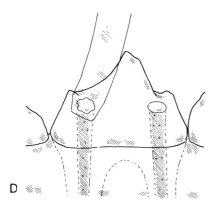

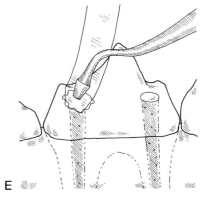

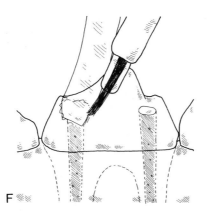

Step 5—Smoothing the Restoration

Substep 1—The restoration is carved with a fine diamond, coated with cocoa butter *(A)*.

Substep 2—The cocoa butter is wiped from the tooth *(B)*.

Substep 3—A coat of varnish or liquid portion of a light-cure resin is applied as a final protective coat *(C)*.

Complications/Cautions

- The tooth conditioner may cause dentinal sensitivity because it is a form of acid etch.
- It is important that the glass ionomer material be applied before the mixture loses its shiny appearance. If this occurs, a new batch of material should be mixed.
- If the glass ionomer restoration crazes, cracks, or falls out, it is usually a problem of moisture *(D)*. Water contamination or overdrying will cause these problems.

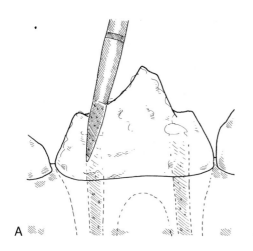

A

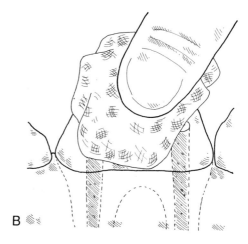

B

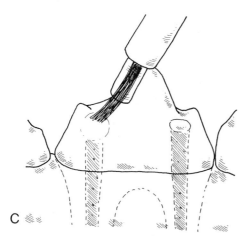

C

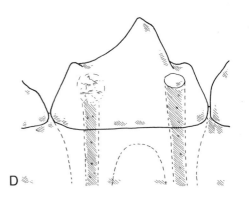

D

Feline Cervical Line Lesions
Etiology

- The pathogenesis of the osteoclastic resorptive lesions on feline teeth is not fully understood.
- Work that has been done shows that the lesions tend to start at the gingival margin or just subgingivally and progress both apically and coronally.
- These lesions have had various names: cervical line lesions, osteoclastic resorption, neck lesion, feline neck lesion, feline caries, and "catvities."

Signs

- They are often not detectable without using an explorer to probe for irregularities of the tooth surface and are commonly covered with hyperplastic gingiva.
- Usually the patient shows signs of discomfort and pain when the lesions are probed.
- This discomfort is sometimes even evident under deep general anesthesia.
- The lesions can be found on all teeth, but molars and premolars are most frequently involved.
- The lesions can be covered with calculus, especially in the molar and premolar teeth.
- Lesions are found on the buccal and lingual surfaces.
- The disease seems to be progressive, and many teeth may be affected and show different stages of destruction at any one time.
- In early stages, lesions can be small enough that they are difficult to detect.

- As they progress, the lesions enlarge, encompassing more and more of the root and crown.
- In advanced lesions an overhang of enamel can be found, with the underlying dentin missing.
- Radiographs often show the affected teeth to be demineralized much more dramatically than appears on visual examination.

Treatment Protocol

Technique for Restoration of Cervical Line Lesion

Step 1—Before restoration is attempted, the tooth should be examined carefully to determine the amount of involvement *(A)*.

- A radiograph is vital to this evaluation.
- It will do the patient little good to restore a tooth whose roots are already being resorbed.

Step 2—Clean the lesion of plaque, hyperplastic gingiva, and any soft dentin that may be present *(B)*.

- This is often difficult to do without penetrating the pulp chamber.
- If the pulp chamber is penetrated, a vital pulp capping or extraction should be performed.

Step 3—The lesion is isolated by packing retraction cord into the sulcus *(C)*.
Step 4—The lesion is pumiced *(D)*.
Step 5—The lesion is rinsed and dried, and a restorative of either glass ionomer or a dentinal bonding agent/acrylic resin is placed.

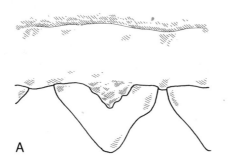

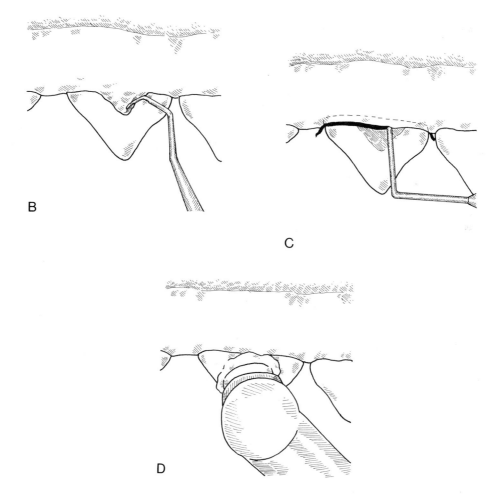

A

B

C

D

Placing a Glass Ionomer Restorative

Substep 1—A dentin conditioner is applied to the neck lesion with a brush *(A)* and, following the manufacturer's instructions, either actively scrubbed or let passively to sit on the surface.

Substep 2—The dentin conditioner is thoroughly washed from the tooth surface *(B)*, and the tooth is dried.

Substep 3—After mixing, the glass io- nomer is inserted into an injection syringe and then into the neck lesion *(C)*.

Substep 4—A Mylar strip is placed over the glass ionomer and tooth *(D)*. Pressure is placed on the Mylar with an instrument such as a condensor, curette, or explorer *(E)*.

Substep 5—The "flashing" (glass ionomer that has flowed out around the Mylar) is coated with varnish or a light-cured unfilled resin *(F)*.

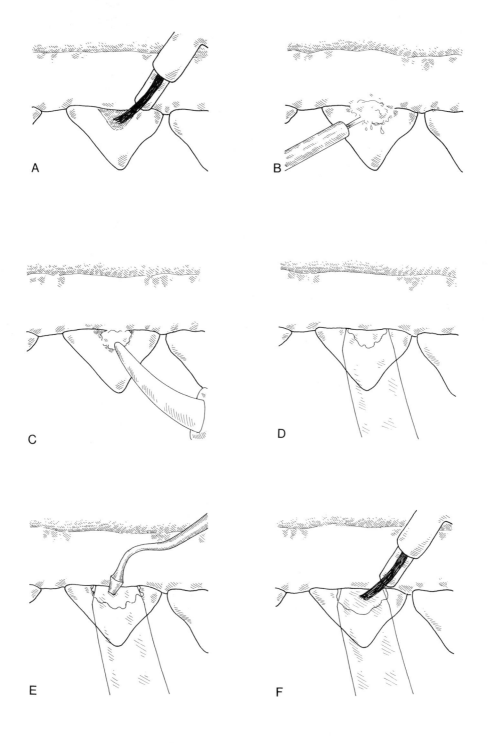

Placing a Glass Ionomer
Restorative *(Continued)*

Substep 6—When the glass ionomer is hard (2 to 3 minutes) the Mylar is removed, and the excess glass ionomer is trimmed away *(A)*.

Substep 7—Excess material is wiped away from the surface *(B)*.

Substep 8—The glass ionomer is recoated with varnish or light-cured unfilled resin *(C)*.

Step 6—Home care will assist in maintaining the patient's oral health.

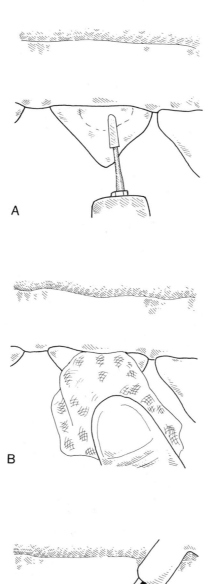

A

B

C

Amalgam

General Comments

- Amalgam is a metal alloy of mercury and silver that may also contain copper, zinc, tin, and other metals.
- Amalgam is mixed with amalgamators, which are mechanical mixing devices that have universally replaced the traditional method of mixing amalgam by mortar and pestle trituration. The mortar is replaced by a capsule that contains the mercury alloy, and a metal or plastic ball of smaller diameter than the capsule serves as the pestle. The capsule is placed in the amalgamator, and when the machine is turned on, the materials are mixed.
- Depending on the alloy, it usually takes from 10 to 30 seconds to mix the amalgam.
- It is important that amalgam be mixed in proper proportions; this is one of the major advantages of the premixed capsules.
- Amalgam is an easy material to work with; it is strong and able to withstand years of wear. Often the tooth will wear around an amalgam restoration, leaving a button of amalgam protruding beyond the worn tooth structure.
- Mercury is a poison, and direct contact with skin should be avoided.
- Amalgam seals by corrosion, and a black edge will be seen around the filled area at a later date. Because black discoloration is normal, clients should be told of its future appearance. Painting a varnish over the area to be restored prior to amalgam placement can minimize discoloration.

Indications

- Final restoration.
- Core buildup for crown.

Contraindication

- Restorations where cosmetics are important.

Materials

- Amalgam in capsule.
- Amalgamator.
- Amalgam carrier.
- Amalgam condensers.
- Amalgam burnishers.
- Amalgam carvers.
- Amalgam finishing cups.
- Amalgam well.

Technique
Step 1—Surface Preparation

Substep 1—The outline and retention of the cavity are prepared using a diamond or carbide bur (A).

Substep 2—Unsupported enamel is chiseled along the margins to remove the enamel overhangs (B).

Substep 3—In areas within 1 mm of the pulp, resinated calcium hydroxide is placed (C). (See indirect pulp cap technique, page 208.)

Substep 4—In deep restorations, a liner glass ionomer may be placed (see section on glass ionomers).

Step 2—Sealing the Dentinal Tubules

- A cavity varnish or dentin adhesive is placed (D).
- Dentin adhesives have been shown to significantly reduce microleakage around amalgam restorations.[9]
- Use only a thin layer over all surfaces and allow to dry prior to placement of the amalgam.

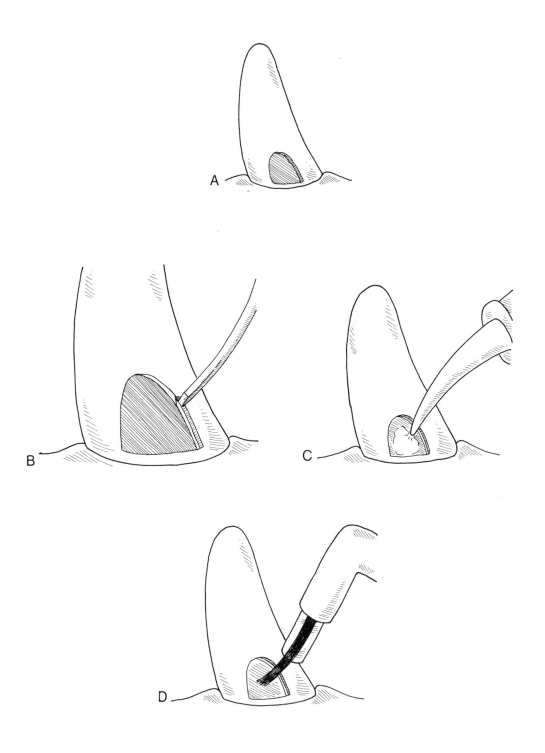

Step 3—Placement of the Restorative Material

Substep 1—The amalgam capsule is activated according to the manufacturer's instructions.

Substep 2—The amalgam is triturated at the time and speed as directed by the manufacturer.

Substep 3—The mixed amalgam pellet is placed in an amalgam well (A). Properly prepared amalgam should appear shiny and "moist." Overmixed amalgam appears chalky and flaky and will not condense. Undermixed amalgam appears nonhomogeneous.

Substep 4—An amalgam carrier is loaded with amalgam from the well (B).

- Caution should be used not to compact the amalgam in the carrier. If it becomes compacted it may be necessary to replace the carrier tip or use a sharp, pointed instrument to dig out the amalgam.

Substep 5—Amalgam is placed in the restoration (C).

Substep 6—The first layer of amalgam is condensed with pressure (D). Smaller condensers are used in the early filling stage, with larger condensers for the final condensing.

Substep 7—Subsequent layers are condensed; pay attention to eliminate voids. A slight overfill is desired; this is taken care of in the next step.

Step 4—Amalgam Carving

- The final anatomic form is created with an amalgam carver. While carving, the operator should carve from tooth surface into the restoration to avoid "scooping" out the amalgam.

Step 5—Burnishing

- The surface of the amalgam is burnished using a burnisher (E).

- Burnishing renders the restoration more corrosion resistant.
- The process is to rub the surface lightly until the surface takes on a velveteen or satin appearance.[4]
- Burnishing is directed from the restorative surface to the tooth surface.[11]
- The restoration may be polished 24 hours after placement (F).

Complications

- Microleakage resulting in penetration of bacteria, bacterial products, soluble ions, and saliva into the gap between the restoration and cavity walls.
- This can result in pulp irritation, inflammation, and necrosis.
- Inherent characteristics of the material such as the lack of chemical adhesion, differences in the coefficients of thermal expansion between the amalgam restoration and tooth structure, and the dimensional changes and surface texture of the amalgam after insertion into the prepared cavity. This can lead to microleakage or tooth fracture.
- Inadequate condensation can result in voids along the cavity margins and in the restorative material.
- Overtrituration (mixing) resulting in overcontraction.
- Overmixing causes amalgam to set before it is placed into the cavity preparation.
- Undertrituration results in high-setting expansion and increased corrosion. If undermixed, the material will be dull and grainy, leading to a weak and rough surface with free mercury.
- Delay in placing the amalgam into the restoration that results in a partial set of the amalgam, weakening the restoration. Depending on the product and amount of trituration, the amalgam begins to solidify in 1 to 5 minutes.
- Careless placement of lining material on the walls that prevents contact of amalgam with tooth structure.[9]

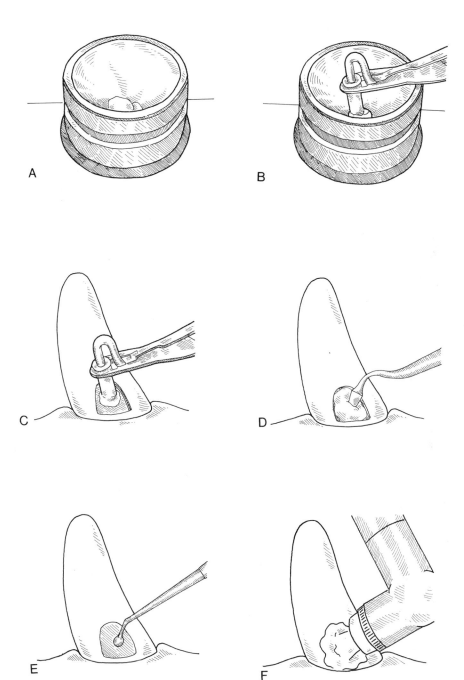

PIN RESTORATION

General Comments

- A pin-retained buildup is formed with pins placed into the dentin and is covered with amalgam, composite, or a glass ionomer.
- If minimal buildup is needed, the pin-retained buildup method may be used.
- In general, the least number of pins possible should be used. They should be placed at least 2 mm from each other, the other walls, and the pulp. At least 1.5 mm of restorative material should cover the pin.[11]

Advantage

- Provides additional retentive surface.

Disadvantages

- Pins weaken tooth structure.
- Restoration will not withstand much lateral force.

Materials

- Power equipment.
- Slow-speed handpiece.
- TMS pin kit—Minikins.*

Technique

Step 1—Appropriate endodontic or restorative preparation is performed (A and B).

*Whaledent, New York, NY 10001

Step 2—With a slow-speed handpiece and bur that comes with the Minikin kit, a hole is drilled in the dentin with one pass (C).

Step 3—The pin is loaded into the pin instrument (D).

Step 4—The pin is seated into the pre-drilled hole (E).

Step 5—When the pin reaches home, the pin will break off at the precut location (F).

Step 6—A restoration is placed with chemical- or light-cure composite resin, a glass ionomer, or amalgam using a previously described technique (G).

Complications/Cautions

- Caution must be used in vital teeth not to penetrate the pulp tissue; this may lead to failure. If penetration occurs, a small amount of calcium hydroxide may be placed in the hole, followed by the permanent restoration. The hole should not be used for the pin.
- Caution must be used to avoid perforation of the periodontal ligament space. If this should occur, a small amount of calcium hydroxide should be placed in the hole, and that hole should not be used for the procedure. Radiographs should follow at 6-month intervals.
- When drilling, caution must be used to make the hole as close to the size of the drill as possible (attempt to avoid wobble).
- Stripping threads of drilled holes will lead to an unstable pin, and the hole should not be used.

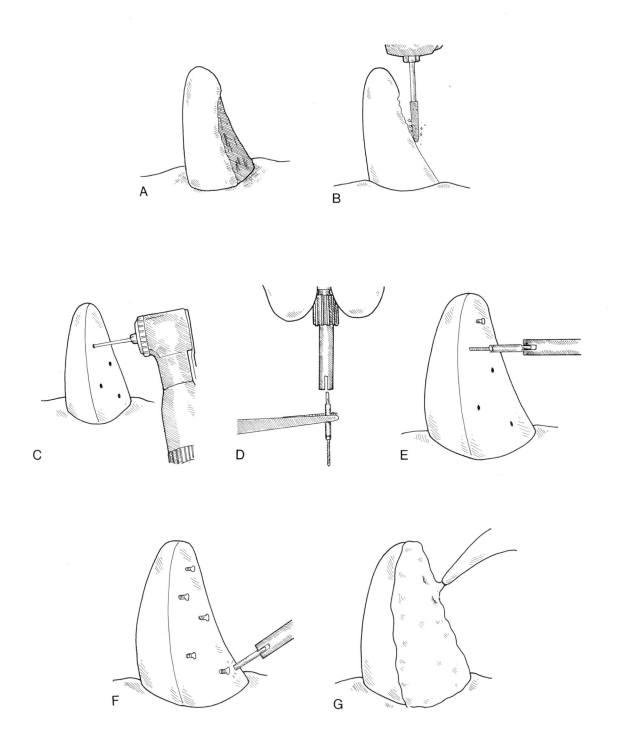

CROWN THERAPY

Crown ("Cap")—General Technique

General Comments

- A crown is an appliance that replaces the function and structure of a damaged tooth and protects the portion of the tooth that remains.
- It can be made to closely match the function and appearance of the tooth.
- The decision to place a crown is determined after careful consideration of the animal's life style and the owner's requirements.
- The replacement crown is termed a full crown if it covers all of the tooth.[12]
- If only a portion of the tooth crown is covered, it is termed a partial crown.
- The material that the crown is made of affects its appearance.
- The margin of the crown is the edge that interfaces with the tooth.
- Maintenance or conservation of tooth structure is the primary concern in crown preparation design. It is unwise to remove more tooth structure than absolutely necessary to create retention and integrity; and at the same time, enough tooth structure must be removed to create adequate space for the restoration.
- The preparation should be designed with a parallel technique of the walls and a 6° taper to increase the resistance of the crown to dislodgment.
- Canine teeth in dogs and cats do not lend themselves to parallel technique as readily as most human teeth because the canines in dogs and cats are conical and not box-like, as in humans.

- Parallelism is accomplished by "stair-stepping" the preparation between the mesial and the distal surfaces in canine teeth.
- Greater retention is achieved when most of the available surface area of the prepared axial wall of the tooth is in contact with the cast restoration.
- It must have adequate occlusal clearance or the restoration will strike other teeth.
- The margin of the restoration must facilitate good hygiene and not create areas for plaque and debris to accumulate, and at the same time, it should be accessible so it can be finished by the veterinarian and the client can maintain it.
- Ideally, the margin placement is on the enamel surface. This is more readily accomplished when aesthetics are not a primary concern.
- If aesthetics are of paramount importance, subgingival placement of the margin is necessary.

Indications

- Enamel hypoplasia or aplasia (dentinal structures are intact, pulp is vital).
- Fractured teeth with damaged pulp, vitality lost, postendodontic therapy.
- Undamaged pulp where the pulp is vital when additional protection is desired.
- A crown should be used when deterioration or damage has left an unstable or inadequate supragingival portion of the crown structure that it is not salvageable by other methods.
- A crown is also used to protect a damaged tooth from further deterioration.

Contraindications

- Thin wall structure; always radiograph before a crown preparation.
- Nonvital tooth without endodontics.
- Endodontically treated tooth where practitioner is unsure of the results.

Objective

- To protect the tooth and to improve the cosmetics and function of the tooth.

Materials

- A crown of semiprecious metal. The least expensive material that should be used will be silver colored. Generally, the cost of the metal is a smaller portion of the total cost of a crown.
- Gold alloy produces a gold colored crown.
- A crown made of a gold alloy is also more malleable, resulting in easier fabrication and placement.
- A tooth-colored crown can be made by fusing porcelain to a metal shell or by using porcelain alone. Porcelain by itself is extremely fragile and its use is limited.[13]
- Porcelain fused to metal can be used to create aesthetic restorations. Unfortunately, this method is more expensive and requires removal of more tooth structure than a metal crown.

Technique

- The technique for crown therapy includes the following basic steps: (1) evaluation for preparation; (2) reduction and margin preparation; (3) taking an impression and casting; (4) manufacture of temporary crown (optional); (5) laboratory orders and manufacture of crown; and (6) cementation of crown.
- The many alternatives and methods that can be used must be selected case by case.

Step 1—Evaluation for Preparation

- The occlusal edge or surface is evaluated for reduction to allow space for the metal in the crown.
- Anticipated wear determines space requirements and crown thickness.
- Allow a minimum of 1.5 mm of space for the areas of increased wear potential and 1 mm of space for the areas of little or no wear potential.[12–14]
- The incisor, premolar, and molar teeth that have occlusal surfaces require additional space allowance on the occlusal surface.
- The canine and premolar teeth without an actual occlusal surface usually require little reduction for space allowance, but do require reduction and beveling of any sharp or thin edges.

Step 2—Reduction and Margin Preparation

- A gingival retraction cord is placed with a cord packer. The purpose of the cord is to isolate the gingiva from the tooth surface. Care must be taken to avoid wrapping the gingival cord in the bur while preparing the tooth surface.
- A tapered coarse diamond bur is used for initial reduction (Table 8–5).
- Either a chamfer or shoulder is created at the gingival edge of the preparation.
- The margin should be placed either 1 mm above or 1 mm below the free gingival margin.

Axial Reduction

- The tooth structure is removed by axial reduction along the long axis of the tooth. The bur is held near parallel to the tooth axis.
- The tooth surface should be reduced attempting to create walls that are near parallel with a 6° slope.
- Undercuts should be avoided, and when looking at the preparation from the coronal surface the entire prepared surface should be visualized.
- If possible, reduction should be made in one pass, moving in a counterclockwise direction around the tooth.
- A level margin all around the tooth should be maintained.
- A stair-step reduction of the canine tooth may be necessary to maintain parallel walls (A).

Margins

Chamfer

Description

- A chamfer is a type of margin created by removing structure to leave a gradual transition to the uncut surface (B). This may be accomplished first by gross reduction with a coarse tapered diamond bur and then creating a finish line with a medium or fine tapered diamond bur.

Advantage

- This type of margin allows for a slip joint and is a good design for gold restorations.

Disadvantages

- The main disadvantage of a chamfer is that it is more difficult to design clearly.

- A chamfer is not a good design for a porcelain or porcelain fused to metal restoration because it does not give enough support to the edge of the porcelain.

Shoulder Joint

Description

- A shoulder joint is a butt joint (C). It is created at the same time as axial reduction using a tapered-cylinder flat-end bur.
- This margin must be used for porcelain restoration to give adequate support to the edge of the restoration.
- A shoulder with an internal bevel is created at the same time as axial reduction using a tapered-cylinder round-end bur (D).

Advantages

- The biggest advantage of this margin is that a definite finish line is created.
- For the beginner, the shoulder is more easily created.
- The diameter of the bur is an easy means by which to measure the amount of reduction performed.

Disadvantage

- Difficult to seal definitively.

Shoulder with External Bevel

Description

- The shoulder is trimmed with a flame or beveled-cylinder diamond bur (E).

Advantage

- Creates a better margin.

Disadvantage

- A steady hand is necessary to avoid destruction of the shoulder.

Additional Comments

- A metal cast crown requires axial reduction of 1 mm all over.
- A porcelain fused to metal crown requires a reduction of 1.5 to 2.0 mm to allow space for the porcelain.

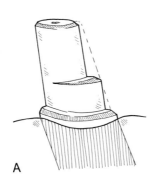

A

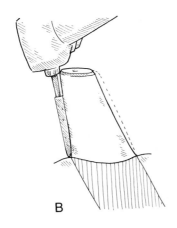

B

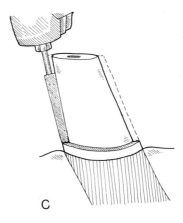

C

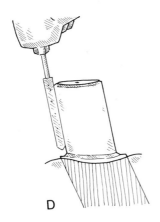

D

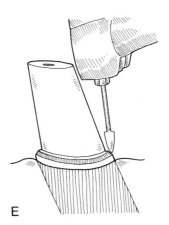

E

Table 8–5. DIAMOND BURS FOR CROWN THERAPY

Bur Type	Use
Tapered flat end	Creates flat shoulder
Long, thin round end	Creates chamfer
Long shank with flame tip	To modify shoulder preparation
Curettage, 55° bevel	Creates shoulder with bevel
12-mm Flame	Creates feather
Stip tipped	Periodontal use for curettage

Step 3—Taking Impressions and Castings

General Comments

- Several types of materials are available for taking impressions for crowns. The alginate impressions, as used for making study models for orthodontics, by themselves are not accurate enough for crown fabrication.

Rubber Base

Description

- These materials are rubber-like in nature and contain large molecules with weak interaction between them that are joined together at certain points to form a three-dimensional network.[2]
- The three kinds of commonly used rubber-based materials for taking impressions are: polysulfide rubber, siloxane polymers, and vinyl polysiloxane.

Polysulfide Rubber

Description

- An impression material supplied as a two-part system, containing a base and a catalyst.

Use

- Impressions for crown, bridge, implant crown.

Advantage

- Good working time (although may be too long for many).

Disadvantages

- Requires thorough mixing.
- Lack of a "snap set"—curing goes on slowly.
- Impressions should be poured after 15 minutes and before 72 hours.
- Messy; unpleasant odor.

Siloxane Polymers

Use

- Crowns and bridges.

Advantage

- Accurate representation of the prepared tooth.

Disadvantage

- Poor ability of dental stone to "wet and flow" into the impression.

Vinyl Polysiloxane Polymers

Description

- These are silicone-addition-type impression materials.
- These impression materials are usually available in different consistencies: light, medium, and heavy body.

Use

- Impressions for crown and bridge.

Advantages

- Accurate reproduction of detail.
- Dimensional stability; prevents longer delay before pouring.
- Excellent elasticity; enables recovery from undercuts.
- Good tear strength reduces the likelihood of impression damage.

Disadvantage

- Decreased wetability; stone does not flow as readily into the impression.

Materials

- Orthodontic trays.
- Large paper mixing pads.
- Large spatulas.

Technique

- The crown is prepared as previously described.
- The retraction cord is pulled from the gingival sulcus just prior to taking the impression.

Step 1—Equal parts of the material are placed on a paper pad.
Step 2—The material is thoroughly mixed.
Step 3—The material is placed into an impression tray.
Step 4—The tray is inserted over the prepared tooth.
Step 5—Once set, the impression material is removed with a snapping movement from the mouth and the cast is poured.

Variation in Technique with Vinyl Polysiloxane Polymers

- The light-bodied material is mixed and placed into a curved-tip syringe.
- The light-bodied material is injected around the prepared tooth and into the subgingival area.
- Equal amounts of the medium-bodied material are placed on the mixing pad, are mixed, and are placed in the impression tray.
- The filled tray is placed over the light-bodied material covering the prepared tooth.
- Once the impression material is set, the tray and impression material are removed, and a cast is poured in standard fashion.

Complications/Cautions

- Organic contaminants on the teeth may cause roughness to the impression or bubbles and voids.
- Roughness may be caused by overdessication of teeth prior to taking the impression.

- Inadequate working time caused by an incorrect base/accelerator ratio, with excess catalyst or ambient temperature and humidity too high.
- Prolonged setting time caused by incorrect base/accelerator ratio, poor storage conditions, or use of outdated materials.
- Poor mixing techniques resulting in an uneven mix, causing uneven curing that may cause distortion, loss of detail, and/or roughness of the impression as well as bubbles or voids.
- Distortion, caused by poor adhesion of impression material to tray, may be avoided by using the tray adhesive that comes with many impression materials.
- Distortion, from partial polymerization, caused by excessive delay in seating the tray in the mouth.
- Distortion and loss of detail due to movement of the tray after it is seated in position.
- Excessive bulk of material may cause marked thermal contraction on cooling, thus causing distortion.
- Loss of detail and/or roughness caused by removing the tray prior to full setting of the impression material.
- Prolonged removal of the tray from the mouth may cause prolonged stress, with distortion and loss of detail of the impression.
- After taking the impression, place the tray with the tray down and impression material up to avoid distortion of the impression.
- Care must be taken to make sure the material is completely set prior to removal from the mouth.

Hydrocolloid/Alginate

Description

- A two-part process is performed where, first, the impression material is warmed and injected around the tooth.
- As the injected material cools and solidifies, an alginate mixture is mixed, placed in a tray, and placed over the solidified material.

Use

- Impressions for crowns.

Advantage

- Superior reproduction of the crown preparation.

Disadvantage

- Requires a boiler pot to heat the hydrocolloid.

Equipment/Instruments

- Boiler pot and thermometer.
- Impression trays.
- Cohere* reversible hydrocolloid.
- Large-gauge injection needles.
- Rubber bowl.
- Large spatula.
- Type II alginate (irreversible hydrocolloid).

---

*Gingi-Pak, Camarillo, CA 93011

Technique

Step 1—The syringe containing the hydrocolloid material is placed in the boiling pot and the water is brought to a boil for 5 minutes.

Step 2—The temperature in the pot is reduced to a constant 140 to 150° F for a minimum of 10 minutes prior to use.

Step 3 (optional)—The teeth may be lighly sprayed with a preimpression release agent.

Step 4—A large-gauge injection needle (that comes with the hydrocolloid) is placed on the syringe and the material is injected around the prepared tooth.

Step 5—Type II alginate is mixed in a rubber bowl and placed into the impression tray.

Step 6—A standard alginate, irreversible hydrocolloid impression is made (see Chapter 9 on taking alginate impressions).

Step 7—Once set, the alginate with the hardened hydrocolloid around the tooth is removed from the mouth, and standard casts are poured.

Complication/Caution

- Care should be taken not to burn the oral cavity by using inadequately tempered hydrocolloid (too hot).

Bite Registration

General Comment

- Bite registration allows the dental laboratory to place the models in proper articulation to avoid occlusal interference.

Indications

- Crown and bridge.
- Orthodontics.

Objective

- To obtain an accurate representation of the occlusion.

Materials

- Vinyl polysiloxane.
- Bite wax.

Technique

Step 1—The patient's vital signs are checked and anesthetic stability confirmed.

Step 2—The patient is extubated. The tongue may be gently "rolled back" over itself and placed into the pharynx. The patient should be observed to make sure that breathing is normal.

Step 3—The impression material of choice (a self-mixing injection-type vinyl polysiloxane sets rapidly and removes operator error in mixing) is placed over the canine and incisor teeth.

- If using a chemical curing material, the cure may be hastened by the use of a hair dryer.
- If using bite wax, the wax may be warmed in warm water or with the hair dryer and placed between the incisors.

Step 4—The bite impression material is carefully removed

Step 5—The tongue is placed back in the normal position, and the patient is reintubated.

Complications

- Respiratory obstruction with the tongue.
- Inaccurate impression.
- Recovery from anesthesia prior to setting of the impression material.

Considerations for Making Casts for Crowns/Bridges

Material Complications

- Poor cleaning of the impression prior to pouring the cast may cause an inferior, rough, or chalky cast.
- Excess water in the impression may cause a distorted cast.
- Premature removal of the cast from the impression may cause breaking of the cast.
- Poor mixing or casting technique may cause bubbles or an inferior cast.
- Contamination of the impression surface or dental stone powder may cause a rough cast.
- Incorrect water/powder ratio for the dental stone may cause distortion of the cast. A hard stone material is preferred over plaster of Paris.

Step 4—Manufacture of Temporary Crown (Optional)

General Comments

- The prepared tooth may be protected until the final cast restoration is returned from the laboratory and placed.
- In veterinary patients, this step can make the difference between a successful restoration and a failure because our patients and clients respond variably to instruction to protect the prepared tooth.
- A temporary restoration must be strong enough to remain in place for the time needed.
- The owner should be able to clean around it to prevent soft tissue inflammation or deterioration of the periodontal health, which could interfere with placement of the final restoration.

Direct Acrylic Technique

Step 1—An alginate impression is taken of the prepared tooth and the surrounding area (A).

Step 2—After unseating the impression, a round-ball carbide bur is used to carve some of the alginate away from the impression of the prepared tooth (B).

Step 3—The alginate is filled with a thin mix of acrylic (C).

Step 4—The tooth and surrounding gingiva are lubricated with petroleum jelly (D) and the alginate with the acrylic is seated in the mouth (E).

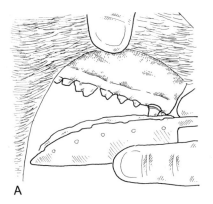

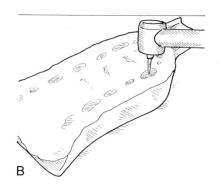

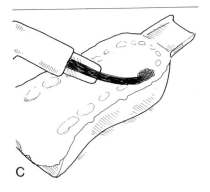

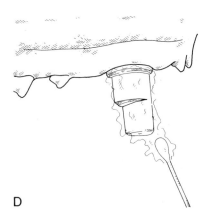

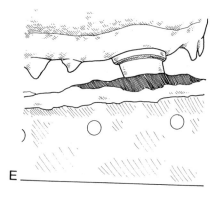

Direct Acrylic Technique *(Continued)*

Step 5—When the acrylic has hardened, the alginate is removed and the acrylic casting is removed from the alginate *(A)*.

Step 6—The casting is trimmed and shaped with acrylic burs in a slow-speed handpiece *(B)*.

Step 7—The acrylic casting is trial fitted and trimmed again or shaped as needed.

• Because the primary function of the temporary restoration is to protect the pre-pared tooth, it is usually better to make it smaller so the patient will not place as much pressure or force on it.

Step 8—Once it fits properly, the restoration can be smoothed with sanding discs and polished with wet pumice on a wheel.

Step 9—A zinc oxide–eugenol temporary cement is applied to cement it in place *(C)*. The restoration is cemented in place *(D)*.

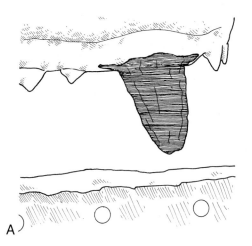

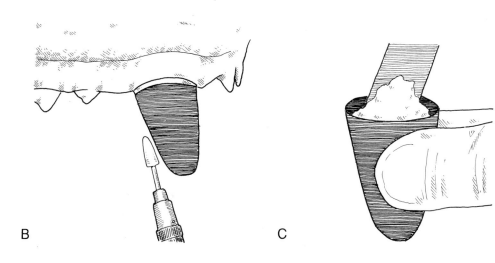

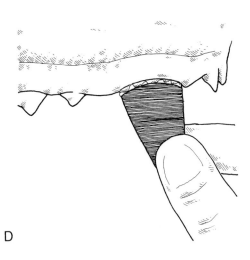

Step 5—Laboratory Orders and Manufacture of Crown

- A written laboratory prescription is sent with the model castings and bite impression registrations.
- The prescription should include type of material to be used for the crown and color with a shade guide.
- The model and new crown are returned from the dental laboratory *(A)*.

Step 6—Trial Placement of the Crown

Substep 1—The temporary crown and filling material are carefully removed, so the shape of the preparation is not altered *(B)*. Clean the surface with a curette *(C)*.

Substep 2—The crown and/or dowel core are checked for proper fit by trial seating on/in the tooth *(D)*.

Substep 3—If there is any binding, remove the casting and brush it with polishing rouge dissolved in chloroform, and reseat the casting. Alternatively, occlusal chalk may be sprayed into the crown and the crown fit over the tooth *(E)*.

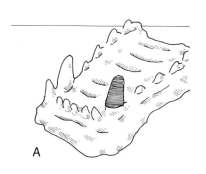

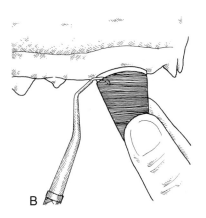

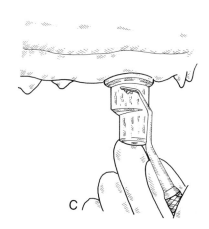

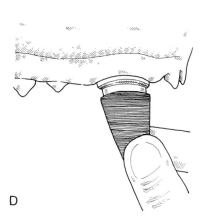

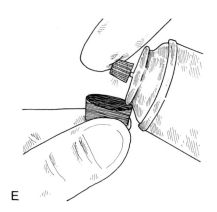

Step 6—Trial Placement of the Crown *(Continued)*

Substep 4—Remove the casting and examine the tooth for residue. Residue *(arrow)* indicates the areas that are binding *(A)*.

Substep 5—Carefully remove some material tooth structure from these spots with a bur and retest *(B)*.

- This process is repeated until the casting seats properly and all the rouge is removed.
- The fit should be snug and the margins smooth.
- Margins are examined with an explorer by pointing the tip toward the gingiva and sliding it down the crown onto the root.
- If the explorer slides over the interface smoothly the crown fits properly.
- This procedure is repeated in several places around the tooth.
- Pumice the inside of the crown with a prophy brush with flour pumice *(C)*.
- Pumice the tooth with a prophy brush *(D)*.

Complications

- Avoid acids, alcoholic solutions, or pure alcohol when placing the crown on a vital tooth.

- When the cement is dry, do not remove any residual cement with sonic or ultrasonic scalers because this may destroy the molecular structure of the cement and thereby weaken the bond and cause loss of the crown.
- Use spatula/hand scaler/curette to remove excess cement.
- If the tooth is damaged to a degree that little structure remains, the surface area is increased with additional cuts of box shapes or grooves, or a combination of the two, in the wall of the tooth.
- Teeth with shortened coronal height may be built up using a dowel-core technique or post-retained buildup, or the crown can be lengthened surgically.
- Although preservation of tooth structure is important, enough space must be made to allow for the thickness of the metal. If the metal is too thin, the restoration will flex or bend under occlusal forces, and the restoration will deteriorate or fail. Bulk can be added at margins where rigidity and reinforcement are needed.

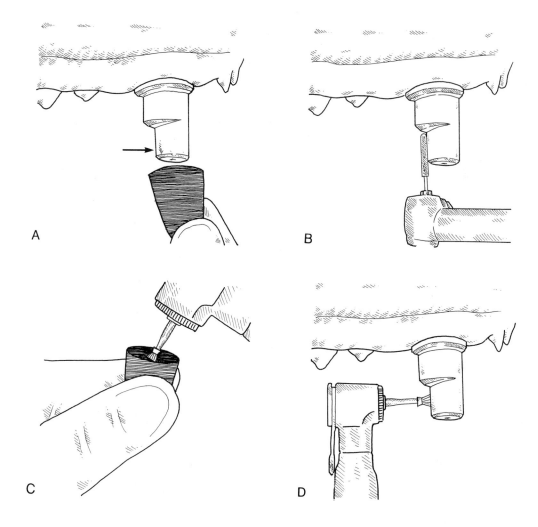

A

B

C

D

Step 7—Cementation of Crown

Technique

Substep 1—The prepared tooth crown is rinsed well with water *(A)*.

Substep 2—The prepared tooth crown is dried according to the type of cement used *(B)*. Some cements require the surface to be bone dry, whereas others (glass ionomers) require a slight amount of moisture (see section on cements).

Substep 3—The manufacturer's directions are followed in mixing the cement *(C)*.

Substep 4—The cement is placed into the crown with a spatula *(D)*.

Substep 5—The crown is seated and held in place firmly until the cement hardens *(E)*.

Substep 6—Excess cement is trimmed from the crown *(F)*.

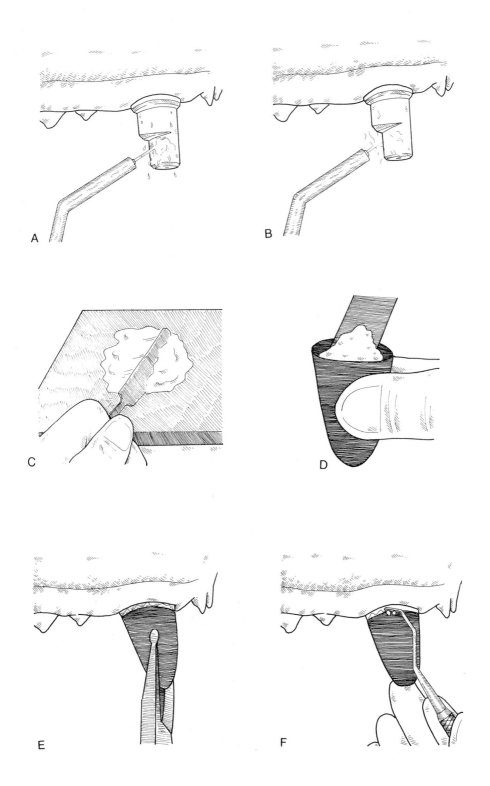

Cementation Materials for Crowns

- Most dental cements have a similar background, and their basic chemistry is derived from a powder, either zinc oxide or aluminum silicate, and a liquid, either phosphoric acid or polyacrylic acid[15] (Table 8–6).
- Cements are also made from composite resins.

Zinc Phosphate

Description

- A mixture of zinc oxide and phosphoric acid.
- This cement has been used for a long time in human dentistry.

Use

- Luting cement for seating permanent prosthesis, crown, or bridge.

Advantage

- One of the primary advantages, its excellent thermal insulation, may not be applicable in veterinary medicine because most of our patients are not fed food with a wide range of temperatures.

Disadvantage

- Very poor adhesive properties limit its use to temporary crowns or techniques that use mechanical retention.

Zinc Oxide–Eugenol

Description

- A mixture of zinc oxide and eugenol.

Use

- As a temporary luting agent for crowns and bridges, or as a temporary filling material.
- Also used as a root canal sealant.

Advantage

- Soothing effect on the pulp.

Disadvantage

- Poor retentive and other physical properties limit its use in veterinary dentistry.

Zinc Polycarboxylate

Description

- The liquid is an aqueous solution of polyacrylic acid and copolymers, whereas the powder is zinc oxide with some magnesium or stannous oxide.
- Stannous fluoride may be added to increase the strength of the cement.

Use

- Luting crowns.
- Must have very clean metal casting for adhesion of cement to crown.

Advantage

- Adhesion to tooth structure.

Disadvantage

- Short working times.

Glass Ionomer

Description

- The glass ionomer cements have been modified to provide radiopacity and handling properties suitable for lining or cementing purposes.

Table 8–6. TABLE CEMENTS

Zinc Phosphate	
Product	Manufacturer
Hy-Bond Zinc Phosphate	Shofu
Zinc Polycarboxylate	
Product	Manufacturer
Durelon	ESPE/Premier
Zinc Oxide-Eugenol	
Product	Manufacturer
Hy-Bond Zinc Oxide Eugenol	Shofu
Glass Ionomers	
Product	Manufacturer
Biocem	L.D. Caulk
Cement/Liner	Parkell
Chem-Fil	Detrey/Dentsply
Ever Bond	Kerr
Fuji Ionomer Type I	Fuji
Lining Cement	G.C. International
Ketac-Cem	ESPE/Premier
Shofu 1	Shofu
Composite Resin Cements	
Product	Manufacturer
Comspan	L.D. Caulk
Conclude	3M
Panavia	J. Morita
Bridge Cements	
Product	Manufacturer
Resin Bonded Bridge Cement	Kerr
MD Bridge Cementation Cement	Den-Mat
Maryland Bridge Adhesive	Getz

Advantages

- Cariostatic activity.
- Bonds to dentin.
- High strength.

Disadvantages

- Dental hypersensitivity reported in humans; may be avoided by using proper technique.
- In vital teeth, pulp sensitivity and possible necrosis caused by chemical irritation from the material and leakage may be a problem.[16]
- Glass ionomers initially have a low pH.

Cautions/Problem Solutions

- The tooth should not be overdried, but rather dried with a gentle stream of air, or simply blotted dry with a gauze pad or cotton pellet.
- Observe mixing ratios recommended by the manufacturer; otherwise, excessive free acid will remain in the tooth structure and cause sensitivity.
- Avoid excessive hydraulic pressure by creating channels in the crown for excess cement to flow out or seating the crown with a slow, steady pressure when cementing it in place.

- Prevent contamination with saliva or water in the early setting stages by using varnish, cocoa butter, or light-cure bonding agent on the marginal surface.
- If recommended with the particular luting agent, use a dentin conditioner prior to placement.

Composite Resin Cements

Description

- Some of the newer products, such as Panavia,* bond chemically to metals, porcelain, tooth enamel, and unetched dentin. Panavia sets in an oxygen-free environment.

Advantage

- Virtually insoluble in water.

Disadvantages

- Irritating to pulp; therefore, pulp must be protected by calcium hydroxide.
- Poor manipulative characteristics; limited working times.

---

*J. Morita USA, Inc., 14712 Bentley Circle, Tustin, CA 92680

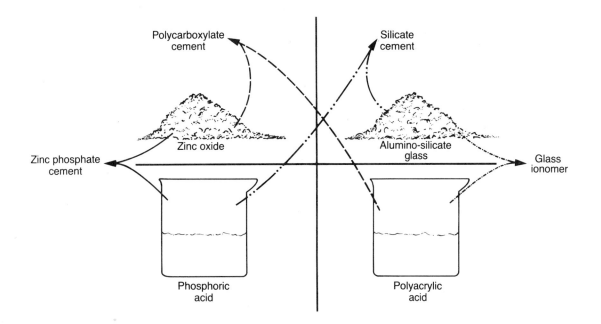

Special Situations

Crown–Dowel-Core Buildup

General Comment

- The minimum distance for dowel length is equal to the crown length.

Indication

- If the crown to be prepared has little remaining retentive surface area, a dowel-core buildup is necessary.

Contraindications

- Vertical root fractures.
- Teeth with inflammatory resorption.
- Teeth subject to excessive forces.

Objective

- To build up a crown to enable restoration of the tooth.

Materials

- Crown preparation instruments and materials.
- Peeso reamers.

Technique

- Prior to axial preparation, the root canal chamber is prepared.

Step 1—The endodontic filling in the coronal portion of the canal is removed *(A)*.

Ideally, two thirds to three quarters of the length of the canal is used *(B)*.

- The natural curve of the canine tooth usually precludes access to the desired two thirds to three quarters length of the root.
- The preparation is extended to the greatest length possible in a straight line.
- If the dentinal wall at the curve is thick, reduction of this area can lengthen the preparation.
- Care is exercised to avoid penetration through the root wall.
- Initially, Peeso reamers are used to remove the gutta percha and to enlarge the canal.
- These reamers have a flexible shank and easily follow the gutta percha.
- The graduated sizes of Peeso reamers offer gradual canal enlargement.
- In mature teeth, the walls are shaped parallel to aid in retention.
- If increased length is required, or the canal is larger than the Peeso reamers, a tapered fissure bur is used.
- Undercuts are carefully avoided.

Step 2—A contrabevel is placed around the periphery of the occlusal portion of the tooth *(C)*.

Step 3—Axial reduction, as with crown preparation previously described.

Step 4—The post is trial fitted *(D)*; there should be no wobble. In long canals, a K-wire or other stainless steel pin should be used and bent to conform to the length of the canal. In this situation, the pin will conform to the natural canal, rather than a track drilled by the Peeso reamer.

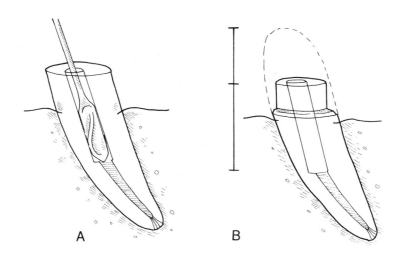

A

B

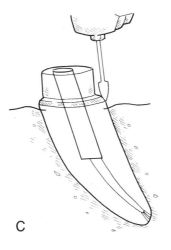

C

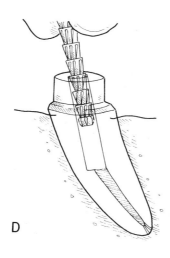

D

Technique (Continued)

Step 5—The cement is mixed and placed on the post (A).

Step 6—The post is placed in the canal and held until the cement sets (B).

Step 7—Core material is mixed according to the manufacturer's instructions and is placed over the post and tooth (C).

Step 8—Once the core material has set, a standard crown preparation is performed (D).

- The axial preparation of these teeth is much the same, except fewer, if any, "stair steps" are needed.

- The shoulder is formed around the tooth and the axial reduction done.

Complications

- Perforation while preparing the root canal for dowel; the treatment is to seal the perforation with calcium hydroxide paste.[17]
- Perforation of the root canal; happens mostly on the mesial side of the tooth curvature.

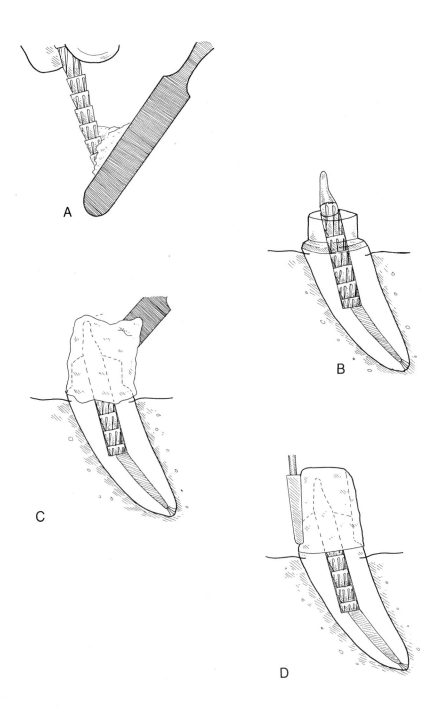

Crown—Dowel Core

- A dowel core is a custom-cast post and coronal buildup.
- One of the strongest methods of crown replacement is the use of a dowel-core casting.
- Ideally, the dowel should be two thirds to three quarters the length of the root and should leave no less than 3 mm of the endodontic filling material at the apex of the tooth.
- The path of insertion becomes important when placing the crown.
- The path of insertion is the line that coincides with the long axis of the preparation.
- This is not necessarily equal to the long axis of the tooth.
- The crown will be placed on the prepared tooth along this line, and no other oral structures can restrict the placement of the crown along this line.
- The path of insertion must always be determined prior to starting the preparation.
- Any retentive grooves or boxes must be oriented in the same direction as the path of insertion.
- The path of insertion of the dowel core and that of the crown do not necessarily need to be the same. The canal is prepared with a Peeso reamer as previously described.

Step 1—The prepared canal is lubricated with a small Peeso reamer and cotton ball covered with petroleum jelly.

Step 2—A plastic sprue, notched or roughened to prevent it from pulling out of the final acrylic pattern, is trimmed to fit into the canal to the apical limit of the dowel preparation.

Step 3—Acrylic is mixed in a dappen dish to a thin consistency.

Step 4—The acrylic is placed in the prepared canal without any voids.

Step 5—A plastic sprue is seated in the canal, and the acrylic is added as needed to encompass the bevel on the occlusal edge of the preparation.

Step 6—As the acrylic reaches a pliable polymerization stage, the pattern is moved in and out of the canal to prevent it from locking.

Step 7—After the acrylic is polymerized, the pattern is removed and the dowel inspected for voids and adequate extension into the canal.

Step 8—If needed, another mix of the acrylic can be used to finish the dowel.

Step 9—When the acrylic has polymerized, seat it and place more acrylic on the tooth around the sprue.

- This acrylic becomes the foundation for the buildup.

Step 10—The pattern is seated in the tooth and shaped to fit the pulp chamber/root canal.

Step 11—The final reduction should closely replicate the desired final form of the dowel.

- The prosthodontic laboratory will use this pattern to cast the post or dowel.

Step 12—The post dowel and core are seated in the tooth, and the gingival retraction cord is placed in the gingival sulcus.

Step 13—An impression is taken (see impression techniques).

- When the impression material has set, it is removed and examined.
- The margin of the preparation must be accurately reproduced and free of flaws.
- The pattern (dowel and core) and impression are sent to a prosthodontic laboratory for preparation of the final castings.

Step 14—Temporary cavity filling material is placed in the coronal orifice of the endodontic canal to protect it until the castings are returned from the laboratory.

Step 15—After the custom dowel and crown are returned from the laboratory, the castings are inspected for fit as with the crown technique.

Step 16—The cement is mixed and placed in the canal and on the dowel.

Step 17—The dowel casting is seated slowly, allowing excess cement to escape, and is held firmly in place until the cement has hardened.

Step 18—Excess cement is removed from the margin.

Step 19—The cast crown is trial seated.

Step 20—The same process of checking fit, precision fitting, and cementing is repeated with the crown casting.

Surgical Crown Lengthening[10]
General Comments

- When teeth are fractured at or near the level of alveolar bone, insufficient crown length may prevent enough retentive surface from being available.
- By decreasing the root length and increasing the crown length, retention may be obtained.

Indications

- Tooth fractured at, near, or below the gingival crest.
- Tooth fractured below the alveolar crest.
- Inadequate retentive coronal surface.
- Gingival tissue overlying coronal surface.

Contraindications

- Patients who will place excessive force on the teeth.
- General health not allowing multiple anesthetic procedures.

Objective

- To expose more tooth surface for crown retention.

Materials

- Materials previously described for crown preparation.
- Oral surgical pack.

Technique

Step 1—The tooth and surrounding tissue are examined for pockets, the depth of keratinized gingiva is measured, and the tooth and surrounding area are "sounded" with an explorer to determine the level of bone and extent of fracture.

Step 2—An inverse-bevel scalloped incision and/or gingivectomy with or without mesial and distal incisions are performed as necessary, as described in Chapter 5. The gingival collar is removed.

Step 3—Using both high-speed and hand instrumentation, bone is carefully removed around the tooth to expose the apical level of the tooth fracture.

Step 4—The bone is smoothed and reshaped.

Step 5—The elevated flap is apically repositioned.

Step 6—The crown margins are prepared, built up if necessary, and finished in routine fashion.

Special Teeth

Canine Teeth

Substep 1—Axial reduction is started on the mesial surface. Reduce it to the desired amount and create a straight surface.

Substep 2—The labial and lingual surfaces are reduced until the prepared surfaces approach the 6° taper.

Substep 3—On the distal surface, the preparation is "stair stepped" to create parallelism with minimal tooth reduction.

- The first "stair step" starts at the gingival edge and extends coronally as the tooth is reduced.
- The shoulder at the gingival edge is as much as 0.5 mm deeper than others in the preparation.
- When the natural shape of the tooth is tapered to the point that parallelism is not achievable, the next "stair step" is cut.
- Moving coronally, parallelism is created to the limits allowable by the natural shape of the tooth without excessive tooth reduction to create a shoulder close to the same dimension as the first shoulder.
- As the preparation is continued coronally, "stair steps" are created as needed.
- With most dog canine teeth, two to three "stair steps" are needed.

Substep 4—The final margin is finished by creating a bevel at the edge of the shoulder.

- This is best done with a flame-shaped diamond bur, using the beveled end of the bur as a gauge for cutting the tooth.
- The bur is held parallel to the tooth, and the beveled end is moved around the shoulder.
- The final bevel on the tooth is approximately the same size as the beveled end of the bur.
- When a fracture has shortened a tooth, fewer "stair steps" are needed.

Molars and Premolars

- The technique used for molars and pre-molars is similar to that used for canines and incisors.

Substep 1—A tapered diamond bur is used for occlusal and axial preparation of premolars and molars.

- Occlusal reduction is performed only in areas that are actually in occlusion.
- Those surfaces or areas in occlusion with the opposing tooth need to be reduced sufficiently to allow 1 to 1.5 mm of clearance between the restoration and the opposing tooth.
- Sharp edges of cusps are reduced and beveled to facilitate the casting process in the laboratory.
- Axial reduction is created with a round-end diamond bur and is initiated by creating a shoulder at the gingival edge.

Substep 2—When the axial reduction is adequate, the edge of the shoulder is beveled with a flame-shaped diamond bur.

- Retention is achieved with creation of parallelism and reduction for space requirements of the crown.
- An adequate approximation of parallelism is easily achieved on the lingual-to-buccal axis.
- The shape of the fourth premolars makes the achievement of parallelism on a mesial-to-distal axis difficult (A).

Substep 3—Additional retention is achieved in endodontically treated teeth by preparing the pulp canals, beginning with the removal of the gutta percha with a Peeso reamer to a depth at least equal to the height of the crown (B and C).

- The canals are prepared with a flat-end tapered diamond bur so the "line of draw" coincides with the long axis of the prepared tooth (D).
- As the bur is moved from one canal to the next, it is held steady so each canal is prepared parallel to the other.

Substep 4—The coronal edge of the canal is expanded or beveled to prevent binding as the restoration is seated.

- The remainder of the preparation is identical to preparations in canine teeth (E and F).

Gingival Retraction

Description

- The gingiva may be retracted away from the tooth by using a gingival retraction cord.
- The cord may be precoated with a hemostatic agent or may be dipped into the hemostatic agent.

Use

- Crown therapy.
- Adhesive restorations close to gingiva.
- Hemorrhage control.

Advantage

- Allows better visualization and working space.

Disadvantage

- Occasionally may interfere with working space.

Materials

- Gingicord,* GingiAid,* GingiBraid.†
- Gingicord packer, Nemitz no. 3.*

Technique

Step 1—The cord is cut to the length of the gingiva to be packed.

Step 2—The cord is packed into the gingival sulcus with a Gingicord packer.

Complications/Cautions

- Care should be taken not to cut the gingiva.
- Excessive hemorrhage may be controlled by pinpoint electrocautery.

---

*GingiPak, Camarillo, CA 93010
†Van R Dental, Los Angeles, CA 90034

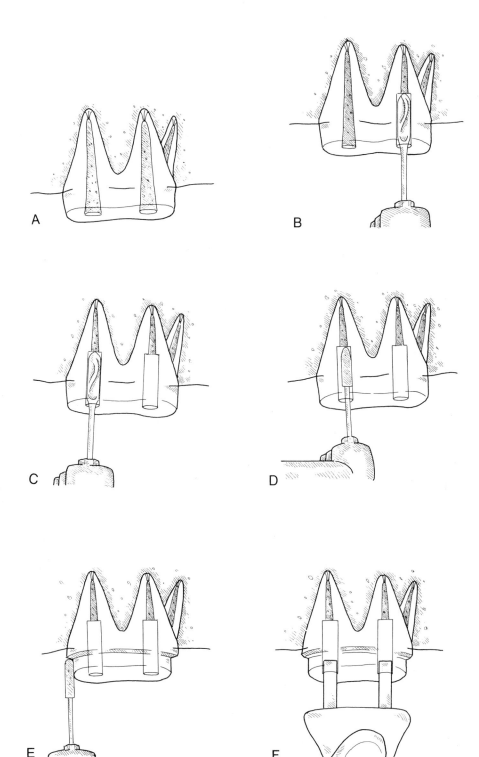

Die Stone

Description

- A harder stone is created by mixing gypsum stone with water, letting it set and dry, and then grinding it again.

Use

- Restorations.

Advantages

- Stone is harder; gives a better chance to remove from the impression without fracture.
- When mixed in proper weight/volume proportions as directed by the manufacturer, it is more accurate.

Materials

- Mixing bowl.
- Spatula.
- Scale.
- Syringe/measuring cup to measure volume.

Technique

- Mix according to instructions used in Chapter 9.

Improving Metal-To-Cement Adhesion

- Roughening the inside of metal crown surface may improve cement adhesion to the metal. This may be accomplished in the office by using a Micro-etcher.*
- Diamond roughening is not a good way to roughen the crown.
- Chemical etching is messy, possibly dangerous, and not a good technique.
- The prosthodontic laboratory may be able to sandblast the crown or bridge. In this case, the restoration may be returned in a liquid environment. The crown is protected in this environment until ready for cementation.

---

*Danville Engineering, 881 Danville Blvd, Danville, CA 94526.

Restorations over Vital Teeth

General Comments

- Restorations placed over vital teeth require special considerations so the pulp tissue is not damaged at the time the restoration is placed or at a later date.
- Lining and base cement materials are used in restorative dentistry as pulp-protection agents (Table 8–7).
- Liners and bases provide insulation under metallic restorative materials and a chemical barrier under plastic restoratives.

Calcium Hydroxide

Description

- Calcium hydroxide lining cements are commonly used to promote pulpal protection and healing.

Advantage

- The alkaline environment encourages remineralization and antibacterial activity.

Disadvantages

- Low strength properties, leading to a weak structure.
- High solubility, leading to resorption of the material.

Table 8–7. LINING/BASE MATERIALS

Calcium Hydroxide Cements	
Product	Manufacturer
Advanced Formula II Dycal	L.D. Caulk
Life	Kerr
Reocap	Vivadent
Reolit	Vivadent
Prisma VLC Dycal	L.D. Caulk
Care	Vivadent

Glass Ionomer Liners	
Product	Manufacturer
Aqua Cem	Detrey/Dentsply
Fuji Dentin Cement	Fuji
Ketac-Bond	ESPE/Premier
Ketac-Cem	ESPE/Premier
Ketac-Silver	ESPE/Premier
Lining Cement	Fuji
Miracle Mix	Fuji
Shofu Base	Shofu
Shofu Lining	Shofu
Zionomer	Den-Mat

Resin-Based Calcium Hydroxide

Description

- Calcium hydroxide is incorporated into a resin base.

Advantage

- Easy to use.

Disadvantage

- Little is known of its relative properties and clinical performance.

BLEACHING OF NONVITAL TEETH

General Comment

- Stained teeth may be whitened by using concentrated hydrogen peroxide solutions.

Indication

- Bleaching of nonvital teeth.

Contraindication

- Is not to be used on vital teeth.

Materials

- Hydrogen peroxide* (active and walking technique).
- Peroxyborate monohydrate† (walking technique).

Techniques[18]

Active Technique

Step 1—Root canal therapy is performed; a liner is placed over the gutta percha in the root canal to prevent penetration of the hydrogen peroxide into the apex.
Step 2—The gingiva is coated with petroleum jelly.

*Superoxol, Union Broach Dental Products, 3640 37th Street, Long Island, NY 11101.
†Amosan

Step 3—A rubber dam is placed over the tooth.
Step 4—A clamp is placed.
Step 5—The rubber dam is ligated with floss.
Step 6—The pulp chamber and surface of the tooth are acid etched for 60 seconds with phosphoric acid.
Step 7—The pulp chamber is thoroughly rinsed with water for 1 minute and dried.
Step 8—Cotton pellets or paper points are saturated with hydrogen peroxide.
Step 9—The saturated paper points or cotton pellets are placed into and around the tooth.
Step 10—Heat is applied to the tooth surface with a heating unit, Heat 'N Touch unit, or hair dryer. Heat should be applied to each surface for 60 seconds.
Step 11—The pellets and cotton points are replaced several times, for a total of four to six cycles.
Step 12—If bleaching is obtained, the pulp chamber is rinsed thoroughly for at least 1 minute with water and dried with paper points.
Step 13—The coronal portion of the canal and the access site are restored.

Walking Technique

Steps 1 through 11—The tooth is prepared as in the active technique.
Step 12—Peroxyborate monohydrate is mixed with 30% hydrogen peroxide to form a thick paste.
Step 13—The paste is placed into the pulp chamber, leaving space for the temporary filling material.
Step 14—A cotton pellet is placed over it.
Step 15—The access opening is sealed with a glass ionomer or zinc phosphate base.
Step 16—The patient is returned for reexamination and replacement of the walking paste as needed.
Step 17—Once the tooth is bleached, a restoration is placed.

Complications

- Leakage of hydrogen peroxide under the rubber dam.
- Irritation/burning of the gingiva.
- Safety goggles must be worn at all times during bleaching procedures by all staff in

the dental area; extremely caustic agents are used.

Aftercare—Follow-up

- Tooth-whitening pastes may be beneficial in keeping the tooth bleached.

References

1. Basrani E. Fractured Teeth. Philadelphia: Lea & Febiger, 1985.
2. Phillips RW. Skinner's Science of Dental Materials (8 ed.). Philadelphia: W.B. Saunders Co., 1982:646.
3. Zwemer TJ. Boucher's Clinical Dental Terminology (3 ed.). St. Louis: C.V. Mosby Co., 1982.
4. Leinfelder KF, Lemons JE. Clinical Restorative Materials and Techniques. Philadelphia: Lea & Febiger, 1989:359.
5. Tholen M. Veterinary restorative dentistry–1: Basic principles. VM/SAC 1983;12:1875–1880.
6. Croll TP. Repair of defective class I composite resin restorations. Quintessence Int 1990;21(9).
7. Eisner ER. Chronic subgingival tooth erosion in cats. Vet Med 1989;84(4):378–387.
8. Emily P. Restoring feline cervical erosion lesions. Vet Forum 1988;10:22–23.
9. Ben-Amar A. Reduction of microleakage around new amalgam restorations. J Am Dent Assoc 1989;119(6):725–728.
10. Limardi RJ. A Surgical Approach for Increasing Crown Length. Presented at the 1990 Meeting, co-sponsored by the Academy of Veterinary Dentistry and the American Veterinary Dental College. Las Vegas: Veterinary Dentistry '90, 1990.
11. Marzouk MA, Simoton AL, Gross RD. Operative Dentistry. St Louis: Ishiyaku, 1985.
12. Shillingburg HT, Sumiya H, Fisher DW. Preparations for Cast Gold Restorations. Berlin: Die Quintessenz, 1974:16, 25, 31, 147.
13. Johnson JF, Phillips RW, Dykema RW. Modern Practice in Crown and Bridge Prosthodontics. Philadelphia: W.B. Saunders Co., 1971:59, 374.
14. Coelho DH, Rieser JM. A Complete Fixed Bridge Procedure. New York: New York University Press, 1963:29, 38.
15. Seluk LW. Sucessful Glass Ionomer Techniques. Palo Alto: Shofu Dental Corporation, 1989.
16. Smith DC, Ruse ND. Acidity of glass ionomer cements during setting and its relation to pulp sensitivity. J Am Dent Assoc 1986;119(5):654–657.
17. Fahrenkrug P. Crowns: Indication, Preparation, Proceedings. Presented at the 1989 Meeting, co-sponsored by the Academy of Veterinary Dentistry and the American Veterinary Dental College. New Orleans: Veterinary Dentistry '89, 1989.
18. Golden AL. Vital and Non Vital Bleaching Techniques. New Orleans: Nabisco, 1988.

chapter 9

DENTAL ORTHODONTICS

OCCLUSAL (BITE) EVALUATION

- Bite evaluation must involve more than just the relationship of the incisors and number of teeth. The entire mouth and dentition must be used to evaluate occlusion properly.

Step 1—Observe the symmetry of the head, face, and dentition.

- The midpoints of the mandibular and maxillary dental arches should be centered over each other and should be in alignment with the midplane of the head.

Step 2—Count the teeth.

- There should be no missing teeth.

Canine Dental Formula
Primary

$$2\left(i\frac{3}{3}\ c\frac{1}{1}\ p\frac{3}{3}\right) = 28$$

Adult

$$2\left(I\frac{3}{3}\ C\frac{1}{1}\ P\frac{4}{4}\ M\frac{2}{3}\right) = 42$$

Feline Dental Formula
Primary

$$2\left(i\frac{3}{3}\ c\frac{1}{1}\ p\frac{3}{2}\right) = 26$$

Adult

$$2\left(I\frac{3}{3}\ C\frac{1}{1}\ P\frac{3}{2}\ M\frac{1}{1}\right) = 30$$

Step 3—Evaluate the occlusion of the incisors (A). The normal incisor occlusion has the large cusp of the lower incisors occluding near the cingulum on the lingual side of the upper incisors (B). The large cusps of the central incisors should be centered with each other. The second and third incisors lose their centered relationship and the large cusp of the third mandibular incisor should be in the interproximal space between the second and third maxillary incisors.

- The incisors should be in an evenly curved line with no rotation.

Step 4—Observe the relationship of the canine teeth (C).

- The mandibular canine tooth should occlude buccal to the gingiva of the maxilla and should divide the space between the maxillary canine tooth and the maxillary third incisor.
- This is the most reliable reference point in the mouth.[1]

Step 5—Observe the relationship of the premolars (D).

- The large cusp on the lower fourth premolar should divide the space between the upper third and fourth premolars.

Step 6—Observe the occlusal plane of the upper and lower arches (E).

- The premolars should interdigitate from the second premolars back to the cusps of the upper fourth premolar with overlapping of the cusp tips.
- The molars should occlude to allow the cusps to function in crushing.
- The premolars and molars should be aligned mesial to distal in a slightly curved line with none of the teeth rotated.

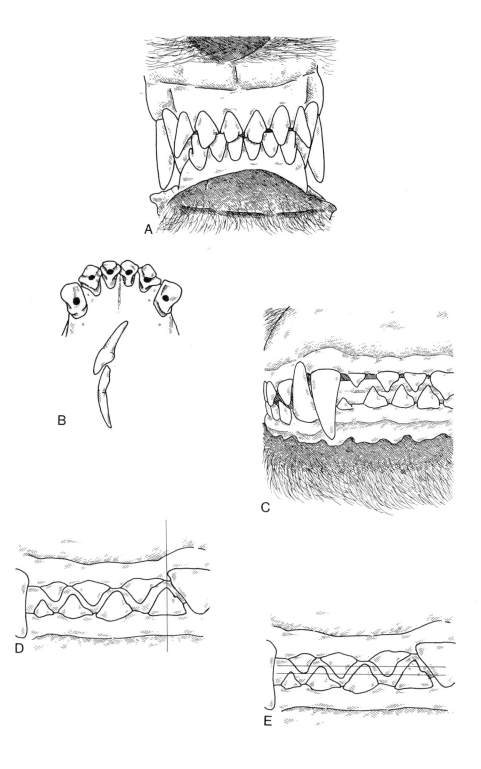

Classes of Occlusion

Normal

- Scissor bite: normal occlusion pattern in which the lower incisors occlude next to the cingulum on the lingual surface of the upper incisors.

Class 1

- Patients with class 1 occlusion have a normal occlusion with one or more teeth out of alignment or rotated.
- Anterior crossbite is a commonly seen abnormal occlusion where one or more of the lower incisors are anterior to the upper incisors and the rest of the teeth occlude normally *(A)*.
- Level bite: An abnormal occlusal pattern where the upper and lower incisors occlude cusp to cusp.
- Base narrow or lingually displaced canine teeth: the tips of the mandibular canine teeth are displaced lingually and occlude on the hard palate *(B)*. Base narrow mandibular canines may also occur in class 2 occlusions.

Class 2

- Patients with class 2 occlusion have the lower premolars and molars positioned behind (distal to) the normal relationship *(C and D)*. This occlusion may be also termed brachygnathism, overshot, retrusive mandible, or distal mandibular excursion.

Class 3

- Patients with class 3 occlusion have the lower premolars and molars positioned ahead (anterior) of the normal relationship *(E)*. This occlusion may also be termed prognathism, undershot, protrusive mandible, or mesial mandibular excursion.

Unclassified

- Wry bite: An abnormal occlusion caused by a difference in length of the two maxillae and mandibles. This abnormal occlusion is reported to be genetically created and can result in a variety of different jaw relationships.

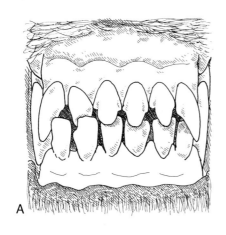

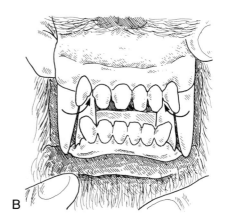

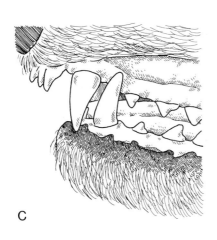

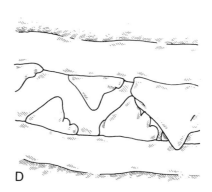

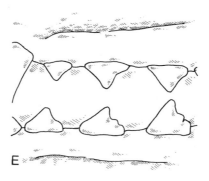

Orthodontic Fundamentals

- Tooth roots are held in the alveolus by the periodontal ligament (PDL) that attaches to the cementum on the tooth and the alveolar bone.
- Osteoclasts and osteoblasts are found in the alveolar bone.
- Forces applied to the crown of the tooth are transmitted by the PDL to the bone.
- Stretching the PDL stimulates the osteoblasts to deposit new bone.
- Compressing the PDL stimulates the osteoclasts to resorb bone.
- The magnitude of the force applied to the crown of the tooth is critical. If the force exceeds the capillary blood pressure in the PDL, then the PDL will necrose or hyalinize and become cell free. Osteoclasts then remove bone in the hyalinized area, and tooth movement continues again.
- Types of movement are created by the way the force is applied to the tooth:
  - Tipping—One part of the tooth moves a greater distance and direction than another (A).
  - Bodily—All parts of the tooth move the same distance in the same direction (B).
  - Rotational—The tooth is rotated around its axis (C).
  - Intrusion—The tooth is moved into the alveolus (D).
  - Extrusion—The tooth is moved out of the alveolus (E).
- Duration of the force also influences the response. The three classes of duration are:
  - Continuous—the force gradually falls (but does not reach zero) between adjustments.
  - Interrupted—The force falls to zero between adjustments.
  - Intermittent—The force falls to zero when a removable appliance is removed and regained when the appliance is replaced.
- Anchorage is resistance to unwanted tooth movement.[2] The object is to create a platform from which an orthodontic force may be exerted that will move the tooth and only minimally move the anchorage (unless one also wants to move the anchorage).
- Once tooth movement to the desired position has been obtained, the tooth or teeth must be maintained in their desired position; in veterinary orthodontics this is usually 2 to 4 weeks. This is known as the retainer period.

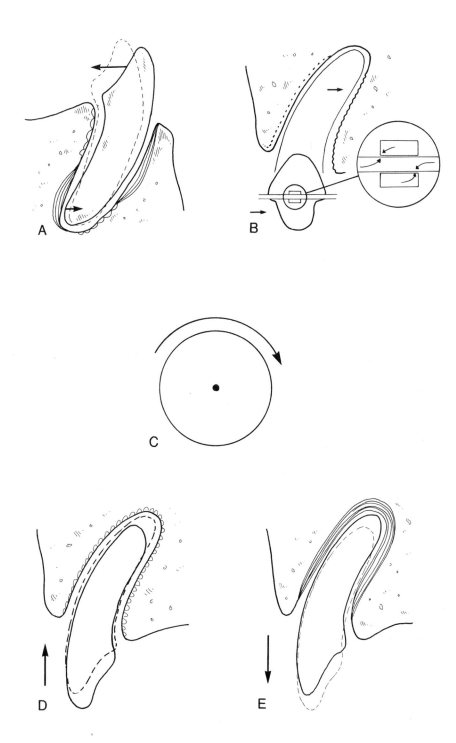

GENERAL ORTHODONTIC TECHNIQUES

Making an Impression

- A good impression and model are necessary for many dental procedures.
- They allow a practitioner to study and measure the oral architecture, to confer with a colleague or laboratory, and to fabricate prostheses and appliances.
- They also are an excellent medical record.
- An impression must be an accurate representation of the structure studied.

Indication

- Any time a model is needed for study, treatment planning, or appliance fabrication.

Contraindication

- Uncooperative patients or patients unable to undergo general anesthesia.

Materials

- Impression tray. Do not use styrofoam cups, cut soft plastic bottles, etc. as trays because they are too unstable.
- Alginate.
- Bowl and spatula.
- Room-temperature water.

Technique

Step 1—Select an impression tray that fits over all the teeth loosely *(A)*.

Step 2—The alginate is "fluffed" by gently rolling or shaking the container *(B)*.

Step 3—The alginate is measured into the mixing bowl with the measuring spoon provided with the alginate *(C)*. The amount will depend upon the size of the tray used. Use trial and error until you know how much alginate a particular tray size needs. Place the alginate in the rubber mixing bowl *(D)*.

Step 4—Measure water with the container provided with the alginate *(E)*. If tap water is too cold or too hot, use water from a storage flask at room temperature to avoid variations in setting time caused by water temperature. Water temperature affects the setting speed of the alginate. Warmer water speeds up the setting time; colder water slows it down. Pour all the water into the bowl with the alginate at the same time *(F)*.

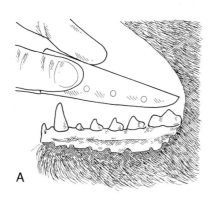

A

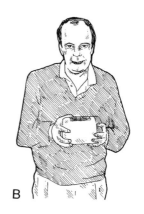

B

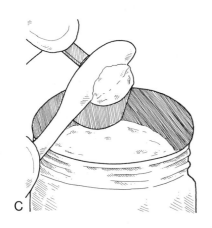

C

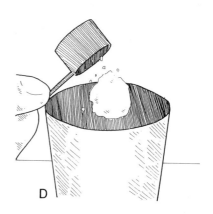

D

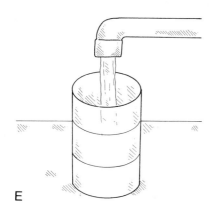

E

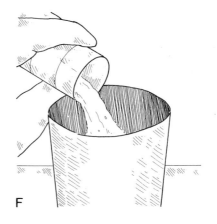

F

Technique (Continued)

Step 5—The alginate and water are mixed with the spatula (A). Incorporate all the powder first by mixing in the center of the bowl. Smooth the mix by spatulating the mixture against the sides of the bowl with the spatula (B). The bowl is held in one hand and the spatula is used to vigorously spread the mixture onto the sides of the bowl. The entire mixing procedure should be completed in 30 to 45 seconds. The mixing is finished when all the lumps are removed and the consistency is homogeneous.

Step 6—The alginate is placed in the tray; be careful not to create air bubbles or voids (C).

- The surface is smoothed and lightly dampened with water.

Step 7—The patient's mouth is held open, and the tray with the alginate is carefully placed in the mouth (D). First contact with the teeth is made in the distal portion of the mouth and the tray is gently rocked forward to incorporate the teeth in the anterior portion of the mouth (E).

- Once the tray is in position it is held steady until the alginate has set. The time is dependent upon the alginate used and the temperature of the water.
- Test the setup by pressing a finger on exposed alginate. When the finger does not stick or leave an indentation the alginate has set.

Step 8—The tray with the alginate is removed from the mouth by firmly snapping it off the teeth (F).

- Examine the impression for voids, flaws, or bubbles. If there is an imperfection in the impression in a critical area, the impression should be retaken. If the model is not going to be poured immediately, wrap the alginate and tray in a damp paper towel (G). (Do not soak the tray and alginate in water because it will absorb water and distort the impression.) Alginate impressions should be poured within 30 minutes.

Step 9—To record the correct articulation, a sheet of bite wax is softened in warm water, placed in the mouth, and the patient is made to bite down on it. Also available are special bite impression materials that may be injected into the occlusal space.

Complications

- Improper mixing will leave lumps and bubbles in the alginate. To prevent this, mix more thoroughly.
- Too thin a mixture will tend to run out of the tray and not stay around the teeth. Follow the manufacturer's instructions on the mix and adjust only if necessary in small amounts.
- Too firm a mixture will not conform to the teeth and mouth well and thus will not give an accurate impression. Correct by using a thinner mix.
- If the tray is not filled properly, voids or bubbles may be incorporated into the impression. Use care and fill the tray completely and smoothly.
- Bubbles can be trapped when the tray is placed in the mouth. To prevent bubbles, it is best to place the tray from distal to anterior slowly.
- Movement while the alginate is setting will cause distortion. Because movement is generally caused by the patient, proper sedation or anesthesia of the patient will prevent this problem.
- The alginate may tear when removed from the mouth. This is especially a problem in the canine teeth, which are further apart at their coronal end than in the gingival area, a configuration causing them to diverge. Slow removal of the impression as well as a slight rotational movement will help to prevent tearing. A minimal tear can be corrected on the model later.
- Alginate will become distorted if the water content changes between the time the impression is taken and the model is poured. It will also become distorted if the tray is not solid.

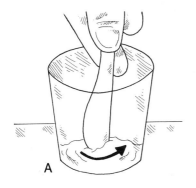

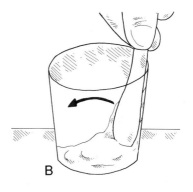

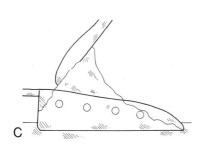

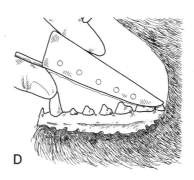

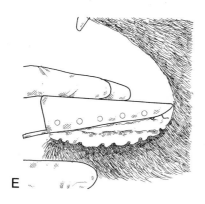

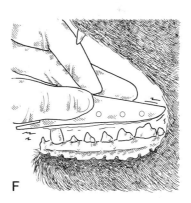

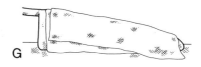

Making a Model

Once the impression is made, a model should be poured as soon as possible.

Indications

- The model is used as part of the medical record.
- With a model, oral structures can be evaluated extraorally, and a treatment plan can be created for orthodontia or crown and bridge fabrication.
- The dental model or a copy of the model may be used to fabricate appliance(s).
- Models may be used to facilitate communication with colleagues or laboratory personnel.
- The model of the patient may be used as a visual aid in discussing the case with the owner and in showing what treatment is indicated and how an appliance will be placed in the mouth.

Materials

- An accurate impression.
- Die stone.
- Mixing bowl and spatula.
- Vibrator.
- Scale.

Technique

Step 1—The stone is measured into the mixing bowl, ideally by weighing (A).

Step 2—Water is measured. All the water is added to the stone in the mixing bowl at one time (B).

Step 3—Start mixing in the center of the bowl (C). After all the water is incorporated into the stone, spatulate the mixture on the sides of the bowl to remove air bubbles and to remove lumps of unmixed powder.

Step 4—The bowl with the stone can be placed on the vibrator to help remove air bubbles (D).

Step 5—Hold the impression under a gentle flow of water from the tap and drain off excess water by holding it upside down. Placing the tray on the vibrator may ensure that excess pools of water have been removed.

Step 6—Place an edge of the tray with the impression onto the vibrator (E).

- Slowly add a small amount of mixed stone in the center of the impression.
- With the aid of the vibrator the stone is made to flow into the voids made by the teeth (F). Go slowly, allowing the stone to move into the voids without trapping air. This is the most critical part of the process.
- For smaller teeth a disposable brush may be used to place a small amount of mixed stone into the individual teeth; avoid bubble formation.

Step 7—After the stone is spread into the intricacies of the impression and any air bubbles have been vibrated out, additional stone is placed on the impression to make the model thick enough to minimize fragility (G).

Step 8—Place the impression with the stone in it on the counter and allow the stone to harden (H).

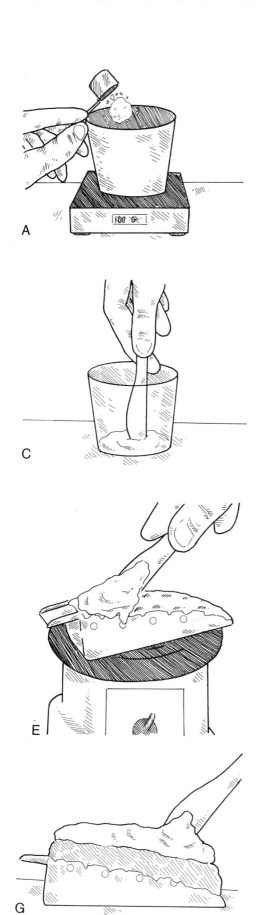

A

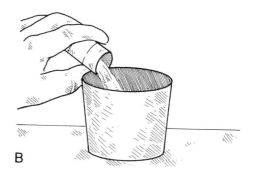

B

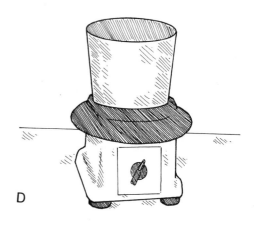

C

D

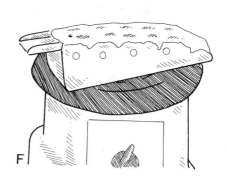

E

F

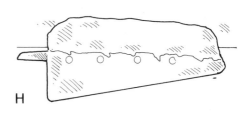

G

H

Technique (Continued)

Step 9—The hardened stone is removed from the alginate impression after 30 to 60 minutes *(A)*.

Step 10—A flat base is made with additional stone so the model will sit firmly and evenly on a counter or table.

- Start by mixing another batch of stone or plaster the same way as previously described.
- Place a layer of the stone onto the bottom of the hardened stone.
- The model is turned over and placed on a flat surface, such as a countertop, and adjusted until it is level with the teeth up.

Step 11—Once the stone has set, excess stone can be trimmed away using a model trimmer.

Step 12—Label the model with the patient and client's name and date it was made.

Step 13—The bite registration previously taken is placed between the models of the upper and lower arches, thus aligning them correctly. The distal ends of the models are trimmed with a model trimmer, and wax is used to position them. To align the models correctly they are placed on a flat surface on their distal ends.

Complications

Incorrect Mix Ratios

- The stone will not flow if the mixture is too thick. Correct by using a thinner mixture, but be aware that changing the proportions from the manufacturer's instructions may cause distortion.
- Too thin a mixture will be weak and not as dimensionally stable. Correct by mixing more thickly.

Inadequate Mixing

- Lumps of unmixed stone will be found in the mix. Mix more thoroughly.

Air Bubbles

- Mixing can incorporate air into the stone mixture. Correct by spatulating against the sides of the bowl more carefully.

- Air can be trapped in the intricacies of the impression. This is usually done when the stone is placed in the impression too rapidly and is not allowed to flow into the small voids of the impression. Correct by placing small amounts of stone on the impression and allowing it to spread slowly using the vibrator.
- In deep voids, such as those made by the canine teeth, a small amount of water left in the void will aid in prevention of trapping air.

Nonrigid Trays

- Allow the impression to become distorted before the stone is poured or set.

Desiccation of the Alginate

- The time between taking the impression and pouring the stone is too long. The stone should be poured quickly after the impression is taken. Wrapping the impression in a damp paper towel until it is poured will diminish this distortion. This will allow the delay of pouring the stone for 30 to 60 minutes.

Fracturing of Crowns on Model Teeth

- This is often caused by trying to remove the stone from the impression too early *(B)*. Slow down, be patient, and work smart, not hard. Even the most patient practitioner will, on occasion, break a crown off as the model is removed from the impression. Most of the time the fractured piece can be placed back in position and cemented. Allow the model and fragment to dry completely.
- After the model is dry the fractured piece can either be cemented on with a glass ionomer cement or with polymethacrylate *(C and D)*.
- For very long teeth with narrow diameters, a small piece of orthodontic wire (24 to 26 gauge) may be placed into the impression prior to pouring the model. This will stiffen the teeth and will prevent fracture.

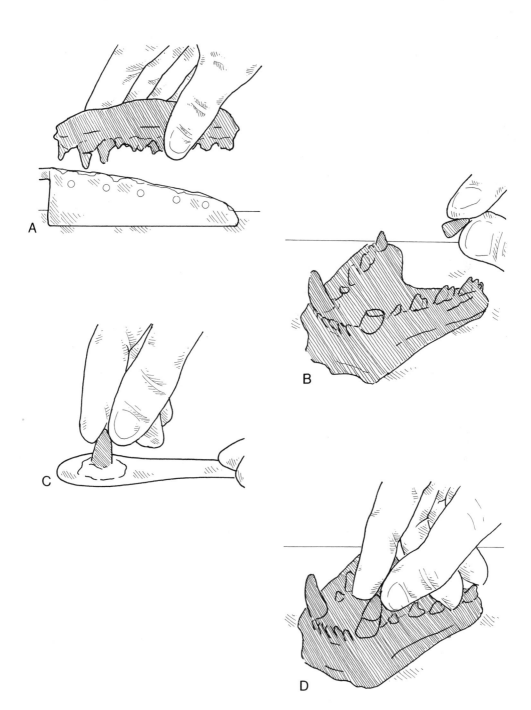

A

B

C

D

Direct Bonding of Band, Brackets, and Buttons

- Brackets or buttons are bonded to teeth for applying forces to achieve orthodontic movement.
- Bands can be used alone for attachment of elastics or arch wires or are incorporated into an appliance for fixation to the teeth.

Indications

- For attaching fixed or removable acrylic or metal appliances.
- Lingual or labial arch wires.
- Attachment of acrylic or metal appliances.
- For orthodontic movement with elastics.

Contraindication

- Patients that cannot be controlled and chew on hard objects.

Materials

- Bands, brackets, and/or buttons.
- Orthodontic bonding agent.
- Spatula.
- College pliers.
- Scaler.
- Flour pumice, prophy cup.

Technique

Step 1—The teeth that are to have brackets attached are scaled to remove any calculus (A).

Step 2—A flour pumice is used to polish and remove any plaque (B).

- Do not use prophy paste because it may contain fluoride, waxes, and glycerin that may inhibit the bond.

Step 3—The bracket or button is chosen and trial placed on the tooth (C). The baseplate should fit flat on the tooth. If it does not fit flat, three-pronged pliers are used to bend the bracket or button baseplate to conform to the tooth surface.

Step 4—Phosphoric acid gel is placed on the tooth for 30 to 60 seconds (D). The time depends on concentration of the acid and whether an "active" or "passive" technique is used. With the active technique, the operator scrubs the tooth surface with a sponge or brush and acid etches for the time period. The passive technique allows the phosphoric acid to coat the tooth undisturbed for the time period. Using active or passive technique and the time period depend on the manufacturer's instructions for the bonding agent. These instructions should be followed exactly.

Step 5—Using a three-way syringe, water is used to rinse off the acid (E). It is best to make sure rinsing is complete by continuing the rinsing for 45 to 60 seconds.

Step 6—The tooth is dried using air from the three-way syringe or a hand-held hair dryer on a low setting (F).

- At this point the area on which the bracket will be placed should have a dull, chalky appearance.
- It is critical that this air be free of moisture and oil.
- If contamination of the prepared tooth surface occurs either by saliva, blood, oil, or other substance, the preparation should begin again from step 2, but cutting the etching time by 75%. This can be thought of as a contest between the operator and the environment! If contamination gets there first, the operator loses.

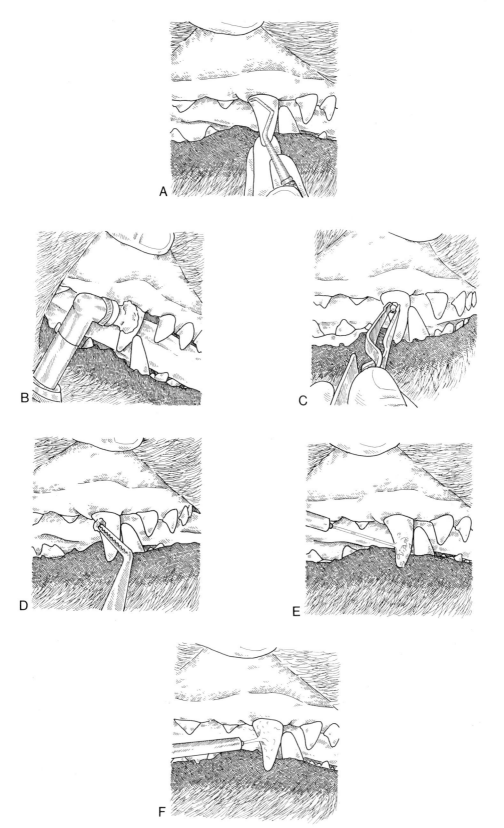

Technique (Continued)

Step 7—The unfilled bonding agent is mixed and applied to the surface of the tooth *(A)* and to the baseplate of the button or bracket *(B)*.

Step 8—The filled bonding agent is mixed *(C)* and is placed on the back side of the bracket *(D)*. (Each manufacturer of bonding agents has specific instructions on the way their products are to be mixed and used. To achieve good results, these instructions should be meticulously followed.)

Step 9—The bracket is placed on the tooth in the position desired and pressed firmly against the tooth; some of the bonding agent extrudes around the edges of the bracket *(E)*.

Step 10—Excess bonding agent is removed with a scaler before it has set *(F)*. Wait to put a force on the bracket until the bonding agent has had the required time to finish polymerizing *(G)*. This time is given in the package insert of the bonding agent.

- Test the strength of the bond by putting pressure on the bracket with college pliers. If the bond is not sufficient it is easier to rebond it while the patient is under anesthesia than to find out in a day or two and require the patient to return to the office for another anesthetic.[2]

Complications

Brackets or Buttons Come Off When Force Is First Applied

- Usually something in the bonding process was not done well.

- The tooth must be clean, etched, and dry.
- No oil can be present.
- The bonding agent must have been mixed properly and placed in a timely manner.

Brackets or Buttons Come Off at a Later Time

- Chewing on hard objects can shear bracket/buttons off, or long hair, carpet yarn, or strings tangled on the appliance will then pull them off.
- Clients must be educated that during the orthodontic treatment the patient must not be allowed to chew on hard objects.

Discoloration of the Tooth When the Brackets Are Removed

- This happens when the brackets are not kept clean; one of the reasons for the practitioner to use progress visits for monitoring the patient during orthodontic treatment.

Aftercare

- Routine progress examinations will be needed to monitor the progress of tooth movement and to make sure good oral hygiene is being properly performed.

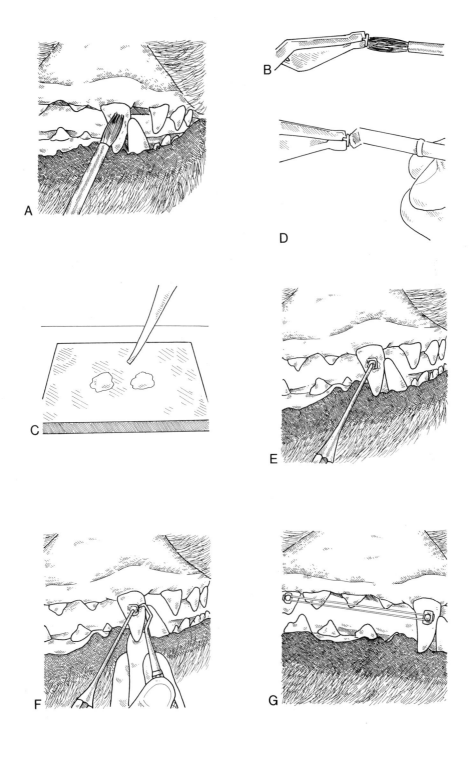

Making Bands

- Orthodontic bands may be used as alternatives to buttons or brackets.
- Because orthodontic bands wrap around the entire tooth, they give more bonding area and are more durable than buttons or brackets.
- The bands may have brackets or buttons soldered onto them or may be incorporated into arch wires.

Indications

- Orthodontic tooth movement.
- Lingual or labial arch wires.
- Attachment of acrylic or metal appliances.

Contraindication

- Poor client/patient compliance with oral hygiene.

Materials

- Patient's dental model.
- Band material; suggested sizes: 0.150" × 0.003", 0.150" × 0.004", 0.180" × 0.005", and 0.180" × 0.006".
- Flux; this should be a flux recommended for orthodontic work.
- Silver solder.
- Gas torch.
- Welder (optional).
- Orthodontic bonding material or luting cement (acrylic, composite resin zinc oxide–eugenol or glass ionomer).

Technique

Step 1—A dental stone model is manufactured as previously described.

Step 2—The band material is contoured to conform to the tooth shape on the model at the location where the band will be placed.

Step 3 (optional)—The band material is clamped in place with hemostats and is removed from the model. The band material may be spot "tack" welded with a welder to hold it in place. The band material is placed back on the model.

Step 4—The ends of the band material are bent along the portion of the band circling the tooth.

Step 5—Excess band material is trimmed.

Step 6—Flux is applied to the band in the area to be soldered.

Step 7—The band is soldered.

- Arch wires or buttons may be soldered or welded onto the band.

Step 8—The tooth to be banded is prepared as for button or bracket placement.

Step 9—The orthodontic bonding cement is mixed and applied to the inside of the band (*A*).

Step 10—The band is placed over the crown of the tooth to be banded (*B*).

Step 11—The band is firmly seated with pliers or a band pusher (*C*). Excess cement is removed with a curette.

Complications

- Excess heat applied to the band may melt and destroy the band.
- Poor cementing technique may cause the band to come off or may create voids that lead to microleakage causing decay, observed as a black stain in the tooth enamel when the band is removed.

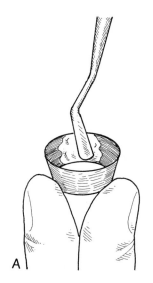

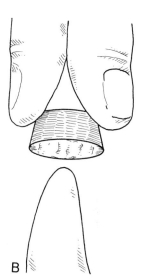

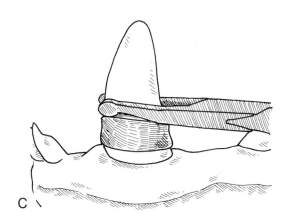

Making Acrylic Appliances

- An acrylic appliance may be manufactured either by a dental laboratory or by the practitioner.[3, 4]

Indications

- Orthodontic tooth movement.
- Splinting of avulsed teeth.
- Splinting of oral fractures.

Contraindications

- Severely infected areas.
- Uncooperative patients that may not allow oral hygiene.

Materials

- Dental model as previously described. It is recommended that a second "working model" be manufactured, whether by taking a second impression on the patient, by pouring two models from the first impression, or by taking an impression of the first model and pouring a second model from this impression.
- "Tin foil substitute"—material to inhibit bonding of acrylic to the working model.
- Rope wax.
- Sticky wax.
- Dental acrylic (denture type material).
- Ruby lab burs.
- Wax-carving instrument.
- Propane or alcohol torch.

Technique

Step 1—The area on the model where the appliance will be built is coated with the tin foil substitute and is allowed to dry (A).

Step 2—Rope wax is placed around the area where the appliance is to be manufactured (B).

Step 3—Any wires such as finger springs, retaining wires, etc. are bent and placed on the model in the desired position (C).

Step 4—Sticky wax is placed by heating a wax-carving instrument and dipping the wax carver into the hardened wax so the wax melts onto the instrument (D) and flows onto the model and wire (E). When the wax cools it will harden and hold the wire in the desired position.

Step 5—The acrylic is placed onto the model.

- Three techniques are used to place the acrylic onto the model.
- Any one or all of the techniques may be used.

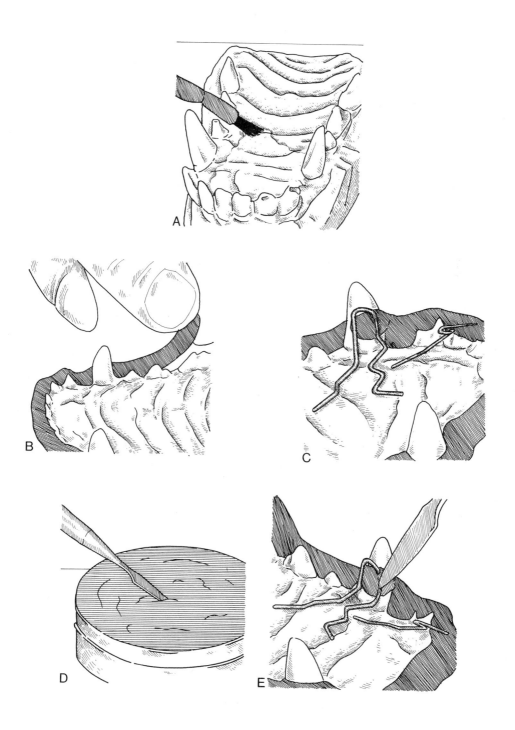

Alternate 1—"Salt and Pepper" Technique

Alternate 1 substep 1— A light coating (1 to 2 mm) of the acrylic powder (polymer) is sprinkled from the container onto the model in the area contained by the rope wax (A).

Alternate 1 substep 2—Drops of the acrylic liquid (monomer) are dropped onto the powder (B). The powder will undergo a color change as the polymer is wetted (the color depends on the brand and shade).

Alternate 1 substep 3—Additional polymer and monomer are added to build up the appliance as desired (C).

Alternate 2—Mixing Technique

Alternate 2 substep 1—The powder is placed in a paper cup (D).

- A rubber bowl used for alginate should not be used because the acrylic will destroy the bowl.
- Specially made glass or rubber bowls are made for this use.

Alternate 2 substep 2—The liquid is added, according to the manufacturer's directions (E).

Alternate 2 substep 3—The liquid and powder are mixed with a spatula (F).

Alternate 2 substep 4—The mixture is poured onto the model (G).

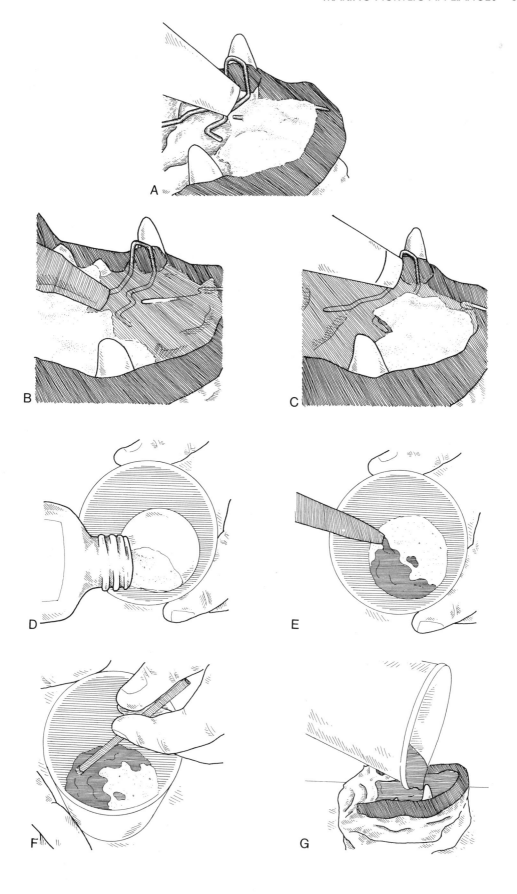

Alternate 3—Brush Method

Alternate 3 substep 1—The polymer and monomer are each placed in dappen dishes (*A*).

Alternate 3 substep 2—A brush is dipped into the polymer (*B*) and then dipped into the monomer (*C*) to obtain a small amount of acrylic on the brush tip. The polymer absorbs the liquid monomer.

Alternate 3 substep 3—The paste of acrylic is carried and placed on the model in the desired location (*D*).

- The brush technique allows a precise placement of the dental acrylic.

Step 6 (optional)—The model and appliance are placed in a pressure pot, and pressure and heat are applied to eliminate air bubbles and make a stronger appliance. Acrylic cured in this manner will be clearer.

Step 7—Once hardened, the appliance is removed from the model.

Step 8—With a lab bur and slow-speed handpiece the appliance is trimmed and shaped.

Step 9 (optional)—The appliance is smoothed with a polishing wheel.

Complications

Appliance Sticking to Model

- Failure to apply adequate amount of tin foil substitute or releasing agent.

Breakage of the Appliance

- The appliance is too thin or needs reinforcing wires.

Breakage of the Model

- Breakage of the model while manufacturing the appliance almost always occurs; therefore, a working model should be used.

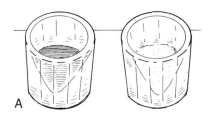

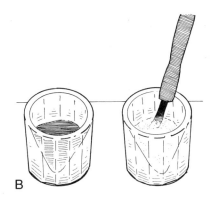

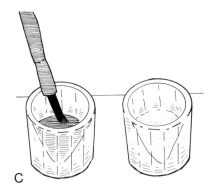

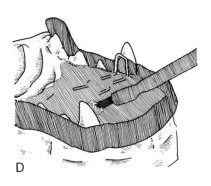

INTERCEPTIVE ORTHODONTICS

- The dental "lock" formed by the lower teeth occluding or locking with the upper teeth affects the growth and development of the bony structures of the jaws.
- By interfering with this "lock," the bony structures are more readily allowed to grow independently of each other and more closely reflect the genetic programing.
- Selective teeth are extracted to allow the mandible or faciomaxillary complex to grow independently.
- A primary tooth may be extracted to create space for an adult tooth to erupt unimpeded.

Indications

- Abnormal occlusion in a young animal prior to the eruption of the adult teeth.
- Treatment is started as early as possible to allow the longest time for correction to occur before the adult teeth erupt.
- Retained deciduous teeth: Any primary tooth that is not lost by the time its homologous adult tooth has erupted.[5-7]

Technique

Step 1—The bite is evaluated and the desired movement identified. For example, in a patient with a class 2 occlusion, the mandible needs to move rostrally.

Step 2—Any primary tooth that is or would inhibit the desired movement is extracted. Care must be taken to extract all the tooth and root and not to damage the developing permanent tooth bud.

- In this situation it is better to extract any primary tooth that the practitioner believes might be hindering growth than to err on the conservative side and extract fewer teeth.

Complications

- If the entire root is not extracted, eruption of the adult tooth may be hindered.
- Careless extraction techniques may damage the adult tooth.

ORTHODONTIC APPLIANCES

- Many types of orthodontic appliances exist; each is custom made for the patient.

General Indication

- The general indication for an orthodontic appliance is to correct a malocclusion that is causing or may lead to discomfort or tooth loss.

General Contraindications

- Ankylosis of teeth.
- Severe periodontal disease.
- Untrained/unsupervised patients.
- Patients whose chewing habits cannot be controlled.
- Clients who will not comply with oral hygiene or oral hygiene examinations.
- The deception of others.

Specific Appliances

Button to Button

- The movement of a tooth or teeth with elastics or "power chain or cords" attached to the teeth with buttons, brackets, or bands.
- Use of buttons bonded to a tooth to secure an elastic is a straightforward way to achieve simple tooth movement of a single tooth or group of teeth (lower incisors).
- The force vector/s is/are determined by where the button is placed on the anchor tooth and the tooth to be moved. These forces must be carefully evaluated to determine the appropriate positions to place the buttons so unwanted movement does not occur.

Objective

- To achieve tooth movement (usually bodily or tipping) using force created by elastics.

Indications

- Minor displacement of teeth.
- Rostral displacement of maxillary canines.
- Rostral tipping or displacement of mandibular canines.
- To tip lower incisors caudally when angled forward.

Contraindication

- See general contraindications to orthodontic appliances.

Materials

- Orthodontic buttons.
- Preferred button: Ormesh Curved Lingual Pad with button.*
- Flour pumice.
- Prophy cups.
- Orthodontic bonding material.
- Scaler or curette.
- Bracket holding forceps or cotton pliers.
- Orthodontic elastics of various sizes/ strengths.
- Grey chain elastic (power cord chain†).
- Scissors.

Technique

- Buttons are bonded to the teeth as previously described.
- One or more buttons are placed on the anchor tooth/teeth.
- Another button is placed on the tooth to be moved or as support for the elastic across the lower incisors.
- Elastic chain (power cord) or orthodontic elastics of appropriate size are placed between the buttons to create the desired force on the tooth/teeth to be moved.
- The initial force on the teeth is determined by the strength of the elastic, or number of holes between the teeth when using grey chain.
- The exact force to be used depends on the type of power chain, age of patient, tooth to be moved, etc. The best guideline is to start with a light force and increase the force in subsequent visits if the desired movement is not being obtained.

---

*Ormco 300-0096, Glendora, CA.
†Ormco 639-0010, Glendora, CA.

Displaced Maxillary Canines

- Occasionally, in male Shetland sheepdogs most often, the maxillary canine is angled rostrally, causing interference with the mandibular canine (*A*).
- The maxillary canine can be displaced mesially; this pattern is associated with a retained primary tooth. This may occur alone or in conjunction with lingually displaced mandibular canines.
- The anchor teeth are the maxillary third, fourth premolar, and first molar.
- The button on the canine tooth must be placed in a location to create the appropriate movement. In an angled tooth, it may be placed closer to the tip of the tooth initially, for more tipping action to move the crown into position. As the crown becomes more perpendicular the button can be replaced to the midtooth area, to achieve a bodily movement into normal position.
- The exact elastic to be used depends on the age of patient, the distance to be moved, etc. The best guideline is to start with a light elastic with a diameter equal to half the distance between the fourth premolar and canine tooth position. In subsequent visits the elastics can be increased in strength (from light to medium or medium to heavy), or a smaller-diameter elastic can be selected if the desired movement is not being obtained.

Advantages

- Less expensive way to move teeth.
- Tolerated well by the animal.
- Elastic size or length can be adjusted easily as the tooth moves.

Disadvantages

- Buttons can be displaced by chewing on hard objects.
- Can create displacement of fourth premolar if used alone as the anchor tooth.

Rostrally Displaced Mandibular Canines

- Seen occasionally where one or more of the lower canines is tilted forward, often interfering with the maxillary lateral incisor and causing displacement or wear of that tooth.
- Buttons are placed in the midtooth area of the canine and buccally or lingually on the third and fourth premolars or lingually on the lower molar for anchorage.
- Orthodontic elastic or grey chain is stretched between the buttons to create a light force (*B*).
- The elastics are changed daily and the size adjusted as tooth movement occurs.
- Grey chain elastic can be adjusted by decreasing the number of links between the buttons. The chain elastic should be replaced at least weekly.

Advantages

- Simple, less expensive movement of a displaced canine tooth.
- Tolerated well by the animal.

Disadvantages

- Dislodgment of the buttons.
- Placing too much force on the teeth with elastics' moving tooth too fast or moving the anchor teeth.
- Difficult to place buttons on small teeth in miniature breeds.

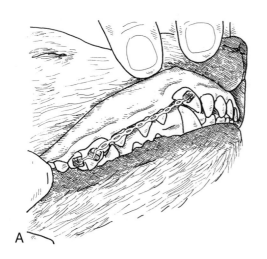

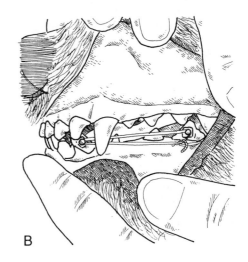

A

B

Caudal Movement of Lower Incisors

- In animals with anterior crossbite, moving the lower incisors caudally alone or in conjunction with movement of the upper incisors forward with an appliance may be needed to achieve a scissors occlusion.
- Buttons are placed on the buccal surface of the lower canines and on each of the second incisors.
- An appropriate-size orthodontic elastic or grey chain is stretched across the incisors from canine to canine (A).
- Another variation of this technique places small brackets on the second lower incisors (B). An orthodontic elastic or elastic cord is placed around both canines. The two strands of elastic stretched between the canine teeth are brought in front of the incisors and are secured in the slot of the brackets. Small amounts of bonding material can be placed on the canines and central incisors to help keep the elastic from slipping.
- The buttons/brackets secure the elastics and keep them from slipping down onto the gingiva.
- Very little force is needed to create the desired movement.
- These techniques should not be used until the permanent canines have a developed root (about 7 months of age); otherwise, these teeth are not secure enough to use as anchor teeth and they may be displaced.

Advantages

- Less expensive method of moving teeth. Casts to design an appliance are not needed.
- Can be easily applied.

Disadvantages

- Buttons can be dislodged.
- Can create excessive crowding of teeth or may displace the canines if too much force is used.

- Does not allow for a retainer period to keep teeth in position. Elastic may be replaced with stainless steel wire placed between the buttons to maintain desired position.

Complications

- Early removal of buttons requiring replacement with another anesthetic procedure.
- Noncompliance of owners to maintain oral hygiene with gingival irritation secondary to debris/hair wrapped around buttons.
- Sliding on incisors of elastic either behind the teeth or down onto gingiva. This is usually corrected by creating a ledge on central incisors with bonding material to hold elastic in place.
- Improper application of elastic by the owner's creating excessive force on teeth and undesirable movement/crowding.

Aftercare

- Home oral hygiene; taking care to keep the buttons and elastics free of hair, lint, etc.
- Recheck appointments every 10 to 14 days to monitor home hygiene and tooth movement.
- Replacement of elastics daily or grey chain as needed.
- Soft food and no chew toys.
- Removal of the buttons or brackets is easily accomplished using pliers. Squeeze the prongs together on brackets or use band-removing pliers for buttons or bands.
- The excess bonding material is removed with the band-removing pliers and/or ultrasonic scaler and the teeth are polished with a fluoride-containing pumice.
- Occasionally, the bands may have to be cut with a high-speed handpiece to remove the bands after orthodontic movement is complete. Eye protection must be worn.

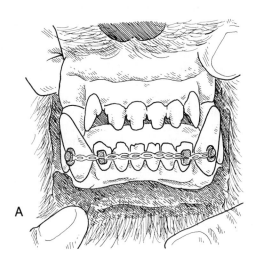

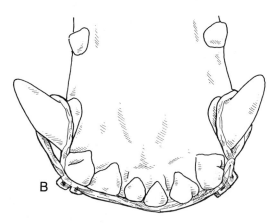

Arch Wires

- Arch wires may be placed on the maxillary or mandibular teeth, on either the palatal/lingual or labial surface.
- Arch wires are held in place by either bands or brackets usually attached to the canine teeth.

Objective

- A wire appliance using various activating forces creating loops, arches, and finger springs is designed to create tooth movement.

Indications

- Anterior crossbite, moving upper incisors forward.
- Anterior crossbite, moving lower incisors back.
- Movement of one or more teeth.
- Depressed mandibular central incisors.[8]

Contraindications

- Teeth so small that wire cannot be maintained in proper position.
- General orthodontic appliance contraindications.

Materials

- Patient's dental model.
- Laboratory-fabricated arch wire.
- Orthodontic wire, welder, solder, etc., if practitioner is capable of manufacturing in office.
- Brackets, bands if not incorporated into appliance.
- Orthodontic bonding material.
- Flour pumice.
- Rubber cups.
- Scaler or curette.

Technique: General

- The technique of manufacturing the arch wire is beyond the scope of this text, and the text begins with a fabricated arch wire.

- Many types of configurations can be used with the arch wire.
- The arch wire with incorporated bands is applied as described in the brackets/band bonding technique.
- Brackets are bonded to the tooth first and the arch wire fitted and secured with ligature wire if using an arch wire by itself.

Arch Wire Elastics

- An arch wire is designed to come across the labial surface of the mandibular incisors and is welded to bands that encircle the canine teeth.
- The arch wire forms the desired position for forward movement of the teeth.
- The arch wire has small hooks over each incisor allowing a small elastic to be placed between the arch wire and the button on the tooth to be moved.
- Buttons or brackets are bonded onto the tooth/teeth to be moved first.
- The appliance is bonded to the canines as previously described under band cementing.
- Once the bonding material is set, elastics are placed between the bracket on the tooth and arch wire (A). The strength of an elastic is measured in ounces and is calibrated at approximately twice the diameter of the elastic. For example, a ⅜" light elastic has 3 ounces of force when stretched to ¾".
- The elastics should be changed daily by the client.

Advantages

- Less expensive appliance to make than expansion devices.
- Can achieve rapid movement of teeth.
- Easy to keep clean.

Disadvantages

- Can cause irritation of upper lip.
- Owner must be able to change small elastics daily.
- Buttons or brackets can be dislodged.
- Arch wire can be bent.
- Arch wire design has to allow space for lower canine to come into normal position.

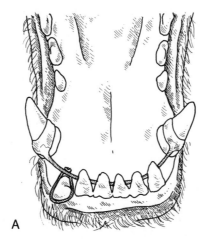

A

Arch Wire Finger Springs

- This technique uses bands around the canine teeth that are linked together with an arch wire that has finger springs soldered onto it to create the desired tooth movement.
- It can be designed to move a single tooth or several teeth.
- This appliance can be adapted to use in the maxilla or mandible, moving incisors forward or caudally.
- The appliance is trial fitted and the finger springs are adjusted with three-prong or appropriate orthodontic pliers so the spring pressure will move the teeth to their desired position (A). A slight overadjustment should be anticipated; however, additional adjustments may be made later on recheck visits.
- The appliance is cemented to the canines following the technique described on pages 358 to 359.
- The active finger spring wires are tucked behind the upper incisors (B). A small ledge of composite resin or bonding material can be placed on the lingual surface of the incisors to keep the wire from slipping forward off the teeth.

Advantages

- Simple appliance to design.
- Less expensive than expansion devices.
- Easy to keep area clean.

Disadvantages

- Spring wires get caught in hair, blankets, and carpet and become bent out of position.
- Laceration of lips/tongue from bent or broken wires.

Labial Arch Wires

- A labial arch wire uses a retention device (usually bands) connected by an arch wire that lies on the labial surface of the teeth (C).
- Springs are formed by loops in the diastema between the canine and lateral incisor.
- Closing these loops gradually with pliers over time creates the desired force to move the teeth.
- This type of arch wire can be used for an anterior crossbite by tipping the lower incisors lingually if there is a space between the incisors and canine teeth.

Advantages

- Easy appliance to design and place.
- Well tolerated by the animal.
- Can act as its own retainer when the desired tooth position is reached.
- Easy to keep clean around it.

Disadvantages

- Cannot be used in dogs with very small incisors.
- Wire can be bent/dislodged by chewing on undesirable objects.

Complications

- Breakage of finger springs.
- Bending of finger springs.
- Hair and carpet getting caught in wires.
- Loss of appliance.

Aftercare

- Rechecks every 10 to 14 days.
- Adjust elastics, finger springs, or loops as needed to maintain orthodontic force.
- After retainer period the appliance is removed using band-removing pliers.
- Excess cement is removed with band-removing pliers or an ultrasonic scaler and the teeth are polished with fluoride-containing pumice.

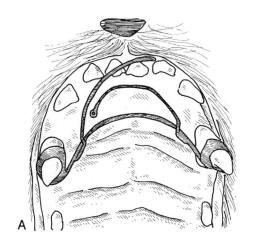

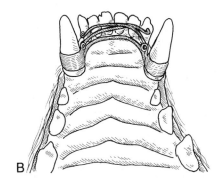

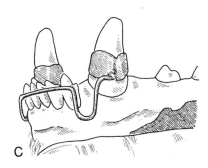

Expansion Devices

- Expansion screws, acrylic plate, or arch wire may be used to expand teeth.
- Small expansion screws can be placed in acrylic appliances or attached to wires and bands to create gradual movement of the teeth by adjusting the screw that directs an orthodontic force on the the teeth to be moved.
- These screws come in various sizes and expansion capabilities.
- The practitioner can either create his or her own appliance with acrylic or wires and bands or send the patient's models to a laboratory to have one fabricated.
- Either removable or fixed appliances can be designed.
- Removable appliances (usually maxillary) are designed with wire loops that lie along the palatal surface of the canines and lateral incisors. Brackets or buttons are bonded to the buccal or labial surface of these teeth near the gingival margin, and small elastics are placed over the wire on the appliance and button/bracket to hold the appliance in place.
- Removable appliances are removed during eating and allow for easier cleaning and oral hygiene.
- Fixed appliances are designed with bands around the canine teeth and are cemented in place.

Objective

- To create gradual tooth movement using an expansion device that places an orthodontic force on the tooth/teeth to be moved.

Indications

- Anterior crossbite, maxillary appliance.
- Lingually displaced mandibular canines.
- Posterior crossbite.

Contraindication

- See general orthodontic appliance contraindications.

Materials

- Worm gear.
- Expansion screws; Unitek # 440–160 Mid-Palatal Suture Expansion Screw.*
- Orthodontic wire; suggested sizes: 0.016″, 0.020″, 0.022″, 0.028″, 0.032″, 0.036″, and 0.040″.
- Buttons/brackets.
- Orthodontic cement/bonding material.
- Flour pumice.
- Rubber cups.
- Patient's models.
- Laboratory-fabricated appliance.
- Adjusting key.

Techniques

Maxillary Acrylic Appliance for Anterior Crossbite

- An acrylic appliance is designed with the expansion screw placed front to back embedded in the acrylic (A). The acrylic is cut so the front half of the screw is in a section of acrylic that will move separately against the incisors to be pushed forward.
- This can be a removable or fixed appliance.
- The expansion screw is adjusted using a small wire key in the hole at the center of the expansion screw that expands the screw, thus putting an increased pressure on the teeth to be moved.
- This screw, adjusted by the owner, gradually moves the teeth into the desired position.
- When the teeth are in place, the appliance is left in place for an additional period of time for the retainer period.

Advantages

- A strong device that does not have loose wires that can be bent or catch on hair, etc.
- Can be designed as a removable appliance for easy cleaning (B).
- Well tolerated by the animal.

---

*Unitek Corporation, 2724 South Peck Road, Monrovia, CA 91016.

- Creates a more uniform, controlled tooth movement.

Disadvantages

- More expensive to manufacture than arch wire.

- Owner must take care of home oral hygiene.
- Owner must be able to make adjustments with wire key.

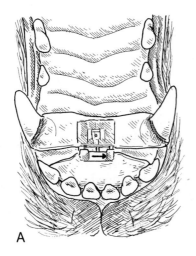

A

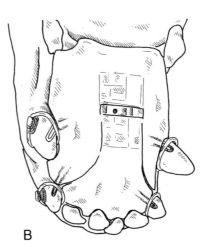

B

Lingually Displaced Mandibular Canines

- This common occlusion problem is usually caused by retained primary canines that do not allow the adult teeth to come into position outside the maxillary arch.
- The pressure caused by the indentation of the mandibular canines on the hard palate can lead to periodontal disease of the maxillary canines, pain, and necrosis of the palatal tissue.
- The expansion screw is placed in a wire support structure with bands around the mandibular canines (A).
- This device can be used effectively when both canines need to be moved out and are located in their normal relationship mesial to distal.
- Variations on the device, such as a wire arm alongside the premolars or placing it at an angle between the canines, have been used to achieve movement of a single canine without shifting position of the other.
- The device is cemented to the canines using the technique described on pages 358 to 359.

Advantages

- Easily designed to create desired movement.
- Well tolerated by the animal.
- Easy to keep clean.
- Cannot be removed easily by the animal.

Disadvantages

- Owner must be able to make the screw adjustments.
- Will not change mesial/distal position of the canine tooth.
- Size of animal may limit its use if there is not enough expansion to achieve desired tooth position.
- Appliance can be dislodged by vigorous chewing on hard objects.

Omega or "W" Wire

- An omega/"W" wire is an orthodontic wire bent in the form of the Greek letter "Ω" or "W"(B). Loops designed in the bends of the "W" create an expansion action of the outer arms when activated.
- The wire is soldered to bands around the canines and can be used to move lingually displaced canine teeth.

- The appliance is trial fitted and the outer arms are activated with three-prong pliers to extend to the desired position of the teeth while the appliance is free from the canines.
- The wire and bands are cemented to the teeth as previously described, collapsing the expanded "W". This creates the force to move the teeth into position.

Advantages

- Easily designed appliance.
- Can be made to fit any size mouth.
- Easy to clean around appliance.

Disadvantages

- Cannot control force as easily; may move teeth too fast.
- Force created may not be sufficient to achieve desired movement.
- Can be dislodged or bent by heavy chewing on hard objects.
- Does not have a retainer function as readily as expansion-screw devices.

Complications

- Noncompliance of owner with home oral hygiene leading to palatal mucosa irritation from acrylic appliance.
- Dislodgment or breakage of appliance.
- Alveolar bone necrosis from rapid movement of teeth.
- Premature removal of appliance with teeth drifting back; leave appliance in place for adequate retainer period.

Aftercare

- Home oral hygiene; daily flushing around appliance.
- Expansion-screw adjustments every 3 to 4 days. (Each turn of the key expands the screw 0.25 mm; therefore, four turns equals 1-mm expansion.)
- Recheck examinations every 10 to 14 days to monitor home oral hygiene and tooth movement.
- Appliance is removed with band-removing pliers, excess cement is removed with band-removing pliers or an ultrasonic scaler, and the teeth are polished with a fluoride-containing pumice.

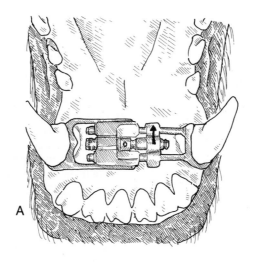

A

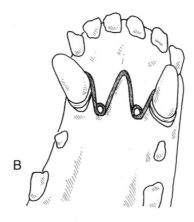

B

Inclined Plane

- Inclined planes are designed of acrylic or cast metal to guide a tooth into a new movement using normal occlusal forces. Every time the animal closes its mouth, the teeth come in contact with the inclined plane and are directed in the desired position.
- They can be used for a variety of tooth movements but are most commonly used for lingually displaced mandibular canines.
- The inclined plane can be designed to allow forward or caudal movement along with buccal movement of the teeth.
- Desired tooth position can be readily achieved with the inclined plane design.
- In mild cases of lingual displacement the palatal gingiva can be used as an inclined plane (see gingival wedge).
- The incline should be created on both sides of the appliance even if only one tooth needs to be corrected. This prevents the shifting of the mandible that may be created if only one canine is guided.

Objective

- To achieve tooth movement using normal occlusal forces against an inclined plane device to direct the tooth into the desired position.

Indications

- Lingual displacement of one or both mandibular canines.
- Caudal displacement of maxillary incisor.

Contraindication

- See general orthodontic appliance contraindications.

Materials

- Patient's models.
- Laboratory-designed inclined plane device.
- Orthodontic cementing materials.
- Flour pumice.
- Rubber cups.

Techniques

Acrylic

- An inclined plane can be designed out of dental acrylic to fit against the hard palate.
- The appliance can be removable or fixed.
- The removable appliance is attached with elastics placed over buttons bonded to the buccal surface of the canines and lateral incisors and wires incorporated into the acrylic that lie along the palatal surface of those teeth.
- The fixed appliance is designed with bands around the maxillary canines and is cemented in place as previously described.
- The inclined plane can be reshaped, as necessary, in the mouth with an acrylic bur in a slow-speed handpiece.
- Periodic adjustments are not needed with these devices because the design of the inclined plane is to create the force necessary to move progressively the tooth into position during natural occlusion.

Advantages

- Acrylic material allows for adjustments, if necessary, during the course of treatment without removing the appliance.
- Less expensive than cast-metal appliance.
- Can be designed as a removable appliance for easy cleaning.

Disadvantages

- Client must maintain good home oral hygiene.
- Appliance must be designed to allow expansion between the maxillary canines for placement of the device and growth in the young animal.
- Acrylic may be fractured by active chewing on hard objects.

Cast Metal

- A cast-metal inclined plane is designed in an appliance with a telescoping bar across the hard palate and bands around the maxillary canines (A).
- The metal inclined plane can be designed to direct the teeth in a number of directions (forward and buccal, or caudal and buccal) (B).
- The appliance is trial fitted and cemented in place as previously described.

Advantages

- The telescoping bar allows for easy placement and continued growth of the animal.
- The appliance is not in direct contact with the hard palate and is easier to keep clean.
- The appliance is well tolerated by the animal.
- Greater appliance strength; therefore, it is less likely to be damaged by larger animals.

Disadvantages

- Adjustments in design require removal and remaking the appliance.
- Discoloration of inside of mandibular canines from contact with some types of metal.
- Wear on the tips of mandibular canines if appliance is in place for a long period of time.
- Teeth must be fully erupted prior to taking the impression to manufacture the appliance.

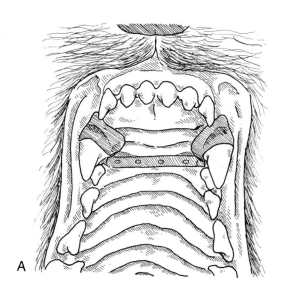

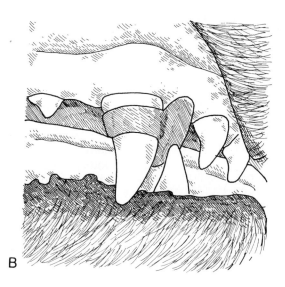

Gingival Wedge

- A wedge can be created in the gingival tissue anterior to the maxillary canine using electrosurgery or a scalpel blade to direct minimally displaced mandibular canines to the outside of the maxillary arch[9] (*A*).
- This technique can be used in animals whose teeth are still erupting, to allow the teeth to come into normal position by the time eruption is complete.

Advantages

- It is not necessary to take impressions and make models to correct the malocclusion.
- Easily performed by any practitioner without additional dental equipment.
- Use in a young animal allows early correction of teeth starting to be displaced.

Disadvantages

- Only effective if mandibular canines are minimally displaced.
- Excessive use of electrosurgery may damage gingiva and create additional sloughing.
- Overaggressive wedging may create permanent change in gingival contour.

Complications

- Premature removal of appliance; prevented by using appropriate cementing material and technique.
- Inadequate appliance design creating incorrect movement or undesired movement; have accurate models and bite impressions for laboratory to work with.
- Inadequate home care by client leading to gingival irritation.

Aftercare

- Recheck examinations every 2 weeks to monitor oral hygiene and tooth movement. Length of treatment depends on the age of the animal and the degree of movement necessary.
- When teeth are in desired position, the appliance is removed using band-removing pliers. Excess cement is removed from the teeth with band-removing pliers or an ultrasonic scaler, and the teeth are polished with a fluoride-containing pumice.

Maryland Bridge

- A cast-metal appliance that uses a variety of forces (expansion screw, elastics) to achieve the desired movement.[10]
- The Maryland bridge concept uses broad coverage of the lingual or palatal surface of the canines (metal "wings") along with cast-metal partial crown covers, to attach the appliance, creating more surface area for cementation and therefore greater retention of the appliance in the mouth.
- Additional circumferential bands over the "wings" provides additional retention.
- The wings, cast crown covers, and band areas cemented in place using a Maryland bridge adhesive or similar luting cement (Comspan,* Panavia†).
- These appliances are very durable in the mouth and are not easily broken or dislodged.

Objective

- To improve retention of an orthodontic appliance to achieve movement of teeth through the use of increased surface contact for cementation.

Indications

- Animals with chewing habits that require a sturdy appliance.
- Animals whose other appliances have been broken or removed by the animal.
- Additional cementation security.

Contraindications

- Poor compliance of owner with follow-up care and rechecks.
- Inability of owner to adjust expansion screws or replace elastics as necessary.

Materials

- Patient's models.
- Laboratory-fabricated appliance.
- Maryland bridge adhesive or luting cement.
- Flour pumice.
- Rubber prophy cups.
- How pliers.
- Scaler or curette.

---

*L. D. Caulk, P.O. Box 359, Milford, DE 19963.
†J. Morita, 14712 Bentley Circle, Tustin, CA 92680.

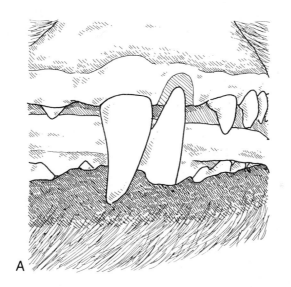

A

Technique

Maxillary Appliance for Anterior Crossbite

- This appliance is cemented to the maxillary canines and incisors following the directions of the cementing product.
- An expansion screw is designed into the appliance to create gradual forward movement of the incisors.

Advantages

- A stronger appliance is beneficial in large dogs that are more likely to break an acrylic appliance.
- There are no wires, buttons, or brackets to be dislodged or caught in hair, chew toys, etc.
- The open design of the cast-metal appliance allows for easy cleaning of the hard palate area and less chance of irritation from deficiencies in home oral hygiene.

Disadvantages

- Increased expense of appliance.
- Must use special luting cements for proper retention.
- Lack of availability; not all laboratories make this style of appliance.

Mandibular Appliance for Anterior Crossbite

- This appliance is cemented to the mandibular canines using the appropriate luting cement and following the instructions included with that particular cement.
- This appliance is designed to use orthodontic elastics across the front of the lower incisors to tip them caudally.
- The elastics are anchored on small hooks incorporated into the canine wings and through a notch in the incisor crown covers (A).
- The elastics are changed daily and the strength of elastic is adjusted as the teeth move into position.

Advantages

- Secure appliance to achieve caudal tipping of the lower incisors.
- Improved attachment and elastics' holding to keep the appliance in place and to prevent gingival damage from slippage.
- The mandibular appliance may be used in conjunction with the maxillary appliance to achieve the desired occlusion in patients with severe anterior crossbite.

Disadvantages

- Increased expense of appliance.
- Must use special luting cements for proper retention.
- Lack of availability; not all laboratories make this style of appliance.

Complications

- Noncompliance of the owner to return for rechecks.
- Discoloration of teeth under wings if cement leaks, staining the tooth surfaces.
- Rare removal of appliance by animal.

Aftercare

- Adjusting elastics or expansion screw as necessary and recheck examination every 2 weeks to monitor tooth movement.
- Removing appliance after proper retainer period. It may be necessary to cut the bands with a diamond bur to facilitate removal. Using an ultrasonic scaler over the wings may help to fracture the cement for removal with band-removing pliers.
- Remaining cement is removed with band-removing pliers or an ultrasonic scaler.

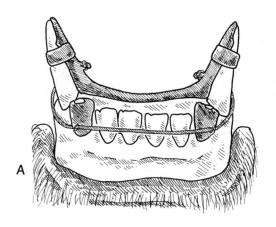

A

LABORATORY PRESCRIPTION (ORTHODONTIC)

- If a dental laboratory is used, a prescription should accompany the models.
- The prescription should order the type of appliance.
- By drawing on the dental chart, the practitioner can indicate the anchorage and type of force to be applied.

References

1. Ross DL. Orthodontics for the dog: bite evaluation, basic concepts, and equipment. Philadelphia: W.B. Saunders Co., 1986:955–966.
2. Proffit WR. Contemporary Orthodontics. St. Louis: C.V. Mosby Co., 1986:579.
3. Wiggs RB. Orthodontics. American Veterinary Dental Society Annual Meeting, St. Louis, 1989.
4. Goldstein GS. The Removable Orthodontic Appliance. American Veterinary Dental Society Annual Meeting, Washington, D.C., 1988.
5. Weigel JP, Dorn AS. Disease of the jaws and abnormal occlusion. In: Harvey CE ed. Veterinary Dentistry. Philadelphia: W.B. Saunders Co., 1985:106–122.
6. Ross D. Veterinary Dentistry. In: Ettinger SJ ed. Veterinary Internal Medicine. Philadelphia: W.B. Saunders Co., 1975:1053–1054.
7. Eisenmenger E, Zetner K. Veterinary Dentistry. Philadelphia: Lea & Febiger, 1985:165.
8. Ross DL. Common Veterinary Orthodontic Indications: Identification and Classifications of Needs. New Orleans: Nabisco, 1988.
9. Goldstein GS. Bite Plates: Removable and Fixed. New Orleans: Nabisco, 1988.
10. Beard GB. Interceptive Orthodontics for Prevention: Maryland Bridges for Correction. New Orleans: Nabisco, 1988.

Dental Lab Prescription

Veterinarian _____ Clinic/Hospital _____

Street Address _____ City _____ State _____ Zip _____ Telephone _____

Patient name/Identification _____ Breed _____ Age _____ Sex _____ .

History:

_____

_____

Diagnosis:

_____

_____

Appliance prescribed:

May we substitute, if a better appliance is available?

☐ Yes, without consultation

☐ Yes, but consult first

☐ No, design as prescribed

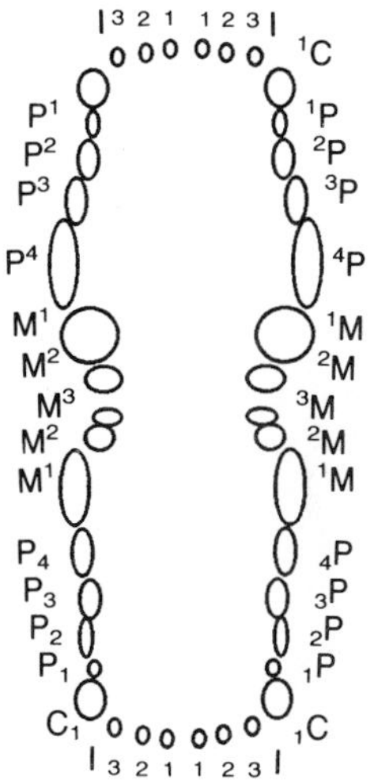

chapter 10

DENTAL ORTHOPEDICS

- Dental techniques may be used to stabilize or assist in the stabilization of the maxillofacial complex, of mandibular fractures, and of luxated teeth.
- Other surgical techniques beyond the scope of this text may need to be used.

SPLINT BONDING

- Bonding with wire splints between teeth is an effective method to achieve stabilization and occlusal alignment of oral structures.
- The strength of the bond limits this method to stabilization of minor components (such as an avulsed tooth or block of teeth with the remainder of the maxillofacial complex or mandible intact or in fractures with other means of stabilization used).

Indications

- Repair maxillary fractures with other stabilization.
- Repair mandibular fractures with other stabilization.
- Stabilize luxated teeth.
- For the surgical correction of malaligned teeth after other fracture repair has been performed.

Contraindication

- Severely fractured and unstable fractures without additional treatment methods.

Objective

- To create stability and proper tooth alignment that leads to fracture healing.

Materials

- 5 mm × 90 mm periodontal splinting material (wire mesh).*
- Orthodontic wire; suggested sizes: 0.016″, 0.020″, 0.022″, 0.028″, 0.032″, 0.036″, and 0.040″.

*Masel, Bristol, PA 19007

- Soft stainless steel orthopedic wire: 18, 20, 24, and 26 gauge.
- Flour pumice (not prophy paste).
- Prophy angle and rubber prophy cups.
- Slow-speed handpiece.
- Orthodontic or light-cured enamel bonding materials.
- Acid-etch materials.

Technique—Avulsed Tooth Fracture

Step 1—Radiographs are taken.
Step 2—The fracture is realigned (A). (In avulsed or fractured teeth, root canal therapy or other treatment may be necessary.)
Step 3—The teeth to be splinted are scaled and polished with a slurry of flour pumice (not prophy paste).
Step 4—A phosphoric acid-etch solution or gel is applied to the enamel surface and after 15 to 30 seconds is rinsed with water for at least 30 to 60 seconds.
Step 5—The surface is air dried.
Step 6—The wire or mesh is bent to lie over the surface to be bonded, is removed, and is set aside (B).
Step 7—A light coat of a liquid, unfilled resin from the orthodontic or composite bonding kit is applied to the teeth to be bonded and to the wire or mesh (C).
Step 8—The filled resin is mixed (if not light cured) and applied to the prepared tooth surface and wire (D).
Step 9—The filled resin is cured with time or light.
Step 10—The bonding is checked for stability by tactile pressure.
Step 11—The bonding material is smoothed as necessary with composite finishing burs (E).

Complications

- Failure to obtain stability; add more wire or rebond.
- Failure to obtain proper occlusion.
- Creation of malocclusion.
- Bonded material preventing the mouth from closing.
- Premature removal of appliance by patient.

Aftercare—Follow-up

- A water pick or curved-tip syringe is used to irrigate debris from between the wire and teeth.
- Radiographs are taken at appropriate intervals.

- When healing has occurred, as determined radiographically and clinically, the appliance is removed with band-removing pliers or a high-speed drill.

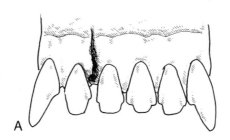

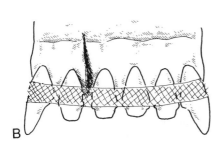

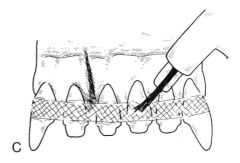

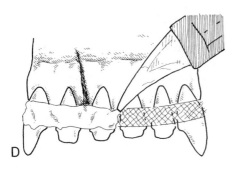

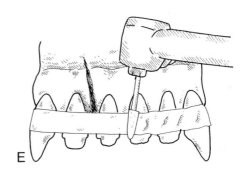

FORMING APPLIANCE IN MOUTH

- Dental acrylics may be cast directly in the oral cavity to create an intraoral splint.

Indications

- Fractured maxillofacial complex.
- Fractured mandible anterior to the first molar.
- Luxated or subluxated teeth.
- To increase stability of other fixation techniques.

Contraindications

- Cases where numerous missing teeth prevent stabilization with the splint.
- Severely comminuted fractures without other techniques.

Objective

- Obtain stability so that healing may occur.

Materials

- Flour pumice (not prophy paste).
- Prophy angle and rubber prophy cups.
- Cold-cure acrylics.
- Petroleum jelly.
- Slow-speed handpiece with acrylic cutting lab burs 75–080, 78–060.*
- Soft stainless steel (surgical or orthodontic) wire; the gauge ranges from 14 to 26, depending on patient and tooth size.

Technique—Mandibular Fracture

Step 1—Appropriate radiographs are taken, malalignments are corrected, and other therapy is performed as indicated (A). The tooth surfaces should be clean.

---

*Brasseler, Savannah, GA 31419

Step 2—The coronal surface of the teeth (usually the canines and larger premolars) may be used for retention of the splint along with wiring techniques. The bonding sites are identified, scaled, and polished with a slurry of flour pumice (B). The oral cavity is rinsed well.

Step 3—The bonding sites are acid etched (see Chapter 8 on acid etching).

Step 4—Wire is bent from tooth to tooth to act as a support for the acrylic (C).

Step 5—A light coat of petroleum jelly is applied to exposed surfaces; be careful to avoid the previously placed wire.

Step 6—A thin layer of the acrylic powder is applied (D).

Step 7—The liquid monomer is dripped onto the powder (E).

Step 8—Additional powder and liquid are alternatively applied until the appliance has been built up for sufficient strength (F).

Step 9—The appliance is trimmed and smoothed.

Step 10—The oral cavity and appliance are inspected for stability and occlusion.

Complications

- Exothermic reaction can burn the oral cavity. This is avoided by using cooler-curing acrylics. Once curing is started, the appliance may be cooled with water spray. This may cause discoloration of the material.
- The tendency of the acrylic material to flow during the setting process into portions of the soft/hard tissue may be missed in fracture cases and may inhibit healing of oral structures.
- Sharp edges may be formed at the margins.
- Stomatitis may occur from food trapping between the appliance and gingiva. This generally will resolve without treatment a few days after the appliance is removed.

Aftercare—Follow-up

- Good oral hygiene must be maintained; owners should be encouraged to flush area twice daily with 0.2% chlorhexidine.

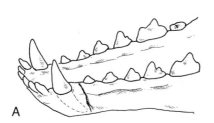

A

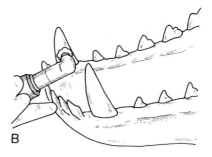

B

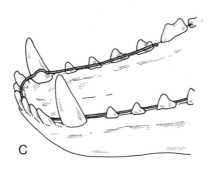

C

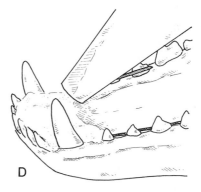

D

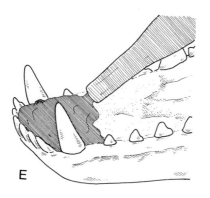

E

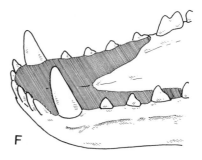

F

APPLIANCE FORMED ON AN ORAL CAST

- This method adds the additional steps of forming a working model (cast) to form the splint.

Indications

- Fractured maxillofacial complex.
- Fractured mandible anterior to the first molar.
- Luxated or subluxated teeth.
- To increase stability of other fixation techniques.

Contraindications

- Cases where numerous missing teeth prevent stabilization of the splint.
- Severely comminuted fractures without other techniques.

Objective

- To obtain stability so that healing may occur.

Materials

- Flour pumice (not prophy paste).
- Prophy angle and rubber prophy cups.
- Impression trays.
- Alginate impression material.
- Rubber bowl.
- Spatula.
- Die stone.
- Rope wax.
- Dental acrylics.
- Slow-speed handpiece with lab burs.
- Soft stainless steel orthopedic wire.
- Orthodontic wire; suggested sizes: 0.016", 0.020", 0.022", 0.028", 0.032", 0.036", and 0.040".

Technique

Step 1—Appropriate radiographs are taken, malalignments are corrected, and other therapy is performed as indicated.

Step 2—The proper impression tray is selected, alginate is mixed, and an impression is taken (see Chapter 9).

Step 3—A stone model is poured (see Chapter 9).

Step 4—An outline of the splint is created on the model with rope wax (see Chapter 9).

Step 5—Bonding sites for wiring the appliance in place are identified.

Step 6—Wire is bent from tooth to tooth to act as a support for the acrylic.

Step 7—A thin layer of the acrylic powder is applied.

Step 8—The liquid monomer is dripped onto the powder.

Step 9—Additional powder and liquid are alternatively applied until the appliance has been built up for sufficient strength.

Step 10—The appliance is trimmed and smoothed.

Step 11—The appliance is trial fitted and inspected for fit.

Step 12—The previously identified bonding sites are cleaned, flour pumiced, and acid etched for 15 to 30 seconds with phosphoric acid gel or solution; then they are rinsed with water for 30 seconds and air dried.

Step 13—The appliance is refitted.

Step 14—Orthodontic bonding material or light-cure restorative material is applied to the appliance and etched teeth to cement the appliance in place.

Complications

- The indirect formation of the cast is a longer procedure and is best suited for a team approach in cases with multiple trauma sites.
- Shifting of the jaw before, during, and after the impression is taken may complicate the installation of the splint.
- Open wounds should be protected from contamination with pumice slurry by the use of a water-soluble sterile lubricant jelly.
- Additional length of time for anesthesia is required to create the cast.

Aftercare—Follow-up

- Client must be instructed on good hygiene techniques. A water pick or other appliance may be used to aid in cleaning the oral cavity.
- Radiographs are taken at appropriate intervals.
- When healing has occurred, as determined radiographically and clinically, the appliance is removed with band-removing pliers or a high-speed drill.

SYMPHYSEAL FRACTURE REPAIR—ANTERIOR CERCLAGE TECHNIQUE

- Symphyseal fractures are common fractures in cats.

Indications

- Fractures of the mandibular symphysis to lateral incisor.

Contraindications

- Osteomyelitis.
- Severe periodontal disease.
- Comminuted fractures.

Objective

- A wire is passed between the skin and bone around both sides of the mandible behind the canine teeth to stabilize and compress the fracture/separation.

Materials

- How pliers.
- 22-gauge soft stainless steel wire.
- Large hypodermic needle (14 to 18 gauge).

Technique

Step 1—The wire is passed into the bore of the needle at the hub (A).

Step 2—The needle is inserted at the ventral midline into the skin of the mandible and is passed along the surface of the bone, directed dorsally to the buccal-distal side of the canine (B).

Step 3—The needle is grasped with orthodontic pliers while the wire is pushed up, but not completely through the needle (C). The needle is removed, leaving the wire between the bone and skin.

Step 4—The needle is reinserted at the ventral midline into the skin of the mandible and directed dorsally to the buccal-distal side of the opposite canine, in similar fashion to the first insertion (D).

Step 5—The wire is inserted into the bore at the tip of the needle (E).

Step 6—The needle is pulled out.

Step 7—While the symphysis is held in proper alignment, the wire is twisted until the mandible is stable (F).

Step 8—The wire is trimmed so that approximately 1/4 inch or 4 twists remain.

Step 9—The wire is gently bent back out of the way, so the sharp edge does not protrude.

Complications

- Breaking the wire by overtwisting. This requires re-wiring.
- Malalignment is prevented by checking the occlusion after the wire is tightened. If the occlusion is not correct, the procedure should be repeated, another technique used, or the patient evaluated for other fractures/TMJ problems.

Aftercare—Follow-up

- The wire is generally removed after 4 to 6 weeks and the jaw checked for stability.

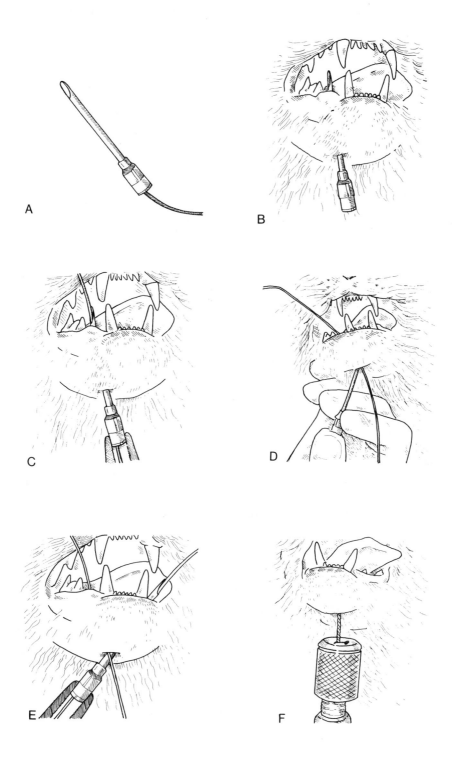

IVY LOOP WIRING TECHNIQUE

- The Ivy loop wiring technique can be used alone or with other fracture stabilization techniques.

Indications

- Fractured maxilla.
- Fractured mandible.
- Used to stabilize intraoral acrylic splints.

Contraindication

- Unstable or comminuted fractures with tooth loss.

Objective

- To place a single wire interdentally stabilizing and aligning adjacent teeth or provide anchorage for an intraoral splint.

Materials

- 24- or 26-gauge soft stainless steel wire.
- How pliers.
- Wire-twisting pliers.

Technique

Step 1—A length of wire is cut and a loop is formed in the middle (A). The ends are twisted together once.

Step 2—The free ends are passed from buccal to palatal/lingual in the interdental space between the two teeth to be stabilized, at the gingival margin (B).

Step 3—One free end is passed rostrally and around the mesial aspect of the first tooth at the interdental space (C).

Step 4—The other free end is passed caudally and around the distal aspect of the second tooth at the interdental space (D). This wire is passed through the preformed loop rostrally and is twisted tight with the other free end (E).

Step 5—The loop can be tightened further and the twisted ends bent to lie flat against the tooth surface.

Step 6—Dental acrylic or composite resin material can be placed over the wire loops for additional security of the wire and to minimize irritation of soft tissue from the loop twists (see splint bonding technique).

Complications

- Loosening wire with gingival irritation/recession.
- Inadequate fixation of fracture if used alone in unstable fractures.

Aftercare—Follow-up

- Home oral hygiene with water pick to keep area clean.
- Follow-up radiographs as necessary to evaluate healing.
- Removal of wire and acrylic when healing is complete.

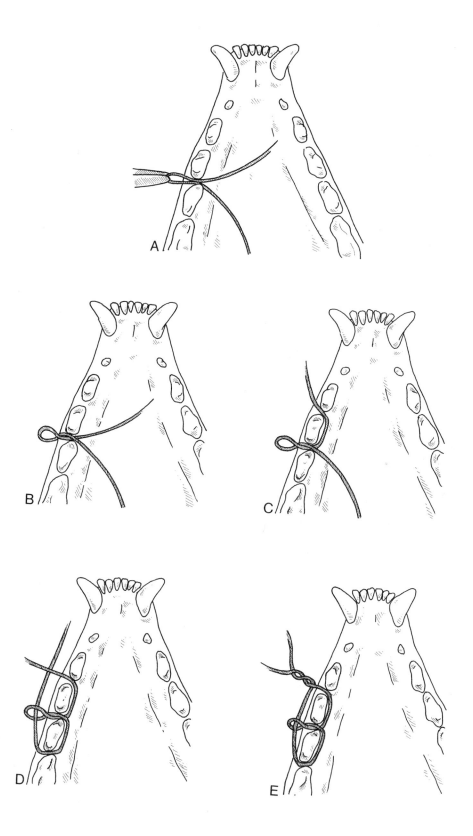

STOUT MULTIPLE LOOP WIRING TECHNIQUE

- Stout wiring technique can be used alone or with other stabilization techniques.
- This technique provides greater support of the dental arch than the Ivy loop technique.

Indications

- Fractured maxilla.
- Fractured incisal bone.
- Fractured mandible.
- To stabilize intraoral acrylic splint.

Contraindication

- Unstable or comminuted fractures with missing teeth.

Objective

- To stabilize several adjacent teeth with an interdental wiring technique.

Materials

- 24- or 26-gauge soft stainless steel wire.
- How pliers.
- Wire-twisting pliers.

Technique

Step 1—A length of wire is cut and pre-stretched to eliminate kinks *(A)*.

Step 2—One end of the wire is passed along the lateral surface of the teeth to be stabilized.

Step 3—The other end is passed around the distal tooth at the interdental space to the medial aspect *(B)*.

Step 4—This end is passed back to the lateral surface at the next interdental space under the buccal wire and looped over this wire and back through the same interdental space *(C)*.

Step 5—The loop formed is twisted tight while the ends of the wire are held taut in place along the teeth *(D)*.

Step 6—This process is repeated until all the teeth to be stabilized are encircled with the wire and the loops tightened *(E)*.

Step 7—The loop twists are bent flat against the tooth surface and can be covered with a dental acrylic or composite resin material for additional security after acid-etch preparation *(F)* (see acid-etch technique, Chapter 8).

Complication

- Loosening of wire with gingival irritation/recession.

Aftercare—Follow-up

- Home oral hygiene with a water pick to keep the area clean.
- Follow-up radiographs as necessary to evaluate healing.
- Removal of wires and acrylic when healing is complete.

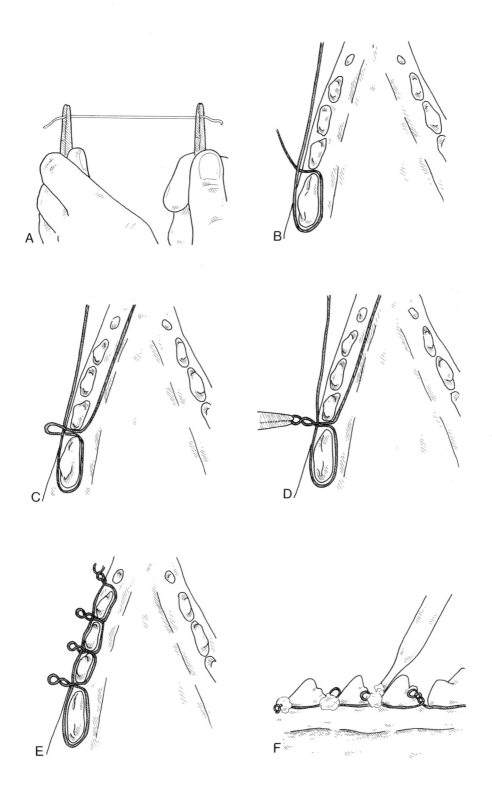

RISDON WIRING TECHNIQUE

- The Risdon technique uses a master wire with auxiliary wires looped around the necks of the teeth and twisted around the master wire.

Indication

- Rostral jaw fractures.

Contraindication

- Lack of good support for teeth (periodontal disease, fractured alveolus, etc.).

Materials

- Various-gauge (18 to 26) soft stainless steel wires.
- How or appropriate orthodontic pliers.

Technique

Step 1—A length of wire is passed around the tooth selected on each side of the jaw to be the distal anchors, leaving equal lengths on the buccal surface *(A)*.

Step 2—The free ends of the wires are twisted together for their entire length *(B)*.

Step 3—The twisted strands from each side are brought together at the midline and are twisted together *(C)*.

Step 4—Secondary wires are wrapped around the individual teeth in each arch and are twisted around the twisted master wire *(D)*.

Complications

- Loosening or breaking of wires, in which case the procedure is repeated or an alternate wiring technique is chosen.
- Irritation of gingiva or soft tissue from loose ends. Orthodontic wax or dental acrylic may be used to cover the sharp points of wire as prevention or treatment.

Aftercare—Follow-up

- Home oral hygiene with a water pick to keep the area clean.
- Follow-up radiographs as necessary to evaluate healing.
- Removal of wires and acrylic when healing is complete.

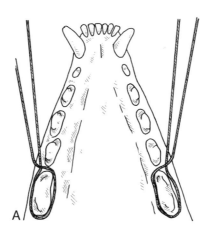

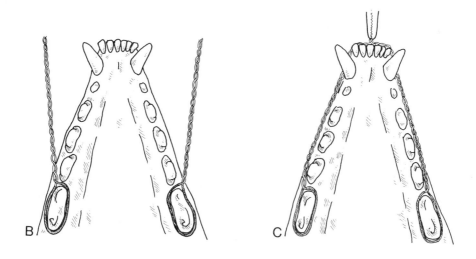

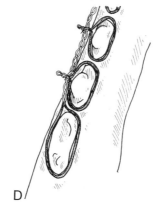

ESSIG WIRING TECHNIQUE

- The Essig wiring technique uses a master wire looped around the teeth involved and twisted, with secondary wires looped around the master wires in the interproximal space and twisted tight.

Indication

- Alveolar fractures with loose or partially avulsed teeth.

Contraindications

- Severe periodontal disease.
- Tooth root fractures without other treatment.
- Missing teeth.

Materials

- Various-gauge (18 to 26) soft stainless steel wires.
- How or appropriate orthodontic pliers.

Technique

Step 1—The master wire is looped around the buccal and lingual surfaces of the teeth (A). If possible, four to five teeth should be used as anchors on each side of the fracture.

Step 2—The master wire is twisted at a site that is out of occlusion (B).

Step 3—The secondary wires are fed through the interproximal space, passing palatally (lingually), looped around the palatal (lingual) portion of the master wire, and passed buccally/labially through the interproximal space and around the buccal/labial portion of the master wire (C).

Step 4—The secondary wires are twisted together (D). Secondary wires are gradually and sequentially tightened until the palatal (lingual) master wire is tight against the teeth.

Step 5—The teeth are examined for stabilization.

Complications

- Overtightening of the wire causing unwanted orthodontic movement.
- Irritation of soft tissues.

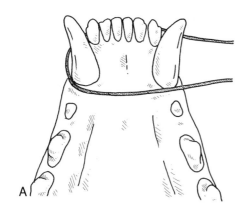

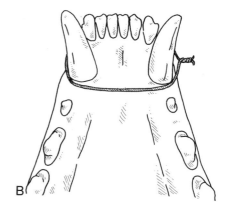

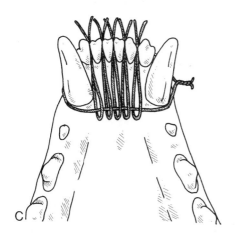

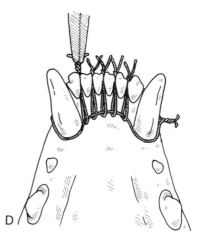

FIGURE-OF-EIGHT WIRING TECHNIQUE

- Wire is wrapped around the canine teeth to provide stabilization in combination with dental acrylics.

Indications

- Mandibular symphysis fracture/separation.
- Avulsion (with root canal therapy) or luxation of the canine tooth.

Contraindications

- Severe periodontal disease.
- Osteomyelitis.
- Failure to perform root canal therapy in the case of avulsed teeth.

Materials

- Various-gauge (18 to 26) soft stainless steel wires.
- How or appropriate orthodontic pliers.
- Acid-etch materials.
- Orthodontic or light-cure acrylics.

Technique

Step 1—The teeth are scaled and polished with flour pumice.

Step 2—The wire is looped from the mesial aspect of one canine (A) to the distal aspect of the opposite canine (B) *(A)*.

Step 3—The wire is looped in a buccal-mesial direction around the opposite canine *(B)*.

Step 4—The wire is directed from canine B back towards the distal aspect of canine A *(C)*.

Step 5—The two ends of the wire are joined together and are twisted on the distal surface *(D)*.

Step 6—The wire and teeth are rinsed and acid etched (see Chapter 8 on acid etching).

Step 7—Dental acrylic and/or composite is placed over the wire and teeth. The acrylic may be placed over the wire and mucosal tissue between the canines.

Step 8—Any rough surfaces are smoothed; then the appliance is polished.

Complications

- Breakage of wire.
- Slippage of wire from bonded teeth.
- Periodontitis from the wire.

Aftercare—Follow-up

- The wire is removed when healing has occurred (6 to 8 weeks)
- Depending on the case, radiographs may be necessary.
- Good oral hygiene must be performed.

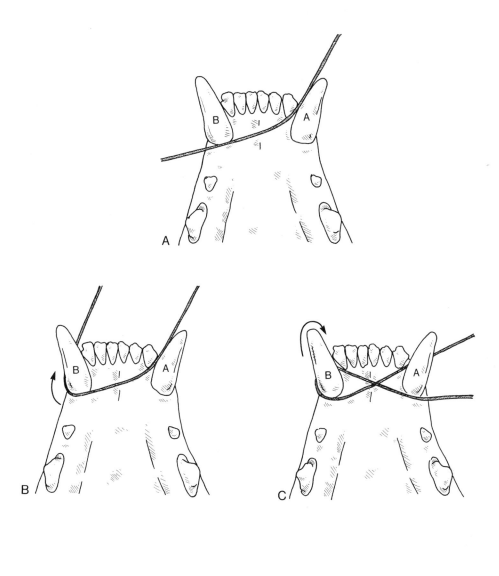

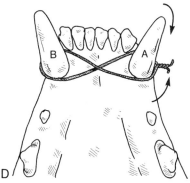

MANUFACTURERS AND SOURCES OF DENTAL MATERIALS

The following is a noncomprehensive list of manufacturers and sources of dental materials. It is included here to provide basic information and is not intended to advertise or endorse these suppliers.

ADDISON BIOLOGICAL LABORATORY, INC.
507 N. Cleveland Avenue
Fayette, MO 65248
Telephone (816) 248-2215
         (800) 311-2530
Products: Maxi/Guard, autogenous biologics, biologics

ALRICH-GIRARD CORP.
3627 N. Andrews Avenue
Oakland Park, FL 33309
Telephone (305) 561-8597
         (800) 654-5705
Products: Electric-motor–driven handpieces, nitrogen-air–driven dental equipment, air scalers, ultrasonic scalers

AMPCO DENTAL EQUIPMENT
1101 Highland Way
Grover City, CA 93433
Telephone (805) 473-0660
         (800) 444-3145
Products: Dental compressers, complete dental systems, handpieces, polishing instruments

ANALYTIC TECHNOLOGY
3301 181st Place
Redmond, WA 98052
Telephone (206) 883-2445
         (800) 428-2808
Product: Touch 'n Heat

ANDERSON DENTAL SERVICES
2054 Running Bridge Ct.
Maryland Heights, MO 63043
Telephone (314) 878-8480
Products: Chairside darkroom, automatic film processor, darkroom safe lights, darkroom chemicals

ARISTA SURGICAL SUPPLY CO., INC.
67 Lexington Avenue
New York, NY 10010
Telephone (212) 679-3694
         (800) 223-1984
Products: Dental and surgical instruments

AVLS
P.O. Box 67127
Lincoln, NE 68506
Telephone (800) 444-3634
Products: Client education aids

BRASSELER USA, INC.
800 King George Blvd.
Savannah, GA 31419
Telephone (912) 925-8525
         (800) 841-4522
Products: 40-mm K-files, hand instruments, burs, diamonds, abrasives

BUFFALO DENTAL MANUFACTURING CO.
575 Underhill Blvd.
Syosset, NY 11791
Telephone (800) 828-0203
Products: Orthodontic bowls, knives, spatulas, vibrators, bench engines, vacuum formers, burs, handpieces

BURNS VETERINARY SUPPLY, INC.
2019 McKenzie, Suite 109
Carrollton, TX 75006
Telephone (214) 620-9941
         (800) 527-7421
Products: Complete veterinary supply distributor; dental products and equipment

BUTLER COMPANY
5000 Brandeton Avenue
Dublin, OH 43017
Telephone (800) 848-5983
Products: Complete veterinary supply distributor; dental products and equipment

CAULK/DENTSPLY
Lakeview and Clark Avenues
Milford, DE 19963
Telephone (302) 422-4511
         (800) 532-2855
Products: Composite restoratives, bases, liners, cements, amalgam restoratives, impression materials

C.D.M.V. INC.
C.P. 608.2999 Choquette
St. Hyacinthe
Quebec, Canada J25 6H5
Telephone (514) 773-6073
Products: Complete veterinary supply distributor, dental products and equipment

CENTRIX, INC.
30 Stran Road
Milford, CT 06460
Telephone (203) 375-8904
            (800) 235-5862
Products: Centrix syringe, bonding agents

CISLAK MANUFACTURING, INC.
5768 W. 77th Street
Burbank, IL 60459
Telephone (708) 458-6163
Products: Hand instruments, feline elevator
kit, sharpening aides, full service dental
supplier

COE LABORATORIES, INC.
3737 W. 127th Street
Chicago, IL 60658
Telephone (800) 323-7063
Products: Impression materials, waxes,
dental materials

COLTEEN/WHALEDENT, INC.
236 Fifth Avenue
New York, NY 10001
Telephone (800) 221-3046
Products: Restorative dentistry supplies,
composites

COLTENE
14 Cane Industrial Drive
Hudson, MA 01749
Telephone (508) 563-3881
            (800) 882-3888
Products: Restorative products, impression
material, composite resins

CORE-VENT CORP.
15821 Ventura Blvd., Suite 420
Encino, CA 91436
Telephone (818) 783-1517
            (800) 551-3838
Products: Implants

COSMEDENT, INC.
5419 N. Sheridan Road
Chicago, IL 60640
Telephone (800) 621-6729
Products: Bonding porcelains, prophy cups,
pastes

COTTRELL, LTD.
7399 S. Tucson Way
Englewood, CO 80112
Telephone (303) 799-9401
            (800) 843-3343
Products: Infection-control products,
disposable plastic trays

CRESCENT DENTAL MANUFACTURING
CO.
7750 W. 47th Street
Lyons, IL 60534
Telephone (312) 447-8050
            (800) 323-8952
Products: Amalgamators, vibrators, prophy
cups

DEN MAT CORP.
P.O. Box 1729
Santa Maria, CA 93456
Telephone (805) 922-8491
            (800) 433-6628
Products: Restorative products, bonding
agents, composites

DENTAL HEALTH PRODUCTS
P.O. Box 355
Youngstown, NY 14174
Telephone (716) 745-9933
            (800) 828-6868
Products: Paper dental products

DENTALAIRE
1820 S. Grande Avenue, Suite D
Santa Ana, CA 92705
Telephone (800) 866-6881
Products and Services: Air compressors,
complete line dental supplies; handpiece
repair

DENTICATOR
11277 Sunrise Park Drive
Cordova, CA 95742
Telephone (916) 638-9303
            (800) 227-3321
Products: Prophy cups, prophy angles

DENVET SALES
11897 Beckett Fall Road
Florissant, MO 63033
Telephone (314) 653-0760
            (800) 523-6640
Products: Electric motor handpieces

DEPPEN ENTERPRISES, INC.
111 St. Matthews Avenue
San Mateo, CA 94401
Telephone (415) 342-2976
Products: Feline extraction forceps, tartar-removal forceps, toothpaste, toothbrushes

EASTMAN KODAK CO.
Health Science Division
Rochester, NY 14650
Telephone (800) 242-2424
Products: Film, radiographic educational aids

ELLMAN DENTAL MANUFACTURING CO.
1135 Railroad Avenue
Hewlett, NY 11557
Telephone (516) 569-1482
          (800) 835-5355
Products: Electrosurgery instruments, rotosonic instruments, burs, dental products

ENGLER ENGINEERING CORPORATION
1099 E. 47th Street
Hialeah, FL 33013
Telephone (305) 688-8581
          (800) 445-8581
Products: Scalers, scaler-polishers, endodontic instruments

FORT DODGE LABORATORIES
800 Fifth Street N.W.
Fort Dodge, IA 50501
Telephone (515) 955-9400
          (800) 383-6343
Products: Chlorhexadine solutions, homecare products, pharmaceuticals

G-C INTERNATIONAL CORP.
7830 East Renfield Road, Suite 12
Scottsdale, AZ 85260
Telephone (602) 948-5854
          (800) 548-9272
Products: Cements, filling materials, glass ionomers, dental instruments, impression materials

GEL KAM INTERNATIONAL
P.O. Box 80004
Dallas, TX 75380
Telephone (800) 527-0222
Products: Stannous fluoride gel

GEORGE TAUB PRODUCTS
277 New York Avenue
Jersey City, NJ 07307
Telephone (201) 798-5353
Products: Die spacers, stains, cavity liners, liquid acrylics, rubber separators, build-up liquids, sealers

GINGI-PAK
P.O. Box 240
Camarillo, CA 93011
Telephone (800) 437-1514
Products: Gingival packing cord, instruments

GOLDEN GATE HANDPIECE REPAIR
1953 Parkside Drive
Concord, CA 94519
Telephone (415) 676-1400
Services: Handpiece repair

GOODWOOD DENTAL ARTS LAB
647 E. Airport Avenue
Baton Rouge, LA 70806
Telephone (504) 928-4239
Services: Full service dental laboratory

HEALTHCO INTERNATIONAL
6555 Sough Kenton Street
Englewood, CO 80111
Telephone (303) 799-4488
          (800) 759-4488
Products: Instruments, equipment, x-ray equipment, impression materials

HENRY SCHEIN, INC.
5 Harbor Park Drive
Port Washington, NY 11050
Telephone (516) 367-9400
          (800) 872-4346
Products: Complete supply of veterinary and veterinary dental products

HU-FRIEDY CO.
3232 N. Rockwell Street
Chicago, IL 60618
Telephone (312) 975-6100
Products: Scalers, probes, dental instruments

HYGENIC
1245 Home Avenue
Akron, OH 44310
Telephone (216) 633-8460
          (800) 321-2135
Products: Heated gutta percha, waxes, acrylics

IMAGE IMPRINTS
P.O. Box 1029
North Hampton, MA 01061
Telephone (413) 586-4439
Products: Imprinted toothbrushes

INTEGRADENT
4206 N. 32nd Street, Suite 1
Phoenix, AZ 85018
Telephone (602) 381-8027
          (800) 822-8027
Products: Full service dental laboratory,
Mann incline plane

INTERPORE
18008 Skypark Circle
Irvine, CA 92714
Telephone (714) 261-3100
          (800) 722-44888
Products: Synthetic bone, implant material

INTERSTATE DENTAL
1500 New Horizon Blvd.
Amityville, NY 11701
Telephone (516) 957-8300
          (800) 645-7171
Products: Dental materials, pharmaceuticals

J. MORITA USA, INC.
14712 Bentley Circle
Tustin, CA 92680
Telephone (714) 544-2854
          (800) 752-9729
Products: Composite resins, dental
adhesives, restorative materials, x-ray
machines, video imaging system

JORGENSEN LABORATORIES
1450 N. VanBuren
Loveland, CO 80538
Telephone (303) 669-2500
Products: Hand instruments

KERR/SYBRON MANUFACTURING CO.
P.O. Box 455
Romulus, MI 48174
Telephone (313) 946-7800
          (800) 521-2854
Products: Composites, impression material,
amalgam laboratory products, endodontic
instruments

KYOCERA INTERNATIONAL
8611 Balboa Avenue
San Diego, CA 92123
Telephone (619) 576-2600
Products: Implants

LAK ENTERPRISES
1794 San Jose Avenue
San Francisco, CA 94112
Telephone (415) 333-2662
          (800) 228-5781
Products: Plastic spatulas, small mixing
bowls, impression trays

LANG DENTAL PRODUCTS
2300 W. Wabansia Avenue
Chicago, IL 60647
Telephone (800) 222-5264
Products: Acrylics

LEE PHARMACEUTICALS
1444 Santa Anita Avenue
South El Monte, CA 91733
Telephone (818) 442-3141
          (800) 423-4173
Products: Restorative and other dental
materials

LESTER DINE
100 Milbar Blvd.
Farmingdale, NY 11735
Telephone (516) 454-6100
Products: Close-up cameras

LORVIC CORP.
8810 Frost Avenue
St. Louis, MO 63134
Telephone (314) 524-7444
Products: Disclosing solution, prophy paste

3M DENTAL PRODUCTS CO.
Building 260-213-009 South, 3M Center
St. Paul, MN 55101
Telephone (612) 733-8283
          (800) 634-2249
Products: Restorative products, adhesive
products, impression materials, finishing
and polishing disks

M & D INTERNATIONAL
517 Maple Avenue
Carpenteria, CA 93013
Telephone (805) 684-4528
Products: X-ray film developer, portable
darkroom

MASEL ORTHODONTICS
2701 Bartrum Road
Bristol, PA 19007-6892
Telephone (215) 785-1600
          (800) 423-8227
Products: Orthodontic instruments,
materials, wire products

MATRIX MEDICAL, INC.
145 Mid County Drive
Orchard Park, NY 14127
Telephone (716) 662-6650
            (800) 847-1000
Products: Dental compressors, anesthesia,
emergency care products

METADENTIA
39-23 62nd Street
Woodside, NY 11377
Telephone (718) 672-4670
            (800) 221-0750
Products: Endodontic instruments,
handpieces

MICROCOPY
3120 Moonstation Road
P.O. Box 3074
Kennesaw, GA 30144
Telephone (404) 425-5715
            (800) 235-1863
Products: X-ray developer, portable
darkroom, diamonds, x-ray numbers

MICROLABS
6998 Sierra Ct.
Dublin, CA 94568
Telephone (415) 829-3611
            (800) 227-0936
Services: Full service dental laboratory

MILTEX INSTRUMENT CO., INC.
6 Ohio Drive
Lake Success, NY 11042
Telephone (516) 775-7100
            (800) 645-8000
Products: Hand instruments, burs, extraction
forceps

MINXRAY
3611 Comercial Avenue
Northbrook, IL 60062
Telephone (708) 564-0323
            (800) 221-2245
Products: Portable radiographic equipment

NEPHRON CORP.
321 E. 25th Street
Tacoma, WA 98421
Telephone (206) 383-1002
            (800) 426-3603
Products: Dental supplies, hand
instruments, burs, diamonds

NOBELPHARMA
51 Sawyer Road, Suite 100
Waltham, MA 02154
Telephone (617) 894-6575
            (800) 447-1160
Products: Implants

NYLABONE PRODUCTS
Box 427
Neptune, NJ 07753
Telephone (201) 988-8400
            (800) 631-2188
Products: Homecare chewing aids

OMNI PRODUCTS
P.O. Box 762
Bountiful, UT 84011-0762
Telephone (800) 777-2972
Products: Diamond burs

OMNI PRODUCTS INTERNATIONAL
P.O. Box 100
Gravette, AR 72736
Telephone (501) 787-5232
            (800) 284-4123
Products: Fluoride gels, rinses, toothbrushes,
implants

ORMCO CORP.
1332 South Lone Hill Avenue
Glendora, CA 91740-5339
Telephone (714) 596-0100
            (800) 854-1741
Products: Orthodontic supplies

ORTHO ORGANIZERS, INC.
1619 S. Rancho Santa Fe Road
San Marcos, CA 92069
Telephone (619) 471-0206
Products: Orthodontic supplies

OSMED, INC.
1669 Placenta Avenue
Costa Mesa, CA 92627
Telephone (714) 568-3417
Products: Synthetic bone

OSSECK VETERINARY EQUIPMENT
1721 Larkin Williams Road
Fenton, MO 63026
Telephone (314) 343-9686
Products: Dental cart (air compressor),
scalers

OXYFRESH USA, INC.
P.O. Box 3723
Spokane, WA 99220-3723
Telephone (509) 924-4999
Products: Homecare products

PARKELL
155 Schmitt Blvd., Box S
Farmingdale, NY 11735
Telephone (516) 249-1134
         (800) 243-7446
Products: Impression materials, bonding
materials, electrosurgical units, ultrasonic
scalers

PEARSON DENTAL
13847 Delsur Street
San Fernando, CA 91340
Telephone (818) 899-1200
         (800) 535-4535
Products: Vibrators, amalgamators, dental
materials, equipment, supplies

PETS VETERINARY DENTAL LAB
P.O. Box 867
Waukesha, WI 53187-9986
Telephone (414) 542-9205
         (800) 558-7734
Services: Full service dental laboratory

PLASDENT
1280 Price Avenue
Pomona, CA 91767
Telephone (714) 620-0289
Products: Plastic trays

PRECISION CERAMIC DENTAL LAB
9591 Central Avenue
Montclair, CA 91763
Telephone (800) 223-6322
Services: Full service dental laboratory

PREMIER/ESPE DENTAL PRODUCTS CO.
Box 111
Norristown, PA 19404
Telephone (800) 523-0440
Products: Glass ionomer restoratives,
cements, dental supplies

PROFESSIONAL DENTAL TECHNOLOGY
P.O. Box 4129
Batesville, AR 72503
Telephone (800) 228-5595
Products: Rotadent electric toothbrush

ROCKY MOUNTAIN ORTHODONTICS
P.O. Box 1887
Denver, CO 80201
Telephone (303) 320-2868
         (800) 525-6375
Products: Orthodontics

RX HONING MACHINE CORPORATION
1301 E. Fifth Street
Mishawaka, IN 46544
Telephone (219) 259-1606
         (800) 346-6464
Products: Sharpening equipment

SAN FRANCISCO DENTAL SUPPLY
1360 Mission Street #300
San Francisco, CA 94103
Telephone (415) 621-8406
         (800) 666-8406
Products: Distributor of dental products

SHOFU DENTAL CORP.
4025 Bohannon Drive
Menlo Park, CA 94025
Telephone (415) 324-0885
Products: Glass ionomers

SHOR-LINE, SCHROER
MANUFACTURING CO.
2221 Campbell Street
Kansas City, MO 64108
Telephone (816) 471-0488
         (800) 444-1579
Products: Scalers, compressors, tables

SPARTIN USA
1725 Larkin Williams Road
Fenton, MO 63026
Telephone (314) 343-8300
Products: Electric scalers

ST. JON LABORATORIES
1656 West 240th Street
Harbor City, CA 90710
Telephone (213) 326-2720
Products: Toothpastes, fluoride foam,
toothbrushes

STAR DENTAL PRODUCTS
1816 Colonial Village Lane
Lancaster, PA 17601
Telephone (717) 291-1161
         (800) 422-7827
Products: Titan-S scaler, handpieces

SUBURBAN SURGICAL CO., INC.
275 Twelfth Street
Wheeling, IL 60090
Telephone (708) 537-9320
　　　　　(800) 323-7366
Products: Compressors, handpieces, tables

SUMMIT HILL LABORATORIES
P.O. Box 535
Navesink, NJ 07752
Telephone (201) 291-3600
　　　　　(800) 922-0722
Products: Ultrasonic scalers, electric motors,
motor packs, electrosurgical units

TELEDYNE-GETZ
1550 Greenleaf Avenue
Elk Grove Village, IL 60007
Telephone (312) 593-3334
　　　　　(800) 323-6650
Products: Alginate, cements, trays, light cure
materials, surgical dressing, prophy cups

THERMAFIL
5001 E. 68th Street
Tulsa, OK 74136
Telephone (800) 662-1202
Products: Endodontic products

TROJAN CAMERA
3540 S. Figueroa Street
Los Angeles, CA 90007
Telephone (818) 908-5301
　　　　　(800) 338-9433
Products: Close-up cameras

ULTRADENT PRODUCTS, INC.
1345 East 3900 South
Salt Lake City, UT 84124
Telephone (801) 277-3203
　　　　　(800) 552-5512
Products: Tissue management products,
impression trays, precomposite materials,
sealant materials, gingival packing cord,
hemostatic solution

ULTRASONIC SERVICES, INC.
7126 Mullins Drive
Houston, TX 77081
Telephone (800) 874-5332
Products: Ultrasonic repair

UNION BROACH DENTAL PRODUCTS
3640 37th Street
Long Island, NY 11101
Telephone (800) 221-1344
Products: K-files, reamers

UNITEK CORPORATION
2724 South Peck Road
Monrovia, CA 91016
Telephone (818) 445-7960
　　　　　(800) 423-3748
Products: Orthodontic supplies (brackets,
etc), radiographic film

UNIVET (USA) LTD.
3095 Kerner Blvd.
San Rafael, CA 94901
Telephone (415) 459-0367
　　　　　(800) 835-3003
Products: General dental supplies

VERATEX/MEDARCO CORP.
P.O. Box 4031
Troy, MI 48007
Telephone (800) 552-8387
Products: Complete supply

VETERINARY COMPANIES OF AMERICA
P.O. Box 148
Topeka, KS 66601
Telephone (800) 982-5722
　　　　　(800) 241-2884
Products: Lymann impression trays,
veterinary distributor

VETERINARY PRODUCTS
LABORATORIES
P.O. Box 34820
Phoenix, AZ 85067-4820
Telephone (604) 285-1667
Products: Homecare products

VETERINARY STAINLESS, INC.
2213 Fairlawn Drive
Carthage, MO 64836
Telephone (417) 358-4716
Products: Dentistry wet/prep stainless-steel
tables

VIVADENT
5130 Commerce Drive
Baldwin Park, CA 91706
Telephone (818) 960-7531
　　　　　(800) 828-3839
Products: Restoratives, ceramics, abrasives,
cosmetic products

WHIP MIX CORP.
361 Farmington Avenue
Louisville, KY 40217
Telephone (502) 637-1451
       (800) 626-5651
Product: Quick-setting dental stone

YOUNG DENTAL MANUFACTURING
13705 Shoreline Court
Earth City, MO 63045
Telephone (314) 344-0010
       (800) 325-1881
Products: Hygiene products

INDEX

Note: Page numbers in *italics* indicate illustrations; those followed by (t) refer to tables.

A

Abrasion, definition of, 19
Abscess(es), apical, definition of, 21
  periapical, definition of, 21
  periodontal, definition of, 21
Abutment, definition of, 21
Acrylics, casting of, in mouth, 392, *393*
Alveolar bone, definition of, 18
Alveolar crest, definition of, 18
Alveolar mucosa, definition of, 18
Alveolitis, in tooth extraction, 184
Alveolus, definition of, 18
Amalgam, orthograde, obturation with, 248, *249*
  restorative, 302–305
    burnishing in, 304, *305*
      instruments for, 83, *83*
    carving in, 304
      instruments for, 83, *83*
    complications of, 304
    general comments on, 302
    indications and contraindications to, 302
    materials for, 302
      placement of, 304, *305*
    sealing dentinal tubules in, 302, *303*
    surface preparation in, 302, *303*
    technique of, 302, *303*, 304, *305*
Amalgam carriers, retrograde, 82, *83*
Amalgam condensers (pluggers), 82, *83*
Amalgam wells, 82
Amalgamators, 82, *83*
Anatomic charting, dental, 10, *11*
Anatomic identification, of teeth, 4
Anatomic terms, definitions of, 18–19
Anchorage, definition of, 21, 344
Ankylosis, in tooth extraction, 184

Anodontia, definition of, 19
Apex, definition of, 18
Apexification, 214–215, *215*
Apexogenesis, 214–215, *215*
Apical, definition of, 19
Apical delta, definition of, 18
Apical foramen, definition of, 18
Appliances, acrylic, maxillary, for anterior crossbite, 376–377, *377*
  formed in mouth, 392, *393*
  Maryland bridge, 382
    techniques of, 384
  orthodontic, 366–385
    acrylic, breakage of, 364
      breakage of model for, 364
      making of, 360, *361*
        brush method in, 364, *365*
        complications of, 364
        mixing technique in, 362, *363*
        salt and pepper technique in, 362, *363*
      sticking to model of, 364
    arch wire, 374
      labial, technique of, 374, *375*
      technique of, elastics in, 372, *373*
        finger springs in, 374, *375*
    button to button, 367, 370
      technique of, 367–368, *369*, 370, *371*
    definition of, 21
    expansion devices in, 376, 378
      technique of, 376–378, *377*, *379*
    inclined plane, 380–382, *381*, *382*, 382
      acrylic, 380
      cast metal, 380–381, *381*
      gingival wedge, 382
      techniques of, 380–382, *381*, *382*
Arch wires, orthodontic, 372, 374
  labial, technique of, 374, *375*

Arch wires (Continued)
  technique of, elastics in, 372, 373
    finger springs in, 374, 375
Arkansas stone, 56
Articulators, 88
Attachment apparatus, definition of, 18
Attrition, definition of, 19
Avulsion, definition of, 20
  splint bonding for, 390, 391

B

Bands, orthodontic, direct bonding of, 354
  making of, 358, 359
Bite. See also Occlusion.
  impression of, definition of, 21
  level, definition of, 20
  open, definition of, 21
  registration of, in impressions and castings,
    314–315
  reverse scissor, definition of, 21
  scissor, 342
  wry, 342
    definition of, 21
Boley gauge, in orthodontics, 90
Bonding, splint, 389–390
  technique of, 389, 390
Bonding agents, application of, 278, 279, 280,
    281
  chemical-cured, 278(t)
  dentin, 278(t)
Bone, hemorrhage of, in tooth extraction,
    treatment of, 182, 183
Bone crushing, for bone hemorrhage, 182
Bone defects, management of, 162–167
  bone grafting in, 166, 167
  general comments on, 162, 163
  ostectomy in, 164, 165
  osteoplasty in, 164, 165
  techniques of, 162–167
Bone grafting, for bone defects, 166, 167
Bone loss, horizontal, definition of, 20
  vertical, definition of, 21
Brachygnathia, definition of, 20
Brackets, orthodontic, breakage of, 356
  direct bonding of, complications of, 356
    technique of, 354, 355, 356, 357
Bridges, impressions and castings in,
    considerations in, 315
Broaches, endodontic, 70, 71
Buccal, definition of, 19
Buccal plate, gingival flap technique with, 192,
    193, 194, 195
Burs, handpiece, 40–47. See also Handpiece
  burs.
Buttons. See also under Appliances.
  orthodontic, breakage of, 356
  direct bonding of, complications of, 356
    technique of, 354, 355, 356, 357

C

Calcium hydroxide, in vital teeth restoration,
    336, 336(t)
  resin-based, 336(t), 337
Calculus, definition of, 20

Calculus (Continued)
  gross, removal of, 110–119. See also Prophy-
    laxis; Scalers.
  missed, detection of, 124, 125
  root planing for, 138
  subgingival, removal of, 120, 121, 122–123,
    123
    complications of, 122, 123
Canal. See Root canal.
Cannules, warmed gutta percha, 76, 77
Cap, definition of, 21
Capping, direct, of pulp, vital pulpotomy
    with, 210, 211, 212, 213
  indirect, of pulp, 208–209, 209
Caries, definition of, 20
Cast. See also Impressions; Models.
  definition of, 21
Cavity, indirect pulp capping for, 208–209, 209
Cement, composite resin, 327
  dental, 326(t), 326–327, 327
Cementoenamel junction, definition of, 18
Cementum, definition of, 18
Ceramic stone, 56
Cerclage, anterior, for symphyseal fracture,
    396, 397
Cervical line, definition of, 19
Cervical line lesions, of feline teeth. See
    Tooth(teeth), feline, cervical line lesions of.
Chisels, 78, 79
Chlorhexidine, for plaque removal, 134
Chloroform dip technique, of obturation, 242,
    243
Chloropercha/eucapercha technique, of
    obturation, 242
Cingulum, definition of, 18
Citric acid, in periodontal therapy, 156
Coagulation, for soft tissue hemorrhage, 182,
    183
Cold pack, for soft tissue hemorrhage, 182
Compressors, in dental equipment, 27–28
  accessories for, 29
  maintenance of, 29, 29
Condensation, obturation with, cold lateral,
    234, 235
  lateral and vertical, 240
  thermomechanical, 246, 247
  vertical, 238, 239, 240, 241
  warm lateral, 236, 237
  with softened gutta percha, 242, 243
Coronal, definition of, 19
Crossbite, anterior, definition of, 19
  mandibular Maryland bridge for, 384
  maxillary acrylic appliance for, 376–377,
    377
  maxillary Maryland bridge for, 384
  posterior, definition of, 21
Crown, definition of, 18, 21
Crown fractures, class A1, of enamel,
    treatment of, 270, 271
  class A2a, of enamel and dentin, treatment
    of, 270, 271
  class A2b, of enamel and dentin, treatment
    of, 270, 271
  class B, of root, treatment of, 270, 271
  vital pulpotomy with direct capping for, 210
Crown-root fracture, treatment of, 270, 271
Crown therapy, 308–337
  cementation in, 324, 325

Crown therapy *(Continued)*
  cementation of crown in, materials for,
    326(t), 326–327, *327*
  contraindications to, 309
  diamond burs for, 310, 312(t)
  die-stone in, 336
  dowel-core build-up in, 328
    complications of, 330
    technique of, 328, *329*, 330, *331*
  dowel-core casting in, 332
  evaluation for preparation in, 309
  general comments on, 308
  gingival retraction in, 334
  impressions and castings in, considerations
    in, 315
    for bite registration, 314–315
    with hydrocolloid/alginate, 314
    with polysulfide rubber, 312
    with rubber base, 312
    with siloxane polymers, 312
    with vinyl polysiloxane polymers, 312
      cautions in, 313
      technique of, 313
  indications for, 308
  laboratory orders in, manufacture of crown
    and, 320, *321*
  margin preparation in, champfer in, 310, *311*
    shoulder joint in, 310, *311*
    shoulder with external bevel in, 310–311,
      311
  materials for, 309
  metal-to-cement adhesion in, improvement
    of, 336
  objective of, 309
  over canine teeth, 333
  over vital teeth, calcium hydroxide in, 336,
    336(t)
    resin-based, 336(t), 337
    general comments on, 336
    lining/base materials in, 336(t)
  placement of crown in, trial, 320, *321*, 322,
    323
    complications of, 322
  reduction in, 310
    axial, 310, *311*
  special situations in, 328–333
  surgical crown lengthening in, 333
  technique of, 309–327
  temporary crown in, direct acrylic technique
    of, 316, *317*, 318, *319*
    general comments on, 316
Curettage, subgingival, 140, *141*
Curettes, 54, *55*
  cleaning and care of, 54
  in dental prophylaxis, techniques of, finger
    rests in, 112, *113*
    instrument-holding, 110, *111*
    working, 114, *115*
  sharpening of, conical stone technique of,
    60, *61*
    moving flat stone-Sharpen-Rite technique
      of, 58, *59*
    moving flat stone technique of, 56–57, *57*
    stationary flat stone technique of, 60, *61*
    stones for, 56
  surgical, 66
  types of, 54, *55*
    Barnhart 1/2, 54
    Barnhart 5/6, 54, *55*

Curettes *(Continued)*
  Columbia 3/4, 54, *55*
  Columbia 13/14, 54, *55*
  posterior, 54
  2R-2L, 54
  4R-4L, 54
  universal, 54, *55*
Cusp, definition of, 18

D

Darkrooms, chairside, 49
  dip tanks for, 49
Dental arch, definition of, 18
Dental chart, canine, *11*
  feline, *13*
  sample of, with disease, 16, *17*
Dental claw, 52, *53*
Dental devices, terminology for, 21
Dental equipment, 23–91
  endodontic, 70–77. See also *Endodontics,
    equipment for.*
  orthodontic, 86–91. See also *Orthodontics,
    equipment and instruments for.*
  periodontal, 50–69. See also *Periodontal equip-
    ment.*
  power, 23–47
    accessories for, 23
    air-driven, 26
      air rheostat controls in, 26
      automatic drain valves in, 28
      automatic/mechanical switching in, 28
      compressors for, accessories with, 29
        maintenance of, 29, *29*
        oil-free/oil-containing, 27
        remote, 27
        tableside, 27
        "whisper-quiet," 28
      electric foot switches in, 26
      experimentation in, plug-in "turnkey"
        units vs., 28–29
      handpieces in, 30–47. See also *Hand-
        pieces.*
      oil-level indicators in, 28, *29*
      three-way syringes in, 28, *29*
      variable features of, 26–29, *29*
    electric motor-driven band, 24–25, *25*
    features of, 23
      foot pedal, 23
      reverse direction, 23
      variable speed, 23
    handpieces in, electric motor, 25, 25–26
      electric motor-driven cable-connected, 25
    uses of, 23
  radiographic, 48–49. See also under *Radiol-
    ogy.*
  restorative, 78–85. See also *Restoration, equip-
    ment and instruments for.*
  selection of, 23
Dental fields, terminology for, 20
Dental hoe, 52, *53*
Dental positioning, terminology for, 19–20
Dental prophylaxis. See *Prophylaxis.*
Dental pulverization, 194–195
  for root tip extraction, 196, *197*
Dental quadrant, definition of, 18
Dental radiology. See *Radiology.*
Dental records, 1–22
  anatomic charting in, 10, *11*

Dental records (*Continued*)
  diagnostics/treatment plan/treatment completed in, 10
  general comments on, 6
  initial oral examination and, 8–9. See also *Oral examination, initial.*
  periodontal charting in, 12, *13–15*
  purpose of, 2
  tooth identification systems in, 2. See also *Tooth identification systems.*
Dental shorthand, of tooth identification, 4
Dental surfaces, terminology for, 19–20
Dental terminology, glossary of, 18–21
  anatomic terms in, 18–19
  dental devices in, 21
  dental fields in, 20
  dental positioning/surfaces in, 19–20
  oral diseases/conditions in, 20–21
Dentin, definition of, 18
  fracture of, treatment of, 270, *271*
Dentinal tubules, sealing of, in restorative amalgam, 302, *303*
Dentistry, restorative/operative, definition of, 19
Diamond burs, for crown therapy, 310, 312(t)
Diastema, definition of, 18
Disclosing solutions, for plaque and calculus detection, 124, *125*
Dressings, in periodontal therapy, 156

E

Edentulous, definition of, 20
Electrocautery, for soft tissue hemorrhage, 182
Elevators, as first-class lever, in single-rooted tooth extraction, 178, *179*
  as wedge lever, in single-rooted tooth extraction, 180, *181*
  dental, 66
    maintenance of, 66
    types of, 66, *67*
  exodontic, 176, *177*
  periosteal, 66
    maintenance of, 66
    types of, 66, *67*
Enamel, definition of, 18
  fracture of, treatment of, 270, *271*
Endo-Ring, 72, *73*
Endocarditis, in tooth extraction, 182
Endodontics, 207–266
  apexification in, 214–215, *215*
  apexogenesis in, 214–215, *215*
  definition of, 19
  equipment for, 70–77
    accessories for, 72, *73*, 74
    automated files in, 74
    bead sterilizers in, 74, *75*
    broaches in, 70, *71*
    canal filling instruments in, 74, *75*, 76, *77*
    cotton pliers in, 70
    Endo-Rings in, 72, *73*
    files in, 70–71, *71*
      cleaning of, 71
      organizers for, 72, *73*
    high-pressure syringe in, 74, *75*
    pluggers in, 74, *75*
      finger, 74, *75*
    reamers in, 70, *71*

Endodontics (*Continued*)
    cleaning of, 71
    spreaders in, 76, *77*
      electrically heated, 76, *77*
    warmed gutta percha cannules in, 76, *77*
  hard tissue formation in, 214–215, *215*
  indirect pulp capping in, 208–209, *209*
  nonsurgical, complications of, 253
  objective of, 208
  root canal in, nonsurgical, 216–253. See also *Root canal, nonsurgical.*
  surgical, 254–265
    complications of, 258
    general comments on, 254
    indications and contraindications to, 254
    materials for, 254
    objective of, 254
    of incisors, 260, *261*
    postoperative care in, 258
    technique of, 255
      access sites in, 256, *257*, 258, *259*
        for canine teeth, 262, *263*
        for double-rooted teeth, 264, *265*
        for incisors, 260, *261*
        for triple-rooted teeth, 264, *265*
      variations of, individual tooth types and, 260–265
  vital pulpotomy in, with direct pulp capping, 210, *211*, 212, *213*
Enzymatic products, for plaque removal, 133
Epithelial attachment, definition of, 18
Erosion, definition of, 20
Essig wiring, technique of, 404, *405*
Exodontics, 173–205. See also *Extraction.*
  contraindications to, 174
  definition of, 19
  dental pulverization in, 194–195
  general comments on, 174
  gingival flap/buccal plate technique in, 192, *193*, 194, *195*
    aftercare for, 194
    complications of, 194
  impacted unerupted imbedded teeth in, treatment of, 204, *205*
  indications for, 174, *175*
  materials for, complicated extraction pack in, 178
    multiroot extraction pack in, 178
    simple single-root extraction pack in, 178
  objectives of, 176, *177*
  oronasal fistula repair in, 198–203
  root-tip fragment extraction in, 196, *197*
Expansion devices, orthodontic, 376, 378
  technique of, 376–378, *377*, *379*
Exploration, periodontal, diagnostic, 128, *129*
  instruments for, 62, *63*
Extraction, instruments for, 66, *67*, 68, *69*
  dental elevators in, 66, *67*
  root tip picks in, 68, *69*
  materials for, complicated pack in, 178
    multiroot pack in, 178
    single-root pack in, 178
  of canine teeth, 185
    complications of, 185
    tongue hanging out of mouth from, 185
    trapping lip from, 185
  of incisors, 178, *179*, 180, *181*
    aftercare for, 184
    complications of, 182–184, *183*

Extraction (*Continued*)
  general comments on, 185
  of molars, mandibular first, 186, *187*, 188, *189*
    mandibular second, 186, *187*, 188, *189*
    mandibular third, 178, *179*, 180, *181*
      aftercare for, 184
      complications of, 182, *183*, 184
      general comments on, 185
    maxillary first, considerations in, 190, *191*
    maxillary second, considerations in, 190, *191*
  of multiple-rooted teeth, 186–191
    complications of, 188
    technique of, 186, *187*, 188, *189*
  of premolars, first, 178, *179*, 180, *181*
    complications of, 182–184
    general comments on, 185
    mandibular second, 186, *187*, 188, *189*
    mandibular third, 186, *187*, 188, *189*
    mandibular fourth, 186, *187*, 188, *189*
    maxillary second, 186, *187*, 188, *189*
    maxillary third, 186, *187*, 188, *189*
    maxillary fourth, considerations in, 190, *191*
  of primary teeth, 196–197
  of retained root tip fragments, 196, *197*
  of simple single-rooted teeth, 178, *179*
    aftercare in, 184
    alveolitis from, 184
    ankylosis from, 184
    cautions in, 185
    complications of, 182–184, *183*
    dental radiology in, 185
    endocarditis from, 182
    fractured root tips from, 182
    fractured socket from, 182, *183*
    gingival tissue tearing from, 184
    hemorrhage from, 182, *183*
    large tooth surface in, 184
    mandibular fracture from, *183*, 183–184
    oronasal fistula from, 184
    painful socket from, 184
    secondary infection from, 183
    technique of, 178, *179*
      first-class lever in, 178, *179*
      wedge lever in, 180, *181*
    tooth cutting site of, 184
  root tip fracture in, 182

F

Facet, definition of, 20
Facial, definition of, 19
Fédération Dentaire Internationale System, of
  tooth numbering, 6, *7*
Figure-of-eight wiring, technique of, 406, *407*
Files, automated, 74
  breakage of, in root canal therapy, 224
  endodontic, 70
    cleaning of, 71
    organizers for, 72, *73*
    types of, 70–71, *71*
Film, processing systems for, 48–49, 102–104.
    See also *Radiology, film-processing
    (development) systems for.*
  location of, 49
  manual, 48

Film (*Continued*)
  mechanical, 48–49, 102–103, *103*
  radiographic, 94, 94(t)
Finger rests, use of, 112, *113*
Finishing strips, for restorative smoothing, 284
Fistula, oronasal, definition of, 21
  in tooth extraction, 184
  repair of, 198, 202
    buccal flap technique of, 198, *199*
    double-flap techniques of, 200, *201*, 202, *203*
    palatal and buccal sliding flap for, 200, *201*
    palatal and labial buccal pedicle flap for, 202, *203*
    single-flap techniques of, 198, *199*
Flap(s), buccal sliding, for oronasal fistula, 198, *199*
  gingival, buccal plate technique with, 192, *193*, 194, *195*
  palatal and buccal sliding, for oronasal fistula, 200, *201*
  palatal and labial buccal pedicle, for oronasal fistula, 202, *203*
  periodontal. See *Periodontal flap techniques.*
Fluoride-based products, for plaque removal, 134
Forceps, calculus-removing, 114, *115*
  extraction, 68
    human, 68
    types of, 68, *69*
    veterinary, 68, *69*
Fracture(s), avulsion, splint bonding for, 390, *391*
  crown. See *Crown fractures.*
  dentin, treatment of, 270, *271*
  enamel, treatment of, 270, *271*
  Essig wiring for, 404, *405*
  figure-of-eight wiring for, 406, *407*
  Ivy loop wiring for, 398, *399*
  mandibular, appliance for, mouth formation of, 392, *393*
    in tooth extraction, *183*, 183–184
  Risdon wiring for, 402, *403*
  root, treatment of, 270, *271*
  root tip, in tooth extraction, 182
  socket, in tooth extraction, 182, *183*
  Stout wiring for, 400, *401*
  symphyseal, repair of, anterior cerclage technique of, 396, *397*
Freeway space, definition of, 20
Frenectomy, mandibular, 142, *143*
Furcation, definition of, 18
Furcation exposure, classification of, 12, *13–15*

G

Gauze sponge, for dental prophylaxis, 132–133
Gels, plaque removal, 133
Gingiva, attached, definition of, 18
  curettage of, 140, *141*
  definition of, 18
  free, definition of, 18
  hyperplastic, definition of, 20
    gingivectomy for, 144
    gingivoplasty for, 146
  retraction of, in crown therapy, 334
  tearing of, in tooth extraction, 184

Gingival flap, buccal plate technique with, 192, *193*, 194, *195*
Gingival groove, free, definition of, 18
Gingival index, classification in, 12, *13–15*
Gingival margin, free, definition of, 18
Gingival sulcus, definition of, 18
Gingivectomy, 144
  complications of, 146
  postsurgical care in, 146
  technique of, 144, *145*, 146, *147*
Gingivoplasty, 146, *147*
Glass ionomer liners, 336(t)
Glass ionomers, crown cementation with, 326(t), 326–327, *327*
  restorative, 286–301
    after root canal therapy, application in, 290, *291*, 292, *293*
      bonding agent application in, 290
      cautions in, 294, *295*
      shaping in, 292, *293*
      smoothing in, 294, *295*
      surface preparation in, 288, *289*
      technique of, 288–295
    for feline cervical line lesions, 298, *299*, 300, *301*
    general comments on, 286–287
    indications and contraindications to, 287
    materials for, 287
    types of, 287(t)
Gnathic, definition of, 18
Grafting, bone. See *Bone grafting.*
Grafting techniques, with free gingival graft, 160, *161*
  with pedicle graft, 158, *159*
Gutta percha, softened, condensation of, obturation with, 242, *243*
  thermoplasticized, obturation with, 250, *251*

H

Haderup system, of tooth identification, 5
Halitosis, definition of, 18
Handpiece burs, high-speed, 40–47
    accessories for, 46, *47*
    bur block for, 46, *47*
    cleaning brush for, 46, *47*
    diamond, 46, *47*
      cleaning stone for, 46, *47*
    fissure, 44, *45*
      tapered, 44, *45*
    flame, 46
    friction grip, changing of, for cap-style handpiece back, 42, *43*
      for overhead chuck-key type, 40, *41*
      replacement of turbine cartridge in, 42
    general considerations in, 44, *45*
    head lengths in, 44, *45*
    inverted-cone, 46, *47*
    multifluted finishing, 46, *47*
    pear-shaped, 46, *47*
    Rotopro, 46, *47*
    round, 44, *45*
    special-use, 46, *47*
  slow-speed, 34, *35*
    high-speed handpiece adapter for, 38, *39*
    latch-type, changing of, 34, *35*
    straight-type, changing of, 34, *35*
    types of, 36
Handpieces, electric motor, *25*, 25–26
    connected to cable driven by, 25
  general maintenance of, 30
  high-speed, 40–47
    burs for, 40–47. See also *Handpiece burs.*
    fiberoptics for, 40
    maintenance of, 40, *41*
    options for, 40
    wrenchless, 40
  slow-speed, 30–39
    autoclavable option for, 30
    burs for, 34, *35*, 36, 38, *39*. See also *Handpiece burs.*
    contra angles for, 32
    discs for, 38, *39*
    drills for, Gates Glidden, 36, *37*
      types of, 36
    green stones for, 38
    mandrels for, 38, *39*
    paste fillers for, 38, *39*
    Peeso reamer for, 36, *37*
    prophy angles for, 30–32, *33*
      circular, 30
      maintenance of, 31–32, *32*
      oscillating, 30–31
    wheels for, 38, *39*
    white stones for, 38, *39*
Hard tissue formation, 214
Hatchets, 78, *79*
Hedström files, 71, *71*
Heidbrink root tip pick, 68, *69*
Hemorrhage, bone, in tooth extraction, treatment of, 182
  persistent, of pulp, treatment of, 226, *227*
  soft tissue, in tooth extraction, treatment of, 182, *183*
Hydrocolloid, with alginate, for impressions and castings, 314
Hyperplasia, gingival, definition of, 20

I

Impression trays, 86, *87*
  custom made, 86
  manufactured, 86
  tray adhesives for, 86
Impressions, definition of, 21
  in orthodontics, 346
    complications of, 348
    technique of, 346, *347*, 348, *349*
Incisal, definition of, 19
Incisal edge, definition of, 18
Incisors, definition of, 19
  extraction of, 178, *179*, 180, *181*
    aftercare for, 184
    complications of, 182–184, *183*
    general comments on, 185
  lower, caudal movement of, button to button appliance for, 370, *371*
  surgical endodontics of, 260, *261*
Inclined plane, orthodontic, 380, 382
    techniques of, 380–382, *381*, *383*
      acrylic, 380
      cast metal, 380–381, *381*
      gingival wedge, 382, *383*
India stone, 56
Infection, secondary, in tooth extraction, 183
Infrabony pocket, definition of, 19

Interdental, definition of, 19
Interproximal, definition of, 19
Interradicular, definition of, 19
Ivy loop wiring, technique of, 398, *399*

J

Jiffy tubes, 84
Juga, definition of, 19

K

K-files, 70, *71*
Kirkland knife, 65, *65*

L

Labial, definition of, 19
Lamina dura, definition of, 19
Ligation, for soft tissue hemorrhage, 182
Light-cure gun, 78–80, *81*
    accessories for, 79–80, *81*
    continuous "on," 78
    fiberoptic cord vs. pistol in, 78
    high-energy output, 78
    light analysis tool for, 80
    multiple tips for, 79
        maintenance of, 80, *81*
    options for, 78
    shield tip for, 80, *81*
Line angle, definition of, 19
Lingual, definition of, 19
Lip, trapping between gum and tooth of,
        canine tooth extraction and, 185
Liquids, plaque removal, 133
Luxation, definition of, 20

M

Mandible, definition of, 19
Mandibular fracture, appliance for, mouth
        formation of, 392, *393*
    in tooth extraction, *183*, 183–184
Mandibular frenectomy, 142, *143*
Manufacturers of dental materials, 409–417
Maryland bridge, 382
    techniques of, 384
Materials, dental, manufacturers and sources
        of, 409–417
Maxilla, definition of, 19
McSpadden method, of obturation, 246, *247*
Medical records, veterinary, general comments
        on, 6
Mental foramen, definition of, 19
Mesial, definition of, 19
Microleakage, in restorative amalgam, 304
    in restorative plastics, 284
Mirrors, periodontal, 62–63
Mobility, classification in, 12, *13–15*
Models, appliance formed on, 394–395
    in orthodontics, air bubbles in, 352
        complications of, 352, *353*
        desiccation of alginate in, 352
        fracture of model crowns in, 352, *353*
        inadequate mixing in, 352

Models *(Continued)*
        incorrect mix ratios in, 352
        indications for, 350
        nonrigid trays in, 352
        technique of, 350, *351*, 352, *353*
Molars, crown therapy for, special
        considerations in, 333
    definition of, 19
    mandibular first, extraction of, 186, *187*, 188,
        189
    mandibular second, extraction of, 186, *187*,
        188, *189*
    mandibular third, extraction of, 178, *179*,
        180, *181*
        aftercare for, 184
        complications of, 182–184, *183*
        general comments on, 185
    maxillary first, extraction of, considerations
        in, 190, *191*
    maxillary second, extraction of, considera-
        tions in, 190, *191*
    surgical endodontics of, considerations in,
        264
Mucogingival line, definition of, 19

N

Neck (cervical line), definition of, 19
Nonadhesive strips, for restorative smoothing,
        284

O

Obturation, 228–253
    application of sealer in, 228, *229*
    application of solid filling material in, 232–
        253
    broken-instrument technique of, 246, *247*
    by cold lateral condensation, 234, *235*
    by custom point fill, 244, *245*
    by lateral and vertical condensation, 240
    by thermomechanical condensation, 246, *247*
    by vertical condensation, 238, *239*, 240, *241*
    by warm lateral condensation, 236, *237*
    chloroform dip technique of, 242, *243*
    chloropercha/eucapercha technique of, 242
    injection filling technique of, 230, *231*
    inverted cone technique of, 248, *249*
    McSpadden method of, 246, *247*
    single-cone technique of, 232, *233*
    spiral filling technique of, 230, *231*
    with orthograde amalgam, 248, *249*
    with softened gutta percha condensation,
        242, *243*
    with thermafil, break-off technique of, 252–
        253
        carrier removal technique of, 253
    with thermoplasticized gutta percha, 250,
        251
Occlusal, definition of, 19
Occlusion, class 1, 342, *343*
    class 2, 342, *343*
    class 3, 342, *343*
    evaluation of, 340, *341*
    normal, 342
    unclassified, 342
Odontalgia, definition of, 21

Odontoblast, definition of, 19
Oligodontia, definition of, 21
Omega wire, 378
Oral disease, terminology for, 20–21
Oral examination, initial, chief complaint in, 8
    client/patient information in, 8
    diet in, 8
    health history in, 8
    home oral hygiene in, 8
    past dental history in, 8
    recording specific findings in, 8–9
Oral surgery, definition of, 19
Orban knife, 65, 65
Oronasal fistula. See Fistula, oronasal.
Orthodontics, 339–387
    appliances in, 360–364, 366–385. See also Appliances, orthodontic.
    bands in, direct bonding of, 354
        making of, 358, 359
    brackets in, breakage of, 356
        direct bonding of, 354
            complications of, 356
            technique of, 354, 355, 356, 357
        removal of, tooth discoloration after, 356
    buttons in, breakage of, 356
        direct bonding of, 354
            complications of, 356
            technique of, 354, 355, 356, 357
    definition of, 19
    equipment and instruments for, 86–91
        articulators in, 88
        Boley gauge in, 90
        impression trays in, 86, 87
        large mixing (buffalo) spatulas in, 87, 87
        pliers in, 90. See also Pliers, orthodontic.
        rubber bowls in, 86, 87
        storage trays in, 90
        vibrators in, 88, 89
        welders in, 88
    fundamentals of, 344, 345
    impressions in, 346
        complications of, 348
        technique of, 346, 347, 348, 349
    interceptive, 366
    laboratory prescription for, 386, 387
    models in, complications of, 352, 353
        indications for, 350
        technique of, 350, 351, 352, 353
    occlusal evaluation in, 340–345. See also under Occlusion.
    retainer period of, 344
    techniques of, 346–365
Orthopedics, dental, 389–407
    anterior cerclage in, 396, 397
    appliance formed on cast in, 394–395
    appliance formed orally in, 392, 393
    Essig wiring in, 404, 405
    figure-of-eight wiring in, 406, 407
    Ivy loop wiring in, 398, 399
    Risdon wiring in, 402, 403
    splint bonding in, 389–390
        technique of, 389, 390
    Stout wiring in, 400, 401
Ostectomy, for bone defects, 164, 165
Osteoplasty, for bone defects, 164, 165
Overbite, definition of, 21

P

Packing, gauze, for bone hemorrhage, 182
Pads, mixing, glass, 84
    paper, 84
Palatal, definition of, 19
Palate, definition of, 19
Palmer notation system, of tooth identification, 2, 3
Pastes, plaque removal, 133
Pellicle, acquired, definition of, 19
Periodontal charting, 12, 13–15
    indices in, 12, 13–15
        furcation exposure in, 12, 13–15
        gingival index in, 12, 13–15
        mobility in, 12, 13–15
        plaque index in, 12, 13–15
Periodontal disease, 106–108, 107, 108(t), 109
    cause of, 106
    stages of, 107, 107–108, 109
    treatment and prevention of, 108, 108(t)
Periodontal equipment, calculus-removal forceps in, 50–51, 51
    curettes in, 54, 55. See also Curettes.
        surgical, 66
    dental claw in, 52, 53
    dental hoe in, 52, 53
    diagnostic, 62–63, 63
        explorers in, 62, 63
        mirrors in, 62–63
        probes in, 62, 63
    fine hand instruments in, 52–61. See also Curettes; Scalers.
        carbon steel, 52
        options in, 52, 53
        replaceable tip, 52, 53
        stainless steel, 52
    large hand instruments in, 52, 53
    periosteal elevators in, 66
        maintenance of, 66, 67
        types of, 66, 67
    scalers in, 53, 53. See also Scalers.
    surgical, 64–66, 65
        knives in, 64
            sharpening of, 65, 65
            types of, 65, 65
        scalpel blades for, 64, 65
        scissors in, 66, 67
Periodontal flap techniques, 148–156
    apically repositioned, 156, 157
    open curettage in, 148, 149
    palatal or lingual surface, for canine teeth, 150, 151
    reverse bevel, 152, 154
        technique of, 152, 153, 154, 155
Periodontal indices, 12, 13–15
    furcation exposure in, 12, 13–15
    gingival index in, 12, 13–15
    mobility in, 12, 13–15
    plaque index in, 12, 13–15
Periodontal ligament, definition of, 19
    tooth root attachment by, 344
Periodontal pocket, definition of, 21
Periodontal therapy, 137–171
    bone defect management in, 162–167. See also Bone defects, management of.
    citric acid in, 156
    dressings in, 156

Periodontal therapy *(Continued)*
    flap techniques in, 148–156. See also *Periodontal flap techniques.*
    general comments on, 138
    gingivectomy in, 144, *145,* 146, *147*
    gingivoplasty in, 146, *147*
    mandibular frenectomy in, 142, *143*
    objectives of, 138
    root planing in, 138, *139*
    soft tissue grafting techniques in, 158–161
        with free gingival graft, 160, *161*
        with pedicle graft, 158, *159*
    splinting in, 168, *169,* 170, *171*
        figure-of-eight wiring technique of, 168, *169*
        lingual wire or pin stabilization technique of, 170, *171*
    subgingival curettage, 140, *141*
Periodontics, definition of, 19
Periodontium, definition of, 19
Pins, restorative, cautions in, 306
    general comments on, 306
    technique of, 306, *307*
Plaque, definition of, 21
    missed, detection of, 124, *125*
    removal of, compounds for, 133–134
    subgingival, removal of, 120, *121*
        complications of, 122, *123*
Plaque index, classification in, 12, *13–15*
Plastics, restorative, 274–286
    complications of, 284
    general comments on, 274
    indications and contraindications to, 274
    materials for, 274
    product options in, 286
    technique of, 274–275
        bonding agent application in, 278, 278(t), *279,* 280, *281*
        restorative agent application in, 280, 280(t), *281*282, 282(t), *283*
        shaping in, 284, *285*
        smoothing in, 284
        surface preparation in, *275,* 275–276, *277*
Pliers, cotton, 70
    orthodontic, 90, *91*
        band/bracket-removing, 90, *91*
        bird beak (loop-forming), 90, *91*
        How, 90, *91*
        three-prong (triple-beaked), 90, *91*
        tweed arch-adjusting, 90, *91*
        tweed loop-forming, 90, *91*
        wire cutting, 90, *91*
Pluggers, 74, *75*
    finger, 74, *75*
Pocket, subgingival, irrigation of, 130, *131*
Polishing, in dental prophylaxis, 126, *127*
Polymers, siloxane, for impressions and castings, 312
    vinyl polysiloxane, for impressions and castings, 312
        cautions in, 313
        technique of, 313
Powders, plaque removal, 133
Premolars, crown therapy for, special considerations in, 333, *334*
    definition of, 19
    first, extraction of, 178, *179,* 180, *181*
        aftercare for, 184
        complications of, 182–184, *183*

Premolars *(Continued)*
    general comments on, 185
    mandibular second, extraction of, 186, *187,* 188, *189*
    mandibular third, extraction of, 186, *187,* 188, *189*
    mandibular fourth, extraction of, 186, *187,* 188, *189*
    maxillary second, extraction of, 186, *187,* 188, *189*
    maxillary third, extraction of, 186, *187,* 188, *189*
    maxillary fourth, extraction of, considerations in, 190, *191*
    surgical endodontics of, access to distal root of, 264
        access to mesial-buccal root of, 264
        access to palatal root of, 264
Pressure, for soft tissue hemorrhage, 182
Probes, periodontal, 62
    color-coded, 62, *63*
    diagnostic, 128, *129*
    notched, 62, *63*
    types of, 62, *63*
Prophylaxis, 105–136
    closed subgingival plaque and calculus removal in, 120, *121*
        complications of, 122, *123*
    detection of missed calculus and plaque in, air technique of, 124, *125*
    disclosing solutions for, 124, *125*
    diagnostics in, periodontal probing/exploring in, 128, *129*
    radiology in, 128
    general comments on, 106, 110
    gross calculus removal in, 110–119
        calculus-removing forceps in, 114, *115*
        power instrumentation in, rotary scaler (rotosonic scaling) in, 118, 118(t)
            sonic, 116, *117,* 118, *119*
            ultrasonic, 114, *115*
        scalers and curettes in, 110
            complications of, 114
            techniques of, finger rests in, 112, *113*
                instrument-holding, 110, *111*
                working, 114, *115*
    home-care instruction in, 132
        care plans for, condition and ability and, 136
        complications of, 134
        techniques of, 132–134
            brushing, 134, *135*
            gauze sponge in, 132–133
            mechanically powered toothbrush in, 132
            toothbrush in, 132
            types of compounds in, 133–134
            water pick in, 133
            wiping, 134, *135*
    oral examination in, 106
    periodontal disease and, 106–108, *107,* 108(t), *109*
    polishing in, 126, *127*
    sulcus/pocket irrigation in, 130, *131*
Prosthesis, definition of, 21
Prosthodontics, definition of, 19
Proximal, definition of, 19
Pulp, definition of, 19

Pulp *(Continued)*
  direct capping of, vital pulpotomy with, 210,
    211, 212, 213
  indirect capping of, 208–209, *209*
  persistent hemorrhage of, treatment of, 226,
    227
Pulp chamber, definition of, 19
Pulpitis, definition of, 21
Pulpotomy, vital, with direct pulp capping,
    210, *211, 212, 213*
Pulverization, dental, 194–195
  for root tip extraction, 196, *197*
Pyorrhea, definition of, 21
Pyrophosphate, for plaque removal, 133

R

Radicular, definition of, 19
Radiology, 93–104
  contraindications to, 94
  dental radiographic units in, 48
  film for, 94, 94(t)
  film-processing (development) systems for,
    48–49, 102–104
    darkrooms in, chairside, 49
      dip tanks for, 49
    hand-tank in, 102, *103*
    large-film processors in, 49
    location of, 49
    manual, 48
    mechanical, 48–49
    one-step rapid, 48, 102
    small-film processors in, 49
    standard veterinary medical solutions in,
      48
    two-step rapid, 48, 102–103, *103*
      complications of, 104
  in dental prophylaxis, 128
  in tooth extraction, 185
  indications for, 94, *95*
  intraoral techniques of, 96
    bisecting angle, 98, *99,* 100
      complications of, 100
    parallel, 96, *97*
  objectives of, 94, *95*
  veterinary medical units in, 48
Reamers, endodontic, 70
  cleaning of, 71
  types of, 70, *71*
Resins, chemical-cured composite, defective
    restorations with, repair of, 286
  types of, 280(t)
Resorption, definition of, 21
Restoration, 267–338
  amalgam for, 302–305. See also *Amalgam, re-
    storative.*
  bleaching in, of nonvital teeth, 337–338
  classification of lesions in, 268, *269,* 270, *271*
    by extent of fracture, 270, *271.* See also
      Crown fractures.
    by location, 268, *269*
  crown therapy in, 308–337. See also *Crown
    therapy.*
  equipment and instruments for, 78–85
    amalgam burnishers in, 83, *83*
    amalgam carvers in, 83, *83*
    amalgam condensers (pluggers) in, 82, *83*
    amalgam wells in, 82

Restoration *(Continued)*
    amalgamators in, 82, *83*
    chisels in, 78, *79*
    curved-tip syringes in, 84–85
    hatchets in, 78, *79*
    jiffy tubes in, 84
    light-cure gun in, 78–80, *81.* See also *Light-
      cure gun.*
    mixing pads in, 84
    mixing spatulas in, 84
    plastic-working (filling), 84
  general comments on, 268
  glass ionomers for, 286–301. See also *Glass
    ionomers.*
  materials for, 272–305. See also specific ma-
    terial; e.g., *Amalgam.*
    general comments on, 272
  of feline cervical line lesion, 296, *297*
  over vital teeth, calcium hydroxide in, 336,
    336(t)
    resin-based, 336(t), 337
    general comments on, 336
    lining/base materials in, 336(t)
  pin, cautions in, 306
    general comments on, 306
    technique of, 306, *307*
  plastics for, 273–286. See also *Plastics.*
  techniques of, cavity preparation, 272
    cutting, 272, *273*
Restorative agent, application of, 280, *281,* 282,
    283
  light cure, application of, 282, *283*
    cautions in, 282
    types of, 282(t)
  resin types of, 280(t)
Risdon wiring, technique of, 402, *403*
Root, attachment to bone of, 344
  definition of, 19
  fenestration of, definition of, 21
  fracture of, treatment of, 270, *271*
Root canal, definition of, 19
  instruments for filling of, 74, *75,* 76, *77*
  lateral (accessory), definition of, 19
  nonsurgical, 216–253
    cleaning and shaping in, complications of,
      224
      objective of, 220
      postoperative care in, 224
      technique of, 220, *221, 222, 223,* 224, *225*
    comments on, 216
    complications of, 253
    coronal access to pulp chamber in, 218,
      219
    glass ionomer restorative after, 288–295.
      See also under *Glass ionomers.*
    indications and contraindications to, 216,
      217
    objective of, 216
    obturation in, 228–253. See also *Obturation.*
    persistent pulp hemorrhage in, treatment
      of, 226, *227*
    postoperative care in, 253
    restoration of coronal access in, 253
Root planing, closed technique of, 138, *139*
Root tip picks, for extractions, 68, *69*
Root tips, fracture of, in tooth extraction, 182
  retained fragments of, extraction of, 196, *197*
Rubber, for impressions and castings, 312

Rubber *(Continued)*
    polysulfide, for impressions and castings, 312
Rubber bowls, 86, *87*
Ruga palatina, definition of, 19

S

Saliva substitutes, for plaque removal, 133
Sanding discs, for restorative smoothing, 284
Sanguinaria-based products, for plaque removal, 133–134
Scalers, 53, *53*
    cleaning and care of, 54
    H6–H7, 54, *55*
    in dental prophylaxis, 110
        techniques of, finger rests in, 112, *113*
            instrument-holding, 110, *111*
            working, 114, *115*
    Jacquette 2Y-3Y, 54, *55*
    maintenance of, 54
    Morse 0–00, 54, *55*
    N135, 54, *55*
    periodontal, sonic, 50, *51*
        ultrasonic, 50
            maintenance of pot/stack model of, 50, *51*
            tip-only replacement model of, 50, *51*
    rotary, for calculus removal, 118, 118(t)
    sharpening of, conical stone technique of, 60, *61*
        moving flat stone-Sharpen-Rite technique of, 58, *59*
        moving flat stone technique of, 56–57, *57*
        stationary flat stone technique of, 60, *61*
        stones for, 56
    sonic, for calculus removal, 116, *117*, 118, *119*
    types of, 54, *55*
    ultrasonic, for calculus removal, 114, *115*
Scalpel blades, periodontal, hawk-billed, 64, *65*
    number 11, 64, *65*
    number 15, 64, *65*
    number 12 and 12B, 64, *65*
    number 15C, 64, *65*
    types of, 64, *65*
Scissors, surgical, 66, *67*
    Goldman Fox number 15, 66, *67*
    LaGrange, 66, *67*
    Minnesota retractor, 66, *67*
Sharpen-Rite technique, of scaler and curette sharpening, 58, *59*
Sharpening stones, Arkansas, 56
    ceramic, 56
    India, 56
Socket, fracture of, in tooth extraction, 182, *183*
    painful, in tooth extraction, 184
Soft tissue, grafting techniques of, with free gingival graft, 160, *161*
        with pedicle graft, 158, *159*
    hemorrhage of, in tooth extraction, treatment of, 182, *183*
Spatulas, large mixing (buffalo), 87, *87*
    mixing, 84
Splint, definition of, 21
Splinting, periodontal, 168, *169*, 170, *171*
        figure-of-eight wiring in, 168, *169*

Splinting *(Continued)*
        lingual wire or pin stabilization in, 170, *171*
Sprays, plaque removal, 133
Spreaders, 76, *77*
    electrically heated, 76, *77*
    finger, 74, *75*
Sterilizers, bead, 74, *75*
Stomatitis, definition of, 21
Stout wiring, technique of, 400, *401*
Sublingual, definition of, 19
Sulcus, subgingival, irrigation of, 130, *131*
Surgical knives, periodontal, 64
        sharpening of, 65, *65*
        types of, 65, *65*
Symphyseal fracture, repair of, anterior cerclage technique of, 396, *397*
Syringes, curved-tip, 84–85
        metal, 85
        plastic, 85
    high-pressure, 74, *75*
    three-way, 28, *29*

T

Thermafil, obturation with, break-off technique of, 252–253
        carrier removal technique of, 253
Tongue, hanging out of mouth of, canine tooth extraction and, 185
Tooth(teeth), anterior, definition of, 18
    canine, crown therapy for, special considerations in, 333
        definition of, 18
        extraction of, 185
        lingually displaced, expansion device for, 378, *379*
        mandibular rostrally displaced, button to button appliance for, 368, *369*
        maxillary displaced, button to button appliance for, 368, *369*
        surgical endodontics of, 262, *263*
    carnassial, definition of, 18
    deciduous, definition of, 18
    discoloration of, from orthodontic brackets, 356
    double-rooted, surgical endodontics of, 264, *265*
    embedded, definition of, 20
    extraction of. See *Extraction.*
    feline, cervical line lesions of, etiology of, 296
        glass ionomer restorative for, 298, *299*, 300, *301*
        restoration for, 296, *297*
        signs of, 296
    fused, definition of, 20
    gemini, definition of, 20
    imbedded, treatment of, 204, *205*
    impacted, definition of, 20
        treatment of, 204, *205*
    incisor. See *Incisors.*
    molar. See *Molars.*
    movement of. See also *Orthodontics.*
        types of, force applied and, 344, *345*
    multiple-rooted, extraction of, 186–191
    nonvital, bleaching of, 337
        active technique of, 337

Tooth(teeth) *(Continued)*
    aftercare in, 338
    complications of, 337–338
    walking technique of, 337
  posterior, definition of, 19
  premolar. See *Premolars.*
  primary, definition of, 19
    extraction of, 196–197
  simple single-rooted, extraction of, complications of, 182–184, *183*
    techniques of, 178, *179*, 180, *181*
  supernumerary, definition of, 21
  triple-rooted, surgical endodontics of, 264, *265*
  unerupted, treatment of, 204, *205*
Tooth cutting, into extraction site, 184
Tooth identification systems, 2
  dental shorthand/anatomic identification, 4
  numerical order (universal tooth numbering system), 4
  Palmer notation, 2, *3*
  Triadan, 2, *3*
Tooth numbering systems, Fédération Dentaire Internationale, 6, *7*
  universal, 4
  Zsigmondy, 6, *7*
Tooth root. See *Root.*
Tooth surface, large, in tooth extraction, 184
Toothbrush, brushing technique with, 134, *135*
  for dental prophylaxis, 132
  mechanically powered, for dental prophylaxis, 132
Triadan system, of tooth identification, 2, *3*

V

Vibrators, 88, *89*
  model trimmer with, 88, *89*

W

W wire, 378
Water pick, for dental homecare, 133
Welders, 88
Wiping, in dental prophylaxis, techniques of, 134, *135*
Wire cutters, orthodontic, 90, *91*
Wires, arch, orthodontic. See *Arch wires.*
  omega, 378
Wiring, Essig technique of, 404, *405*
  figure-of-eight technique of, 406, *407*
  Ivy loop, 398, *399*
  Risdon technique of, 402, *403*
  Stout technique of, 400, *401*

Z

Zinc ascorbate, for plaque removal, 134
Zinc oxide-eugenol, crown cementation with, 326, 326(t), *327*
Zinc phosphate, crown cementation with, 326, 326(t), *327*
Zinc polycarboxylate, crown cementation with, 326, 326(t), *327*
Zsigmondy system, of tooth numbering, 6, *7*